NINTH EDITION

STUDY GUIDE FOR ESSENTIALS OF NURSING RESEARCH

Appraising Evidence for Nursing Practice

Denise F. Polit, PhD, FAAN

President, Humanalysis, Inc.,
Saratoga Springs, New York
and Professor,
Griffith University School of Nursing,
Brisbane, Australia
www.denisepolit.com

Cheryl Tatano Beck, DNSc, CNM, FAAN

Distinguished Professor
School of Nursing
University of Connecticut
Storrs, Connecticut

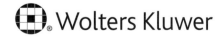 Wolters Kluwer

Philadelphia • Baltimore • New York • London
Buenos Aires • Hong Kong • Sydney • Tokyo

Acquisitions Editor: Christina C. Burns
Director of Product Development: Jennifer K. Forestieri
Development Editor: Meredith L. Brittain
Editorial Assistant: Hilari Bowman
Production Project Manager: Marian Bellus
Design Coordinator: Joan Wendt
Illustration Coordinator: Jennifer Clements
Manufacturing Coordinator: Karin Duffield
Prepress Vendor: Absolute Service, Inc.

Ninth Edition

9 8 7 6 5 4 3 2 1

Printed in China

978-1-4963-5469-3

LWW.com

Preface

This *Study Guide* has been prepared to complement the ninth edition of *Essentials of Nursing Research: Appraising Evidence for Nursing Practice*. It contains material designed to further bridge the gap between the passive reading of abstract materials and the active development of skills needed to critique studies and use the findings in practice.

This guide provides you with opportunities to reinforce the acquisition of basic research skills through systematic learning exercises—some of which are designed to be fun. Please note that some of the articles that are mentioned in the exercises appear on thePoint website and are identified by ☀-. Another important feature is that the appendices include eight research reports in their entirety. We deliberately selected some studies that are directly relevant to evidence-based practice (EBP), such as a study on the results of an EBP implementation project, and two systematic reviews. There are activities in each chapter of this *Study Guide* (the Application Exercises) geared around these studies.

The *Study Guide* consists of 18 chapters—one chapter corresponding to every chapter in the textbook. Each of the 18 chapters (with a few exceptions) consists of four sections:

- **A. Fill in the Blanks.** Terms and concepts presented in the textbook are reinforced by having you complete each sentence. All answers are at the back of the book (Appendix I) for easy reference and cross-checking.
- **B. Matching Exercises.** Further reinforcement for key new terms is offered in a matching exercise, which often involves matching the concrete (e.g., an actual research hypothesis) with the abstract (e.g., the term for a specific type of hypothesis). Again, answers are at the back of the book (Appendix I).
- **C. Study Questions.** Each chapter contains two to five short individual exercises relevant to the materials in the textbook. The answers to select study questions are at the back of the book (Appendix I).
- **D. Application Exercises.** These exercises are geared specifically to help you read, comprehend, and critique nursing studies. In each chapter, the application exercises focus on two of the studies in the appendices, and for each study, there are two sets of questions—*Questions of Fact* and *Questions for Discussion*.
  - **Questions of Fact** will help you read the report and find specific types of information related to the content covered in the textbook. For these questions, there are "right" answers, which we provide at the back of the book (Appendix I). For example, a question might ask: How many people participated in this study?
  - **Questions for Discussion**, by contrast, require an assessment of the merits of various features of the study. For example, a question might ask: Were there

enough people participating in this study? The second set of questions can be the basis for classroom discussions.

We hope that you will find these activities rewarding, enjoyable, and useful in your effort to develop skills for evidence-based nursing practice.

Denise F. Polit
Cheryl Tatano Beck

Contents

PART 1

Overview of Nursing Research and Its Role in Evidence-Based Practice

CHAPTER 1

Introduction to Nursing Research in an Evidence-Based Practice Environment

A. FILL IN THE BLANKS

How many terms have your learned in this chapter? Fill in the blanks in the sentences below to find out. You can have fun with this section by doing it with a friend. Who is the first one to complete the sentence?

1. A _____ is a world view, a way of looking at natural phenomena.

2. The world view that holds that there are multiple interpretations of reality is _____.

3. _____ is the world view that assumes that there is an orderly reality that can be studied objectively.

4. Research designed to solve a pressing practical problem is _____ (as opposed to basic) research.

5. Nurses in practice settings often read and evaluate studies in the context of a journal _____.

6. Research designed to inform nursing practice is referred to as _____ nursing research.

7. The degree to which research findings can be applied to people who did not participate in a study concerns its _____.

8. Many studies seek to understand determinants of phenomena and are referred to as _____-probing studies.

9. A principle that is believed to be true without proof or verification is a(n) _____.

10. _____ evidence is rooted in objective reality and is gathered through the senses.

11. The positivist assumption that phenomena are not random but rather have antecedent causes is called _____.

12. _____ is the repeating of a study to determine if findings can be upheld with a new group of people.

13. The techniques used by researchers to structure a study are called research _____.

14. The type of research that analyzes narrative, subjective materials is _____ research.

15. The scientific method involves procedures to enhance objectivity and reduce _____ that could distort the results.

16. _____ research involves the collection and analysis of numeric information and is associated with the traditional scientific method.

17. One purpose of qualitative inquiry when a new phenomenon is discovered through in-depth scrutiny is called _____.

18. The purpose of research that seeks to understand the underlying causes or full nature of a phenomenon, often involving the use of theories, is _____.

19. In terms of an EBP-related purpose, studies with a _____ purpose seek to identify effective treatments for addressing health problems.

20. In terms of an EBP-related purpose, studies with a _____ purpose seek to understand how clients feel about illness and health.

B. MATCHING EXERCISES

Match each statement in Set B with one of the paradigms in Set A. Indicate the letter corresponding to the appropriate response next to each entry in Set B.

SET A

a. Positivist/postpositivist paradigm

b. Constructivist paradigm

c. Neither paradigm

d. Both paradigms

SET B   RESPONSES

1. Assumes that reality exists and that it can be objectively studied and known   _____

2. Subjectivity in inquiries is considered inevitable and desirable.   _____

3. Inquiries rely on external (empirical) evidence collected through human senses.   _____

4. Assumes reality is a construction and that many constructions are possible   _____

5. Method of inquiry relies primarily on collecting and analyzing quantitative information.   _____

6. Method of inquiry relies primarily on collecting and analyzing narrative, qualitative information.   _____

7. Provides an overarching framework for inquiries undertaken by nurse researchers   _____

8. Inquiries give rise to emerging interpretations that are grounded in people's experiences.   _____

9. Inquiries are not constrained by ethical issues. _____

10. Inquiries focus on discrete, specific concepts while attempting to control others. _____

C. STUDY QUESTIONS

1. Why is it important for nurses who will never conduct their own research to understand research methods?

2. What are some potential consequences to the nursing profession if nurses stopped conducting their own research?

3. Below are descriptions of several research problems. Indicate whether you think the problem is best suited to a qualitative or quantitative approach and explain your rationale.

   a. What is the decision-making process of patients with AIDS seeking treatment?

   b. What effect does room temperature have on the colonization rate of bacteria in urinary catheters?

   c. What are sources of daily stress among nursing home residents, and what do these stressors mean to the residents?

   d. Does therapeutic touch affect the vital signs of hospitalized patients?

   e. What is the meaning of *hope* among patients with stage IV cancer?

   f. What are the effects of a formal exercise program on high blood pressure and cholesterol levels of middle-aged men?

   g. What are the health care needs of the homeless, and what barriers do they face in having those needs met?

4. What are some of the limitations of quantitative research? What are some of the limitations of qualitative research? Which approach seems best suited to address problems in which you might be interested? Why is that?

D. APPLICATION EXERCISES

Exercise D.1: Study in Appendix A

Read the abstract and introduction to the report by Stephens and colleagues ("Smartphone technology and text messaging for weight loss in young adults") in Appendix A on pages 113–120 and then answer the following questions:

Questions of Fact

a. Does this report describe an example of "disciplined research"?

b. Is this a qualitative or quantitative study?

c. What is the underlying paradigm of the study?

d. Does the study involve the collection of empirical evidence?

e. Is this study applied or basic research?

f. Could this study be described as *cause probing*?

   g. Is the specific purpose of this study identification, description, exploration, prediction/control, and/or explanation?

   h. Does this study have an EBP-focused purpose, such as a one related to therapy (treatment), diagnosis, prognosis, etc.?

Questions for Discussion

   a. How relevant is this study to the actual practice of nursing?

   b. Could this study have been conducted as *either* a quantitative *or* qualitative study? Why or why not?

Exercise D.2: Study in Appendix B

Read the abstract and introduction to the report by Cricco-Lizza ("Rooting for the breast") in Appendix B on pages 121–130 and then answer the following questions:

Questions of Fact

   a. Does this report describe an example of "disciplined research"?

   b. Is this a qualitative or quantitative study?

   c. What is the underlying paradigm of the research?

   d. Does the study involve the collection of empirical evidence?

   e. Is this study applied or basic research?

   f. Could this study be described as *cause probing*?

   g. Is the specific purpose of this study identification, description, exploration, prediction/control, and/or explanation?

   h. Does this study have an EBP-focused purpose, such as one related to therapy (treatment), diagnosis, prognosis, etc.?

Questions for Discussion

   a. How relevant is this study to the actual practice of nursing?

   b. Could this study have been conducted as *either* a quantitative *or* qualitative study? Why or why not?

   c. Which of the two studies cited in these exercises (the one in Appendix A or Appendix B) is of greater interest and/or relevance to you personally? Why?

CHAPTER 2

Fundamentals of Evidence-Based Nursing Practice

A. FILL IN THE BLANKS

How many terms have you learned in this chapter? Fill in the blanks in the sentences below to find out. You can have fun with this section by doing it with a friend. Who is the first one to complete the sentence?

1. A clinical practice _____, based on rigorous systematic evidence, is an important tool for evidence-based care.

2. _____ reviews of randomized controlled trials (RCTs) are at the pinnacle of many evidence hierarchies.

3. When a new protocol or guideline is developed in an EBP project, it should be _____ tested to evaluate its utility before being fully implemented.

4. The _____ Collaboration is an important keystone of EBP.

5. When asking clinical questions, the "O" component refers to the _____.

6. When asking clinical questions, the "P" component refers to the _____.

7. An individual RCT study would be level II on an evidence hierarchy for _____ questions.

8. The _____ instrument is an important tool for appraising clinical guidelines.

9. _____ is the acronym for the four-component scheme for asking well-worded clinical questions.

10. _____ is the type of systematic review that involves statistical integration of quantitative research findings.

11. When asking clinical questions, the "C" component refers to the _____.

12. A(n) _____ is a ranked arrangement of the worth of various types of evidence.

13. When asking clinical questions, the "I" component refers to the _____.

7

14. The integration of multiple qualitative studies can be achieved in a
_____.

15. _____ refers to the conscientious use of the best current evidence when making decisions about patient care.

16. Three types of efforts use systematic methods of solving health problems: research, evidence-based practice, and _____, which involves the analysis of existing information to improve performance.

B. MATCHING EXERCISES

Match each of the statements in Set B with the appropriate phrase in Set A. Indicate the letter(s) corresponding to your response next to each of the statements in Set B.

SET A

a. Research utilization (RU)

b. Evidence-based practice (EBP)

c. Neither RU nor EBP

d. Both RU and EBP

SET B   RESPONSES

1. Has been easily achieved in nursing   _____

2. Evidence hierarchies were developed within this context.   _____

3. Is useful only to nurses in academic environments   _____

4. Integrates research findings with clinical expertise and
client inputs   _____

5. Has given rise to models developed by nurses for guiding
the process   _____

6. Always begins with a knowledge-focused trigger   _____

7. The CURN project focused on this   _____

8. Sackett and Cochrane were prominent proponents   _____

C. STUDY QUESTIONS

1. For each of the following research questions, identify the component that is underlined as either the P, I, C, or O component.

   a. Among community-dwelling elders, does <u>fear of falling</u> affect their quality of life?

   b. Does amount of social support among <u>women with multiple sclerosis</u> affect disability to a greater degree than illness duration?

   c. Among children age 5 to 10 years, does participation in the Metropolitan Youth Fitness Initiative result in better cardiovascular fitness than participation in <u>routine school play activities</u>?

    d. Does <u>chronic stress</u> contribute to fatigue among patients with a traumatic head injury?

    e. Among older adults in a long-term care setting, does a reminiscence program reduce <u>depressive symptoms</u>?

    f. Among <u>clients undergoing methadone maintenance therapy</u>, are men more likely than women to be heavy cigarette smokers?

    g. Does <u>family involvement in diabetes management</u> affect glucose control among immigrants with Type 2 diabetes?

    h. Among hospitalized adult patients, is greater nurse staffing levels associated with shorter <u>lengths of hospital stay</u>?

    i. Is music a more effective treatment than <u>normal hospital sounds</u> in reducing pain in women in labor?

    j. Does self-concept affect <u>dietary intake</u> in moderately obese adults?

2. For each of the following clinical questions, fill in the blank (use your imagination!) for the component that is missing. Do not be concerned with whether the question has been addressed by researchers. The exercise is meant to encourage you to be brave about asking clinical questions and to help you get in the habit of asking them. There are no right or wrong answers.

    a. Among _____ (P), does intensive exercise (I) affect peak oxygen consumption (O)?

    b. Does _____ (I) reduce cigarette smoking (O) in high school students (P)?

    c. Does fatigue (I) have a bigger effect than _____ (C) on ability to cope (O) in patients undergoing chemotherapy (P)?

    d. Among patients with a chronic health problem (P), does _____ (I) affect their quality of life (O)?

    e. Among caregivers of patients with Alzheimer's disease, do the age and income level of the caregiver (I) affect _____ (O)?

    f. Among adolescent males (P), does/do _____ (I) affect decisions to be sexually abstinent?

    g. Among cognitively impaired elders being relocated to a nursing home (P), does the person's involvement in the decision to relocate (I) affect _____ (O)?

    h. Among _____ (P), does smoking history (I) affect perceptions of acute coronary syndrome (O)?

3. Think about a nursing procedure that you have learned. What is the basis for this procedure? Examine whether the procedure is based on scientific evidence indicating that the procedure is effective. If it is not based on scientific evidence, on what is it based, and why do you think scientific evidence was not used?

4. Identify the factors in your own clinical setting that you think facilitate or inhibit research utilization and evidence-based practice (or, in an educational setting, the factors that promote or inhibit a climate in which EBP is valued).

5. Read one of the following articles and identify the steps of the Iowa Model (or an alternative model of EBP) that are represented in the projects described.

   • Brown, C. G. (2014). The Iowa Model of Evidence-Based Practice to Promote Quality Care: An illustrated example in oncology nursing. *Clinical Journal of Oncology Nursing, 18*, 157–159.

   • Farrington, M., Bruene, D., & Wagner, M. (2015). Pain management prior to nasogastric tube placement: Atomized lidocaine. *ORL-Head and Neck Nursing, 33*, 8–16.

   • *Harrison, M., Graham, I., van den Hoek, J., Dogherty, E., Carley, M., & Angus, V. (2013). Guideline adaptation and implementation planning: A prospective observational study. *Implementation Science, 8*, 49.

   • Ireland, S., Kirkpatrick, H., Boblin, S., & Robertson, K. (2013). The real world journey of implementing fall prevention best practices in three acute care hospitals: A case study. *Worldviews on Evidence-Based Nursing, 10*, 95–103.

   • *Shaw, R. J., Kaufman, M. A., Bosworth, H. B., Weiner, B. J., Zullig, L. L., Lee, S. Y., . . . Jackson, G. L. (2013). Organizational factors associated with readiness to implement and translate a primary care based telemedicine behavioral program to improve blood pressure control: The HTN-IMPROVE study. *Implementation Science, 8*, 106.

D. APPLICATION EXERCISES

Exercise D.1: Study in Appendix C

Read the abstract and introduction to the report by Yackel and colleagues ("Nurse-facilitated depression screening program") in Appendix C on pages 131–138 and then answer the following questions:

Questions of Fact

a. What was the purpose of this EBP project?

b. What was the setting for implementing this project?

c. Which EBP model was used as a framework for this project?

d. Did the project have a problem-focused or knowledge-focused trigger?

e. Who were the team members in this study, and what were their affiliations?

f. What, if anything, did the report say about the implementation potential of this project?

g. Was a pilot study undertaken?

h. Did this project involve an evaluation of the project's success?

---

*A link to this open-access journal article is provided in the Internet Resources section on the textbook's thePoint website.

Questions for Discussion

a. What might be a clinical foreground question that was used in seeking relevant evidence in preparing for this project? Identify the PIO or PICO components of your question.

b. What are some of the praiseworthy aspects of this project? What could the team members have done differently to improve the project?

Exercise D.2: Study in Appendix G

Read the abstract and introduction (from the beginning to the "Methods" section) of the report by Chase and colleagues ("Effectiveness of medication adherence interventions") in Appendix G on pages 177–186 and then answer the following questions:

Questions of Fact

a. Is this report a systematic review? If yes, what type of systematic review was it? Is this an example of pre-appraised evidence?

b. Where on the evidence hierarchy shown in Figure 2.1 of the textbook would this study belong?

c. What is the stated purpose of this study?

Questions for Discussion

a. What might be a clinical foreground question that was used in seeking relevant evidence in preparing for this project? Identify the PIO or PICO components of your question.

b. What are some of the steps would you need to undertake if you were interested in using this meta-analysis as a basis for an EBP project in your own practice setting?

Key Concepts and Steps in Quantitative and Qualitative Research

A. FILL IN THE BLANKS

How many terms have you learned in this chapter? Fill in the blanks in the sentences below to find out. You can have fun with this section by doing it with a friend. Who is the first one to complete the sentence?

1. Another name for outcome variable is _____ variable.

2. To get access to a site and its inhabitants is to gain _____ into the site.

3. Information gathered in a study is called _____.

4. A _____ is a subset of a population from whom data are gathered.

5. The _____ definition indicates how a variable will be measured or observed.

6. A systematic, abstract explanation of phenomena is a(n) _____.

7. Quantitative researchers perform _____ analyses of their data.

8. Some qualitative researchers do not undertake an upfront _____ review to avoid having their conceptualization influenced by the work of others.

9. Researchers typically use a(n) _____ design in qualitative studies.

10. The type of research that involves an intervention is called _____ research.

11. In medical literature, a study that tests the effect of an intervention is a clinical _____.

12. The qualitative research tradition that focuses on lived experiences is _____.

13. A type of qualitative research that focuses on the study of cultures is _____.

14. Data _____ is a principle used to decide when to stop sampling in a qualitative study.

15. The _____ is the entire aggregate of people in which a researcher is interested (the "P" in PICO).

16. A qualitative tradition that focuses on social psychological processes within a social setting is called _____ theory.

17. A(n) _____ is a somewhat more complex abstraction than a concept.

18. If the independent variable is the cause, the dependent variable is the _____.

19. A research _____ is the basic architecture of a study.

20. A relationship in which one variable directly induces changes in another is a _____ relationship.

21. Qualitative analyses usually involve a search for recurrent _____.

22. In quantitative research, a concept is usually referred to as a(n) _____.

23. A person who provides information to researchers in a study is often called a _____ in a quantitative study.

24. A(n) _____ is a characteristic or quality that takes on different values—that is, that differs from one person or object to another.

25. The presumed influence on a dependent variable is the _____ variable.

26. A(n) _____ is a bond, connection, or pattern of association between variables.

27. Another name for nonexperimental research, often used in the medical literature, is _____ research.

B. MATCHING EXERCISES

1. Match each statement in Set B with one of the paradigms in Set A. Indicate the letter corresponding to the appropriate response next to each entry in Set B.

SET A

a. Term used in quantitative research
b. Term used in qualitative research
c. Term used in both qualitative and quantitative research

SET B   RESPONSES

 1. Subject   _____
 2. Study participant   _____
 3. Informant   _____
 4. Variable   _____
 5. Phenomenon   _____
 6. Saturation   _____
 7. Theory   _____
 8. Data   _____
 9. Emergent design   _____
10. Data analysis   _____

2. Match each term in Set B with one of the terms in Set A. Indicate the letter corresponding to your response next to each item in Set B.

SET A

a. Independent variable

b. Dependent variable

c. Either/both

d. Neither

SET B   **RESPONSES**

1. The variable that is the presumed effect   _____

2. The variable involved in a cause-and-effect relationship   _____

3. The variable that is the presumed cause   _____

4. The variable, "length of stay in hospital"   _____

5. The variable that requires an operational definition   _____

6. The variable that is the main outcome of interest in the study _____

7. The variable that is constant   _____

8. The variable in a grounded theory study   _____

3. Match each activity in Set B with one of the options in Set A. Indicate the letter corresponding to your response next to each item in Set B.

SET A

a. An activity in quantitative research

b. An activity in qualitative research

c. An activity in both/either qualitative and/or quantitative research

d. An activity in neither quantitative nor qualitative research

SET B   **RESPONSES**

1. Choosing between an experimental and nonexperimental design   _____

2. Ending data collection once saturation has been achieved   _____

3. Developing or evaluating measuring instruments   _____

4. Doing a literature review   _____

5. Collecting and analyzing data concurrently   _____

6. Taking steps to ensure protection of human rights   _____

7. Developing strategies to avoid data collection   _____

8. Disseminating research results   _____

9. Analyzing the data for major themes or categories   _____

10. Formulating hypotheses to be tested statistically   _____

C. STUDY QUESTIONS

1. Suggest operational definitions for the following concepts.

  a. Stress:

  b. Prematurity of infants:

  c. Fatigue:

  d. Pain:

  e. Prolonged labor:

  f. Dyspnea:

2. In each of the following research questions, identify the independent variable (IV) and dependent or outcome variable (DV).

  a. Does assertiveness training improve the effectiveness of psychiatric nurses?

  Independent: _____

  Dependent: _____

  b. Does the postural positioning of patients affect their respiratory function?

  Independent: _____

  Dependent: _____

  c. Is the psychological well-being of patients affected by the amount of touch received from nursing staff?

  Independent: _____

  Dependent: _____

  d. Is the incidence of decubitus reduced by more frequent turnings of patients?

  Independent: _____

  Dependent: _____

  e. Are people who were abused as children more likely than others to abuse their own children?

  Independent: _____

  Dependent: _____

  f. Is tolerance for pain related to a patient's age and gender?

  Independent: _____

  Dependent: _____

  g. Are the number of prenatal visits of pregnant women associated with labor and delivery outcomes?

  Independent: _____

  Dependent: _____

  h. Are levels of depression higher among children who experience the death of a sibling than among other children?

  Independent: _____

  Dependent: _____

  i. Is compliance with a medical regimen higher among women than among men?

  Independent: _____

  Dependent: _____

    j. Does participating in a support group enhance coping among family caregivers of patients with AIDS?

        Independent: _____

        Dependent: _____

    k. Is hearing acuity of the elderly affected by the time of day?

        Independent: _____

        Dependent: _____

    l. Does home birth affect the parents' satisfaction with the childbirth experience?

        Independent: _____

        Dependent: _____

    m. Does a neutropenic diet in the outpatient setting decrease the positive blood cultures associated with chemotherapy-induced neutropenia?

        Independent: _____

        Dependent: _____

3. Below is a list of variables. For each, think of a research question for which the variable would be the independent variable and a second for which it would be the dependent variable. For example, take the variable "birth weight of infants." We might ask, "Does the age of the mother affect the birth weight of her infant?" (dependent variable). Alternatively, our research question might be, "Does the birth weight of infants (independent variable) affect their sensorimotor development at 6 months of age?" HINT: For the dependent variable problem, ask yourself, What factors might affect, influence, or cause this variable? For the independent variable, ask yourself, What factors does *this* variable influence, cause, or affect—what might be the consequences of this variable?

    a. Body temperature

        Independent: _____

        Dependent: _____

    b. Amount of sleep

        Independent: _____

        Dependent: _____

    c. Frequency of practicing breast self-examination

        Independent: _____

        Dependent: _____

    d. Level of hopefulness in patients with cancer

        Independent: _____

        Dependent: _____

    e. Stress among victims of domestic violence

        Independent: _____

        Dependent: _____

4. Look at the table of contents of a recent issue of *Nursing Research* or another nursing research journal. Pick out a study title (without looking at the abstract or study description at the beginning) that implies that a relationship between variables was studied. Indicate what you think the independent and dependent variable might be and what the title suggests about the nature of the relationship (i.e., causal or not).

5. Describe what is wrong with the following statements:

   a. Koretsky's experimental study was conducted within the ethnographic tradition.

   b. Forman's experimental study examined the effect of relaxation therapy (the dependent variable) on pain (the independent variable) in patients with cancer.

   c. Strohl's grounded theory study of the caregiving process for caretakers of patients with dementia was a clinical trial.

   d. In Aldrich's phenomenological study of the meaning of futility among patients with AIDS, participants received an intervention designed to sustain hope.

   e. In her experimental study, Bokan developed her data collection plan after she introduced her intervention to a group of patients.

6. Which qualitative research tradition do you think would be most appropriate for the following research questions? Justify your response:

   a. How do the health beliefs and customs of Chinese immigrants influence their health-seeking behavior?

   b. What is the lived experience of being a recovering alcoholic?

   c. What is the process by which husbands adapt to the sudden loss of their wives?

D. APPLICATION EXERCISES

Exercise D.1: Study in Appendix D

Read the abstract, introduction, and first few subsection of the "Methods" section of the report by Eckhardt and colleagues ("Fatigue in the presence of coronary heart disease") in Appendix D on pages 139–150 and then answer the following questions:

Questions of Fact

a. Who were the researchers and what are their credentials and affiliation?

b. Who were the study participants?

c. What were the site and setting for this study?

d. What is the independent variable (or variables) in this study? What is the dependent variable (or variables)? Did the report actually use the terms *independent variable* or *dependent variable*?

e. How was *fatigue* operationally defined? Was a conceptual definition provided?

f. Were the data in this study quantitative or qualitative?

g. Were any relationships under investigation? What type of relationship?

  h. Is this an experimental or nonexperimental study?

  i. Was there any intervention? If so, what is it?

  j. Did the study involve statistical analysis of data?

Questions for Discussion

  a. How relevant is this study to the actual practice of nursing?

  b. How good a job did the researchers do in summarizing their study in the abstract?

  c. How long do you estimate it took for this study to be completed?

Exercise D.2: Study in Appendix F

Read the abstract and introduction to the report by Cummings ("Sharing a traumatic event") in Appendix F on pages 169–176 and then answer the following questions:

Questions of Fact

  a. Who was the researcher and what are her credentials and affiliation?

  b. Who were the study participants?

  c. In what type of setting did the study take place?

  d. What were the key concepts in this study?

  e. Were there any *independent variables* or *dependent variables* in this study?

  f. Were the data in this study quantitative or qualitative?

  g. Were any relationships under investigation?

  h. Could the study be described as an ethnographic, phenomenologic, or grounded theory study?

  i. Is this an experimental or nonexperimental study?

  j. Does the study involve an intervention? If so, what is it?

  k. Did the study involve statistical analysis of data? Did the study involve qualitative analysis of data?

Questions for Discussion

  a. How relevant is this study to the actual practice of nursing?

  b. How good a job did the researcher do in summarizing her study in the abstract?

  c. How long do you estimate it took for this study to be completed?

  d. Which of the two studies cited in these exercises (the one in Appendix D or Appendix F) is of greater interest and/or relevance to you personally? Why?

Reading and Critiquing Research Articles

A. FILL IN THE BLANKS

How many terms have you learned in this chapter? Fill in the blanks in the sentences below to find out. You can have fun with this section by doing it with a friend. Who is the first one to complete the sentence?

1. A _____ is an influence that results in a distortion or error.
2. "The lived experience of caring for a dying spouse" is an example of the section of a research report called the _____.
3. The process of reflecting critically on one's self, used by many qualitative researchers, is _____.
4. One conventional _____ of statistical significance (*p* value) is .05.
5. Qualitative researchers strive to ensure that their findings are _____, which includes enhancing credibility, authenticity, and dependability.
6. If the results of a statistical test indicated a probability of .001, the results would be statistically _____.
7. _____ is the format used to structure most research reports.
8. To address biases stemming from *awareness*, researchers may use a procedure that is usually called _____.
9. A summary of a study, also known as a(n) _____, appears at the beginning of a report.
10. A(n) _____ variable is a variable that is extraneous to the research question but that needs to be controlled.
11. Research reports are most likely to be accessed as _____ articles.
12. Quantitative researchers strive for findings that are reliable and _____.
13. A(n) _____ is a conclusion drawn from the evidence in a study that takes into account the research methods used.
14. _____ is a criterion for evaluating study evidence (mostly in quantitative study) that concerns the accuracy and consistency of information.

15. Research _____ is used by researchers to hold constant outside influences on the dependent variable so that the relationship under study can be better understood.

16. _____ is a strategy used by quantitative researchers to reduce bias and involves having aspects of the study established by chance rather than by personal choices.

17. _____ is to qualitative research what generalizability is to quantitative research.

B. MATCHING EXERCISES

Match each statement in Set B with one of the report sections in Set A. Indicate the letter corresponding to the appropriate response next to each entry in Set B.

SET A

a. Abstract

b. Introduction

c. Method

d. Results

e. Discussion

SET B   RESPONSES

1. Describes the research design   _____

2. In quantitative studies, presents findings from
statistical analyses   _____

3. Identifies the research questions or hypotheses   _____

4. Presents a brief summary of the major features of the study   _____

5. Provides information on how study participants
were selected   _____

6. Offers an interpretation of the study findings   _____

7. In qualitative studies, describes the themes or categories that
emerged from the data   _____

8. Presents a rationale for the significance of the study   _____

9. Describes how the research data were collected   _____

10. Identifies the study's main limitations   _____

11. This sentence would appear there: "The purpose of this
study was to explore the process by which patients cope
with a cancer diagnosis."   _____

12. Includes raw data, in the form of excerpts from participants,
in qualitative reports   _____

C. STUDY QUESTIONS

1. Why are qualitative research reports typically easier to read than quantitative research reports?

_____

_____

_____

2. Read the following "traditional" (1 paragraph) abstract for a study by Hansen and colleagues (2015) and rewrite it as a "new style" abstract with these specific headings: Background, Objective, Methods, Results, Conclusions.

Research on symptom distress experienced by patients with end-stage liver disease at the end of life is limited. The aims of the study were to describe presence, frequency, severity, and distress of symptoms in patients with end-stage liver disease toward the end of life and to describe the variability in psychological and physical symptom distress between and within patients over time. This study used a prospective, longitudinal descriptive design. Data were collected from 20 patients once a month for up to 6 months. Participants completed the Memorial Symptom Assessment Scale, which reports a total score, a Global Distress Index score, and a psychological and a physical distress score. Patients reported lack of energy, pain, difficulty sleeping, and feeling drowsy as the most frequent, severe, and distressing symptoms. Global Distress Index mean scores (measured on a 1 to 4 scale) ranged from 2.6 to 2.9 across time. There was notable variability in psychological and physical distress scores between and within patients across time. Gaining knowledge about the prevalent symptoms experienced by patients with end-stage liver disease and the trajectory of these symptoms is crucial for designing interventions that optimize well-being in patients with end-stage liver disease as they are approaching death.

Hansen, L., Leo, M., Chang, M., Zaman, A., Naugler, W., & Schwartz, J. (2015). Symptom distress in patients with end-stage liver disease toward the end of life. _Gastroenterology Nursing, 38,_ 201–210.

3. Read the titles of the journal articles appearing in the most recent issue of the journal _Nursing Research_ (or another nursing research journal). Evaluate the titles of the articles in terms of length and adequacy in communicating essential information about the studies.

4. Below is a brief abstract of a fictitious study, followed by a critique. Do you agree with the critique? Can you add other comments relevant to issues discussed in Chapter 4 of the textbook?

FICTITIOUS STUDY

Solomons (2017) prepared the following abstract for her study.

Abstract. Family members often experience considerable anxiety while their loved ones are in surgery. This study examined the effectiveness of a nursing intervention that involved providing oral intraoperative progress reports to family members. Surgical patients undergoing elective procedures were selected to either have family members receive the intervention or to not have them receive it. The findings indicated that the family members in the intervention group were less anxious than family members who received usual care.

CRITIQUE OF THE FICTITIOUS ABSTRACT

This brief abstract provides a general overview of the nature of Solomons' study. It indicates a rationale for the study (the high anxiety level of surgical patients' family members) and summarizes what the researcher did. However, the abstract could have provided more information while still staying within a 100- or 125-word guideline (the abstract only contains 77 words). For example, the abstract could have better described the nature of the intervention (e.g., At what point during the operation was information given to family members? How much detail was provided? etc.). For a reader to have a preliminary assessment of the worth of the study—and therefore to make a decision about whether to read the entire report—more information about the methods would have been helpful. For example, the abstract should have indicated how many families were in the sample, how anxiety was measured, and whether group differences were statistically significant. Also missing is information about how families were allocated to receive the intervention—that is, was *randomness* used? Some indication of the study's implications might also have enhanced the usefulness of the abstract.

D. APPLICATION EXERCISES

Exercise D.1: Study in Appendix A

Read the abstract and introduction to the report by Stephens and colleagues ("Smartphone technology and text messaging for weight loss in young adults") in Appendix A on pages 113–120 and then answer the following questions:

Questions of Fact

a. Does the structure of this article follow the IMRAD format?

b. Does the abstract summarize information about the study purpose, how the study was done, what the key findings were, and what the findings mean?

c. Skim the Method section. Is the presentation in the active or passive voice?

d. Is this study experimental or nonexperimental?

e. Was the principle of *randomness* used in this study?

Questions for Discussion

a. What parts of the abstract were most difficult to understand? Identify words that you consider to be research "jargon."

b. Comment on the organization *within* the Method section of this report.

Exercise D.2: Study in Appendix E

Read the abstract and introduction to the report by Byrne and colleagues ("Care transition experiences") in Appendix E on pages 151–168 and then answer the following questions:

Questions of Fact

a. Does the structure of this article follow the IMRAD format?

b. Does the abstract include information about the study purpose, how the study was done, what the findings were, and what the findings mean?

c. Skim the Design and Methods section. Is the presentation in the active or passive voice?

d. Is the study in one of the three main qualitative traditions described in Chapter 3? If so, which tradition?

Questions for Discussion

a. What parts of the abstract were most difficult to understand?

b. Comment on the organization *within* the Results section of this report.

c. Compare the level of difficulty of the abstracts for the two studies used in these exercises—that is, the studies in Appendices A and E. Why do you think the level of difficulty differs?

Ethics in Research

A. FILL IN THE BLANKS

How many terms have you learned in this chapter? Fill in the blanks in the sentences below to find out. You can have fun with this section by doing it with a friend. Who is the first one to complete the sentence?

1. Most disciplines have developed formal _____ of ethics.

2. _____ is the best method of protecting participants' confidentiality but is not always possible.

3. Researchers should conduct a _____/benefit assessment to evaluate the ethical aspects of their research plan.

4. _____ is a major ethical principle concerning maximizing benefits of research.

5. _____ refers to the type of consent procedure that may be required in qualitative research involving multiple points of data collection.

6. A(n) _____ is a payment sometimes offered to participants as an incentive to take part in a study.

7. The _____ *Report* is the basis for ethical regulations for studies funded by the U.S. government.

8. The return of a questionnaire is often assumed to demonstrate _____ consent.

9. Informal agreement to participate in a study (e.g., by minors) is called _____.

10. Participants' privacy is often protected by _____ procedures, even though the researchers know participants' identities.

11. People can make informed decisions about research participation when there is full _____ of relevant information.

12. A(n) _____ is a formal institutional committee (in the United States) that reviews the ethical aspects of a study.

13. A conflict between the rights of participants and the demands for rigorous research creates an ethical _____.

14. Prisoners and children involved in research are examples of _____.

15. _____ procedures offer prospective participants information needed to make a reasonable decision about study participation.

24

Study Guide for Essentials of Nursing Research: Appraising Evidence for Nursing Practice, 9e

16. _____ sessions at the conclusion of a study offers participants an opportunity to learn more about a study, ask questions, and air complaints.

17. A risk no greater than those ordinarily experienced in everyday life is called a(n) _____ risk in research parlance.

B. MATCHING EXERCISES

Match each description in Set B with one of the procedures used to protect human subjects listed in Set A. Indicate the letter corresponding to the appropriate response next to each entry in Set B.

SET A

a. Freedom from harm or exploitation

b. Informed consent

c. Anonymity

d. Confidentiality

SET B   RESPONSES

1. A questionnaire distributed by mail bears an identification number in one corner. Respondents are assured their responses will not be individually divulged.   _____

2. Hospitalized children included in a study, and their parents, are told the study's aims and procedures. Parents are asked to sign an authorization.   _____

3. Participants in a study in which the same people will participate twice by completing questionnaires are asked to place their own four-digit identification number on the questionnaire and to memorize the number for use in the next round. Participants are assured their answers will remain private.   _____

4. Study participants in an in-depth study of family members' coping with a natural disaster renegotiate the terms of their participation at successive interviews.   _____

5. The psychological consequences of a recent mastectomy are being studied. In the interviews, sensitive questions are carefully worded. After the interview, debriefing with the respondent is used to assess the need for psychological support.   _____

6. Women interviewed in the above study (question 5) are told that the information they provide will not be individually divulged.   _____

7. Subjects who volunteered for an experimental treatment for AIDS are warned of potential side effects and are asked to sign an agreement.   _____

8. After determining that a new intervention resulted in participant discomfort, the researcher discontinued the study.   _____

9. Unmarked questionnaires are distributed to a class of nursing students. The instructions indicate that responses will not be individually divulged. _____

10. The researcher assures participants that they will be interviewed at a single point in time and adheres to this promise. _____

11. A questionnaire distributed to a sample of nursing students includes a statement indicating that completion and submission of the questionnaire will be construed as voluntary participation in a study. _____

12. The names, ages, and occupations of study participants whose interviews are excerpted in the research report are not revealed. _____

C. STUDY QUESTIONS

1. Below are brief descriptions of several studies. Suggest some ethical dilemmas that could emerge for each.

   a. A study of coping behaviors among rape victims

   b. An unobtrusive observational study of fathers' behaviors in the delivery room

   c. An interview study of the determinants of heroin addiction

   d. A study of dependence among children with developmental delays

   e. An investigation of verbal interactions among patients with schizophrenia

   f. A study of the effects of a new drug on humans

   g. A study of the relationship between sleeping patterns and acting-out behaviors in hospitalized psychiatric patients

2. Evaluate the ethical aspects of one or more of the following studies using the critiquing guidelines in Box 5.2 in the textbook and available on thePoint. Pay special attention (if relevant) to the manner in which the participants' heightened vulnerability was handled.

   • *Claro, H. G., de Oliveira, M. A., Bourdreaux, J. T., Fernandes, I. F., Pinho, P. H., & Tarifa, R. R. (2015). Drug use, mental health and problems related to crime and violence: Cross-sectional study. *Revista Latino-Americana de Enfermagem*, *23*, 1173–1180.

   • Gonzalez-Guarda, R. M., Cummings, A. M., Pino, K., Malhotra, K., Becerra, M. M., & Lopez, J. E. (2014). Perceptions of adolescents, parents, and school personnel from a predominantly Cuban American community regarding dating and teen dating violence prevention. *Research in Nursing & Health*, *37*, 117–127.

   • *Olsson, M., Carlström, E., Marklund, B., Helldin, L., & Hjärthag, F. (2015). Assessment of distress and quality of life: A comparison of self-assessments by outpatients with a schizopsychotic illness and the clinical judgment of nurses. *Archives of Psychiatric Nursing*, *29*, 284–289.

   • Yeo, S., & Logan, J. G. (2014). Preventing obesity: Exercise and daily activities of low-income pregnant women. *The Journal of Perinatal & Neonatal Nursing*, *28*, 17–25.

---

*A link to this open-access journal article is provided in the Internet Resources section on the textbook's thePoint website.

3. In the textbook, an actual study with ethical problems was described—that is, the Tuskegee study of syphilis among black men. Identify which ethical principles were transgressed in this study (do an Internet search for more information about the Tuskegee experiment, if desired).

4. Below is a brief description of the ethical aspects of a fictitious study, followed by a critique. Do you agree with the critique? Can you add other comments relevant to the ethical dimensions of the study?

FICTITIOUS STUDY

Walsh conducted an in-depth study of nursing home residents to explore whether their perceptions about personal control over decision making differed from the perceptions of the nursing staff. The investigator studied 25 nurse–patient dyads to assess whether there were differing perceptions and experiences regarding control over activities of daily living, such as arising, eating, and dressing. All of the nurses in the study were employed by the nursing home in which the patients resided. Because the nursing home had no institutional review board (IRB), and because Walsh's study was not funded by an organization that required IRB approval, the project was not formally reviewed. Walsh sought permission to conduct the study from the nursing home administrator. She also obtained the consent of the legal guardian or responsible family member of each patient. All study participants were fully informed about the nature of the study. The researcher assured the nurses and the legal guardians and family members of the patients of the confidentiality of the information and obtained their consent in writing. Data were gathered primarily through in-depth interviews with the patients and the nurses, at separate times. The researcher also observed interactions between the patients and nurses. The findings from the study suggested that patients perceived that they had more control over all aspects of the activities of daily living (except eating) than the nurses perceived that they had. Excerpts from the interviews were used verbatim in the research report, but Walsh did not divulge the location of the nursing home, and she used fictitious names for all participants.

CRITIQUE OF THE FICTITIOUS STUDY

Walsh did a reasonably good job of adhering to ethical principles in the conduct of her research. She obtained written permission to conduct the study from the nursing home administrator, and she obtained informed consent from the nurse participants and the legal guardians or family members of the patients. The study participants were not put at risk in any way, and the patients who participated may actually have enjoyed the opportunity to have a conversation with the researcher. Walsh also took appropriate steps to maintain the confidentiality of participants. It is still unclear, however, whether the patients knowingly and willingly participated in the research. Nursing home residents are a vulnerable group. They may not have been aware of their right to refuse to be interviewed without fear of repercussion. Walsh could have enhanced the ethical aspects of the study by taking more vigorous steps to obtain the informed, voluntary consent of the nursing home residents themselves or to exclude patients who could not reasonably be expected to understand the researcher's request. Given the vulnerability of the group, Walsh should have pursued opportunities for a formal review with an institution with which she was affiliated—or she should have established her own review panel composed of peers and interested lay people to review the ethical dimensions of her project. Debriefing sessions with study participants might also have been appropriate.

D. APPLICATION EXERCISES

Exercise D.1: Study in Appendix D

Read the Method section of the report by Eckhardt and colleagues ("Fatigue in the presence of coronary heart disease") in Appendix D on pages 139–150 and then answer the following questions:

Questions of Fact

a. Does the report indicate that the study procedures were reviewed by an IRB or other similar institutional human subjects group?

b. Would the participants in this study be considered a "vulnerable group"?

c. Were participants subjected to any physical harm or discomfort or psychological distress as part of the study? What efforts did the researchers make to minimize harm and maximize good?

d. Were participants deceived in any way?

e. Were participants coerced into participating in the study?

f. Were appropriate informed consent procedures used? Was there full disclosure?

g. Does the report discuss steps that were taken to protect the privacy and confidentiality of study participants? Were data collected anonymously?

Questions for Discussion

a. Do you think the benefits of this research outweighed the costs to participants—what is the overall risk/benefit ratio?

b. Do you consider that the researchers took adequate steps to protect study participants? If not, what else could they have done?

c. The report did not indicate that the participants were paid a stipend. Do you think they should have been?

d. Is there any evidence of discrimination in this study, with regard to people recruited to participate?

e. How comfortable would you feel about having a parent or grandparent participate in this study?

Exercise D.2: Study in Appendix B

Read the Method section of the report by Cricco-Lizza ("Rooting for the breast") in Appendix B on pages 121–130 and then answer the following questions:

Questions of Fact

a. Does the report indicate that the study procedures were reviewed by an IRB or other similar institutional human subjects group?

b. Would the study participants in this study be considered a "vulnerable group"?

c. Were participants subjected to any physical harm or discomfort or psychological distress as part of this study? What efforts did the researchers make to minimize harm and maximize good?

d. Were participants deceived in any way?

e. Were participants coerced into participating in the study?

f. Were appropriate informed consent procedures used? Was there full disclosure? Was process consent used?

g. Does the report discuss steps that were taken to protect the privacy and confidentiality of study participants?

Questions for Discussion

a. Do you think the benefits of this research outweighed the costs to participants—what is the overall risk/benefit ratio?

b. Do you consider that the researchers took adequate steps to protect the study participants? If not, what else could they have done?

c. Comment on the fact that some of the interviews with the mothers were conducted in the presence of other family members.

PART 2

Preliminary Steps in Quantitative and Qualitative Research

Research Problems, Research Questions, and Hypotheses

A. FILL IN THE BLANKS

How many terms have you learned in this chapter? Fill in the blanks in the sentences below to find out. You can have fun with this section by doing it with a friend. Who is the first one to complete the sentence?

1. A research _____ is an enigmatic or troubling condition.
2. A(n) _____ in a quantitative study states an aim and indicates the key study variables and the population of interest.
3. A research _____ is what researchers wish to answer through a systematic study.
4. A(n) _____ is a statement of the researcher's prediction about variables in the study.
5. Hypotheses predict a(n) _____ between the independent and dependent variables.
6. Hypotheses are typically put to a statistical _____.
7. A hypothesis stipulates the expected relationship between a(n) _____ variable and a dependent variable.
8. A research hypothesis in which the specific nature of the predicted relationship is not stipulated is a(n) _____ hypothesis.
9. The results of hypothesis testing never constitute _____ that a hypothesis is or is not correct.
10. Hypotheses typically involve at least _____ variables.
11. The *actual* hypothesis of an investigator is the _____ hypothesis.
12. The hypothesis that posits the absence of a relationship between variables is called a(n) _____ hypothesis.

B. MATCHING EXERCISES

1. Match each sentence in Set B with one of the phrases listed in Set A. Indicate the letter corresponding to the appropriate response next to each entry in Set B.

SET A

a. Statement of purpose—qualitative study

b. Statement of purpose—quantitative study

c. Not a statement of purpose for a research study

SET B   RESPONSES

1. The purpose of this study is to test whether the removal of physical restraints results in behavioral changes in elderly patients.   _____

2. The purpose of this project is to facilitate the transition from hospital to home among women who have just given birth.   _____

3. The goal of this project is to explore the process by which an elderly person adjusts to placement in a nursing home.   _____

4. The investigation was designed to describe the prevalence of smoking, alcohol use, and drug use among urban preadolescents aged 10 to 12 years.   _____

5. The study's purpose was to describe the nature of touch used by parents in touching their preterm infants.   _____

6. The goal is to develop guidelines for spiritually related nursing interventions.   _____

7. The purpose of this project is to examine the relationship between social support and the use of over-the-counter medications among community-dwelling elders.   _____

8. The purpose is to develop an in-depth understanding of patients' feelings of powerlessness in hospital settings.   _____

2. Match each sentence in Set B with one of the phrases listed in Set A. Indicate the letter corresponding to the appropriate response next to each entry in Set B.

SET A

a. Research hypothesis—directional

b. Research hypothesis—nondirectional

c. Null hypothesis

d. Not a testable hypothesis as stated

SET B   RESPONSES

1. First-born infants have higher concentrations of estrogens and progesterone in umbilical cord blood than do later born infants.   _____

2. There is no relationship between women's participation in prenatal classes and the health outcomes of their infants.   _____

3. Many nursing students are interested in obtaining advanced degrees. _____

4. Functional disability after a cardiac event is higher among patients with comorbidities than among those without comorbidities. _____

5. A person's income is related to his or her difficulty in accessing health care. _____

6. Glaucoma can be effectively screened by means of tonometry. _____

7. Higher noise levels result in increased anxiety among hospitalized patients. _____

8. Media exposure regarding the health hazards of smoking is unrelated to a person's smoking habits. _____

9. Patients' compliance with their medication regimens is related to their perception of the consequences of noncompliance. _____

10. Many patients delay seeking health care for symptoms of myocardial infarction because they are afraid. _____

11. Patients from hospitals in urban and rural areas differ with respect to their level of satisfaction with their nursing care. _____

12. A cancer patient's degree of hopefulness regarding the future is unrelated to his or her religiosity. _____

13. The degree of attachment between infants and their mothers is associated with the infant's status as low birth weight or normal birth weight. _____

14. The presence of homonymous hemianopia in stroke patients negatively affects their length of stay in hospital. _____

15. Adjustment to hemodialysis does not vary by the patient's gender. _____

C. STUDY QUESTIONS

1. Below is a list of general topics that could be investigated. Develop at least one research question for each, making sure that some are questions that could be addressed through qualitative research and others are ones that could be addressed through quantitative research. (HINT: For quantitative research questions, think of these concepts as potential independent or dependent variables, then ask, "What might cause or affect this variable (outcome)?" and "What might be the consequences or effects of this variable on other outcomes?" This should lead to some ideas for research questions.)

   a. Patient comfort _____.

   b. Psychiatric patients' readmission rates _____.

   c. Anxiety in hospitalized children _____.

   d. Elevated blood pressure _____.

   e. Incidence of sexually transmitted diseases (STDs) _____.

   f. Patient cooperativeness in the recovery room _____.

   g. Caregiver stress _____.

   h. Mother–infant bonding _____.

   i. Menstrual irregularities _____.

2. Below are five nondirectional hypotheses. Restate each one as a directional hypothesis. Your hypotheses do not need to be "right"—this exercise is designed to encourage familiarity with wording hypotheses.

NONDIRECTIONAL	DIRECTIONAL
a. Tactile stimulation is associated with comparable physiological arousal as verbal stimulation among infants with congenital heart disease.	a.
b. The risk of hypoglycemia in term newborns is related to the infant's birth weight.	b.
c. The use of isotonic sodium chloride solution before endotracheal suctioning is related to oxygen saturation.	c.
d. Fluid balance is related to degree of success in weaning older adults from mechanical ventilation.	d.
e. Nurses administer the same amount of narcotic analgesics to male and female patients.	e.

3. Below are five research hypotheses. Reword them as null hypotheses.

RESEARCH HYPOTHESIS	NULL HYPOTHESIS
a. First-time blood donors experience greater anxiety during the donation than donors who have given blood previously.	a.
b. Nurses who initiate more conversation with patients are rated as more effective in their nursing care by patients than those who initiate less conversation.	b.
c. Surgical patients who give high ratings to the informativeness of nursing communications experience less preoperative stress than do patients who give low ratings.	c.
d. Appendectomy patients who are pregnant are more likely to experience peritoneal infection than female patients who are not pregnant.	d.
e. Women who give birth by cesarean delivery are more likely to experience postpartum depression than women who give birth vaginally.	e.

4. In study questions C.2 and C.3, 10 research hypotheses were provided. Identify the independent and dependent (outcome) variables in each.

INDEPENDENT VARIABLE(S)	DEPENDENT (OUTCOME) VARIABLE(S)
2a	
2b	
2c	
2d	
2e	
3a	
3b	
3c	
3d	
3e	

5. Below are five statements that are *not* testable research hypotheses as currently stated. Suggest modifications to these statements that would make them testable hypotheses.

ORIGINAL STATEMENT	HYPOTHESIS
a. Relaxation therapy is effective in reducing hypertension.	a.
b. The use of bilingual health care staff produces high utilization rates of health care facilities by ethnic minorities.	b.
c. Nursing students are affected in their choice of clinical specialization by interactions with nursing faculty.	c.
d. Sexually active teenagers have a high rate of using male methods of contraception.	d.
e. In-use intravenous solutions become contaminated within 48 hours.	e.

D. APPLICATION EXERCISES

Exercise D.1: Study in Appendix D

Read the abstract and introduction to the report by Eckhardt and colleagues ("Fatigue in the presence of coronary heart disease") in Appendix D on pages 139–150 and then answer the following questions:

Questions of Fact

a. In which paragraph(s) of this report is the research problem stated? Summarize the problem in a sentence or two.

b. Did the researchers present a statement of purpose? If so, what *verb* did they use in the purpose statement, and is that verb consistent with the type of research that was undertaken?

c. Did the researchers specify a research question? If so, was it well-stated? If not, indicate what the question was.

d. Did the researchers specify hypotheses? If there are hypotheses, were they appropriately worded? Are they directional or nondirectional? Simple or complex? Research or null? If no hypotheses were stated, what would one be?

e. Were any hypotheses *tested* in this study?

Questions for Discussion

a. Did the researchers do an adequate job of describing the research problem? Suggest ways in which the problem statement could be improved.

b. Comment on the significance of the study's research problem for nursing.

c. Did the researchers adequately explain the study purpose, research questions, and/or hypotheses? Were they well-worded?

Exercise D.2: Study in Appendix B

Read the abstract and introduction to the report by Cricco-Lizza ("Rooting for the breast") in Appendix B on pages 121–130 and then answer the following questions:

Questions of Fact

a. In which paragraph(s) of this report is the research problem stated? Summarize the problem in a sentence or two.

b. Did the researchers present a statement of purpose? If so, what *verb* did they use in the purpose statement, and is that verb consistent with the type of research that was undertaken?

c. Did the researcher specify a research question? If so, was it well-stated? If not, indicate what the question was.

d. Did Cricco-Lizza specify hypotheses? If there are hypotheses, were they appropriately worded? Are they directional or nondirectional? Simple or complex? Research or null?

e. Were any hypotheses *tested*?

Questions for Discussion

a. Did the researchers do an adequate job of describing the research problem? Suggest ways in which the problem statement could be improved.

b. Comment on the significance of the study's research problem for nursing.

c. Did the researcher adequately explain the study purpose, research questions, and/or hypotheses? Were they well-worded?

CHAPTER 7

Finding and Reviewing Evidence in the Literature

A. FILL IN THE BLANKS

How many terms have you learned in this chapter? Fill in the blanks in the sentences below to find out. You can have fun with this section by doing it with a friend. Who is the first one to complete the sentence?

1. A research journal article written by the researchers who conducted a study is a(n) _____ source for a research review.

2. Descriptions of studies written by someone other than the investigators are considered _____ sources.

3. The _____ approach is a search strategy sometimes called "footnote chasing."

4. When a reviewer identifies a pivotal study and then searches forward for studies that cited that pivotal study, the strategy is called the _____ approach.

5. A major resource for finding research reports are _____ databases.

6. A feature called _____ allows people to search for topics using their own words, rather than needing to know subject codes in the database.

7. When doing a database search, one begins with one or more _____.

8. _____ is an especially important bibliographic database for nurses and the allied health professions.

9. Examples of _____ operators include "AND" and "OR."

10. The controlled vocabulary used to code entries in MEDLINE is called _____.

11. The MEDLINE database can be accessed for free through _____.

12. If a researcher has been prominent in an area, it is useful to do a(n) _____ search in bibliographic databases.

B. MATCHING EXERCISES

Match each statement in Set B with one of the types of databases listed in Set A. Indicate the letter corresponding to the appropriate response next to each entry in Set B.

SET A

a. CINAHL

b. MEDLINE

c. Neither CINAHL nor MEDLINE

d. Both CINAHL and MEDLINE

SET B   RESPONSES

1. An important bibliographic database for nurses   _____

2. Can be accessed on the Internet through PubMed   _____

3. Does not allow the use of truncation symbols   _____

4. Uses MeSH to index entries   _____

5. Focuses on nursing and allied health   _____

6. Does not provide abstracts, only citations   _____

7. Has over 24 million records

8. The articles in the appendices to this *Study Guide* could be
retrieved in this database.   _____

C. STUDY QUESTIONS

1. Below are several research questions. Indicate one or more keywords that you would use to begin a literature search on this topic.

RESEARCH QUESTIONS   KEYWORDS

a. What is the lived experience of being a survivor
of a fatal automobile crash?   _____

b. Does contingency contracting improve patient
compliance with a treatment regimen?   _____

c. What is the decision-making process for a woman
considering having an abortion?   _____

d. Is a special intervention for patients with spinal cord injury
effective in reducing the risk of pressure ulcers?   _____

e. Do children raised on vegetarian diets have different
growth patterns than other children?   _____

f. What is the course of appetite loss among patients
undergoing chemotherapy?   _____

g. What is the effect of alcohol skin preparation before insulin
injection on the incidence of local and systemic infection?   _____

h. Are bottle-fed babies introduced to solid foods sooner
than breastfed babies?   _____

2. Below are fictitious excerpts from research literature reviews. Each excerpt has a stylistic problem. Change each sentence to make it acceptable stylistically, inventing citations if necessary.

ORIGINAL   **REVISED**

a. Most elderly people do not eat a balanced diet.   _____

b. Patient characteristics have a significant impact on
nursing workload.   _____

c. A child's conception of appropriate sick role behavior
changes as the child grows older.   _____

d. Home birth poses many potential dangers.   _____

e. Multiple sclerosis results in considerable anxiety to the
family of the patients.   _____

f. Studies have proved that most nurses prefer not to work
the night shift.   _____

g. Life changes are the major cause of stress in adults.   _____

h. Stroke rehabilitation programs are most effective when
they involve the patients' families.   _____

i. It has been proved that psychiatric outpatients have
higher than average rates of accidental deaths and suicides.   _____

j. The traditional pelvic examination is sufficiently unpleasant
to many women that they avoid having the examination.   _____

3. Read the following research report (or read another article of your choosing):

- Oakley-Girvan, I., Londono, C., Canchola, A., & Watkins Davis, S. (2016). Text messaging may improve abnormal mammogram follow-up in Latinas. *Oncology Nursing Forum, 43,* 36–43.

Use the brief protocol in Figure 7.4 on page 115 in the textbook and complete as much information as you can about the report.

4. Read the literature review section from a research article appearing in a nursing journal in the early 2000s (some possibilities are suggested below). Search the literature for more recent research on the topic of the article and update the original researchers' review section. If possible, use the descendancy approach as one of your search strategies. (Don't forget to incorporate in your review the findings from the cited research article itself.) Here are some possible articles:

- Allen Furr, L., Binkley, C. J., McCurren, C., & Carrico, R. (2004). Factors affecting quality of oral care in intensive care units. *Journal of Advanced Nursing, 48,* 454–462.

- Lindseth, G., & Bird-Baker, M. Y. (2004). Risk factors for cholelithiasis in pregnancy. *Research in Nursing & Health, 27,* 382–391.

- Redeker, N. S., Ruggiero, J. S., & Hedges, C. (2004). Sleep is related to physical function and emotional well-being after cardiac surgery. *Nursing Research, 53,* 154–162.

- Winterbottom, A., & Harcourt, D. (2004). Patients' experience of the diagnosis and treatment of skin cancer. *Journal of Advanced Nursing, 48,* 226–233.

D. APPLICATION EXERCISES

Exercise D.1: Study in Appendix G

Read the abstract, introduction, and the first subsection under "Methods" of the report by Chase and colleagues ("Effectiveness of medication adherence interventions") in Appendix G on pages 177–186 and then answer the following questions:

Questions of Fact

a. What type of research review did the investigators undertake?

b. Did the researchers begin with a problem statement? Summarize the problem in two or three sentences.

c. Did the researchers provide a statement of purpose? If so, what was it?

d. Which bibliographic databases did the researchers search?

e. What keywords were used in the search?

f. Did the reviewers use the ancestry approach in their search for studies?

g. Did the researchers restrict their search to English language reports?

h. How many studies ultimately were included in the review?

i. Were the studies included in the review qualitative, quantitative, or both?

Questions for Discussion

a. Did the researchers do an adequate job of explaining the problem and their purpose in undertaking the review?

b. Did the researchers appear to do a thorough job in their search for relevant studies?

c. Certain studies that were initially retrieved were eliminated. Do you think the researchers provided a sound rationale for their decisions?

Exercise D.2: Study in Appendix H

Read the following abstract, introduction, and Study Design and Methods sections of the report by Beck ("A metaethnography of traumatic childbirth") in Appendix H on pages 187–198 and then answer the following questions:

Questions of Fact

a. What type of research review did Beck undertake?

b. What was the purpose of this research review?

c. Did Beck's review involve a systematic search for evidence in bibliographic databases?

d. How many studies were included in the metasynthesis?

e. Which qualitative research traditions were represented in the review?

Questions for Discussion

a. Did Beck do an adequate job of explaining the problem and the study purpose?

b. Should Beck have searched for and included other qualitative studies on birth trauma? If yes, what would have been her keywords?

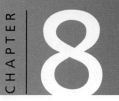

CHAPTER 8

Theoretical and Conceptual Frameworks

A. FILL IN THE BLANKS

How many terms have you learned in this chapter? Fill in the blanks in the sentences below to find out. You can have fun with this section by doing it with a friend. Who is the first one to complete the sentence?

1. The conceptual underpinnings of a study is known as its _____.

2. Abstractions assembled because of their relevance to a core theme form a(n) _____ model.

3. A(n) _____ theory thoroughly accounts for or describes a phenomenon.

4. A theory that focuses on a specific aspect of human experience is sometimes called _____ range.

5. A schematic _____ is a mechanism for representing concepts with a minimal use of words.

6. The four elements in conceptual models of nursing are _____, _____, _____, and _____.

7. The originator of the Health Promotion Model is Nola _____.

8. _____ is the originator of the Humanbecoming paradigm.

9. Roy conceptualized the _____ Model of nursing.

10. A construct that was fully conceptualized by Bandura and that is a key mediator in many models of health behavior is _____.

11. The Transtheoretical Model involves a construct called _____ of _____, which concerns a person's motivational readiness to modify behavior.

12. According to the Theory of _____ _____, a person's intention to act in a certain way determines their actual behavior.

43

B. MATCHING EXERCISES

1. Match each statement from Set B with one of the phrases in Set A. Indicate the letter corresponding to your response next to each of the statements in Set B.

SET A

a. Classic theory

b. Conceptual model

c. Schematic model

d. Neither a, b, nor c

e. a, b, *and* c

SET B   RESPONSES

1. Makes minimal use of language   _____

2. Uses concepts as building blocks   _____

3. Is often a product of grounded theory studies   _____

4. Can be used as a basis for generating hypotheses   _____

5. Can be proved through empirical testing   _____

6. Incorporates a system of propositions that assert
relationships among variables   _____

7. Consists of interrelated concepts organized in a rational
scheme but does not specify formal relationships
among the concepts   _____

8. Exists in nature and is awaiting scientific discovery   _____

2. Match each model from Set B with one of the theorists in Set A. Indicate the letter corresponding to your response next to each of the statements in Set B.

SET A

a. Bandura

b. Pender

c. Roy

d. Prochaska

e. Mishel

f. Ajzen

SET B   RESPONSES

1. Adaptation Model   _____

2. Transtheoretical Model   _____

3. Uncertainty in Illness Theory   _____

4. Social Cognitive Theory   _____

5. Health Promotion Model   _____

6. Theory of Planned Behavior   _____

C. STUDY QUESTIONS

1. Read some recent issues of a nursing research journal. Identify at least three different theories cited by nurse researchers in these research reports.

2. Select one of the research questions/problems listed below. Could the selected problem be developed within one of the models or theories discussed in this chapter? Defend your answer.

   a. What are the factors contributing to perceptions of fatigue among patients with congestive heart failure?

   b. What effect does the presence of the father in the delivery room have on the mother's satisfaction with the childbirth experience?

   c. The purpose of the study is to explore why some women fail to perform breast self-examination regularly.

   d. What are the factors that lead to poorer health among low-income children than higher income children?

3. Suggest an important health outcome that could be studied using the Health Promotion Model. Identify another theory described in this chapter that could be used to explain or predict the same outcome. Which theory or model do you think would do a better job? Why?

4. Read the following open-access article (a link is provided in the Internet Resources section on thePoint website) and then assess the following:

   a. What evidence do the researchers offer to substantiate that their grounded theory is a good fit with their data?

   b. To what extent is it clear or unclear in the article that symbolic interactionism was a theoretical underpinning of the study?

      • Panpanit, L., Carolan-Olah, M., & McCann, T. (2015). A qualitative study of older adults seeking appropriate treatment to self-manage their chronic pain in rural northeast Thailand. *BMC Geriatrics, 15,* 166.

D. APPLICATION EXERCISES

Exercise D.1: Study in Appendix D

Read the abstract and introduction (all of the material before "Methods") of the article by Eckhardt and colleagues ("Fatigue in the presence of coronary heart disease") in Appendix D on pages 139–150 and then answer the following questions:

Questions of Fact

a. Did the study by Eckhardt and colleagues involve a conceptual or theoretical framework? What is it called?

b. Is this framework one of the models of nursing cited in the textbook? Is it related to one of those models?

c. Was the theory thoroughly described?

d. Did the researchers adapt the theory? In what way was it adapted?

e. Does the report include a schematic model?

f. What are the key concepts in the model?

g. Did this model indicate relationships among the concepts?

h. Did the report present conceptual definitions of key concepts?

i. Did the report explicitly present hypotheses deduced from the framework?

Questions for Discussion

a. Did the link between the problem and the framework seem contrived? Did the hypotheses (if any) naturally flow from the framework?

b. Do you think any aspects of the research would have been different without the framework?

c. Would you describe this study as a model-testing inquiry or do you think the model was used more as an organizing framework?

Exercise D.2: Study in Appendix E

Read the report by Byrne and colleagues ("Care transition experiences") in Appendix E on pages 151–168 and then answer the following questions:

Questions of Fact

a. Did this article describe a conceptual or theoretical framework for the study? What is it called?

b. Did the study result in the generation of a theory? What was it called?

c. Did the report include a schematic model? If so, what are the key concepts in the framework?

d. Did the report explicitly present hypotheses deduced from the framework? Did the researchers undertake hypothesis-testing statistical analyses?

Questions for Discussion

a. Does the research problem naturally flow from the framework? Does the link between the problem and the framework seem contrived?

b. Do you think any aspects of the research would have been different without the framework?

c. How good a job do you feel the researchers did in tying the perspectives of the framework into the presentation of the findings and the discussion of the results?

PART 3

Designs and Methods for Quantitative and Qualitative Nursing Research

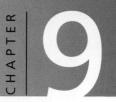
Quantitative Research Design

A. FILL IN THE BLANKS

How many terms have you learned in this chapter? Fill in the blanks in the sentences below to find out. You can have fun with this section by doing it with a friend. Who is the first one to complete the sentence?

1. Good research design in quantitative studies involves achieving four types of _____.

2. A(n) _____ design refers to a study design in which the same subjects are exposed to two or more conditions in random order.

3. The loss of subjects from a study over time is called _____.

4. A key threat to internal validity, stemming from preexisting group differences is the _____ threat.

5. The allocation of subjects to groups by chance is called _____ assignment.

6. Researchers use the strategy of _____ (or masking) to guard against expectation biases.

7. Techniques of research _____ include randomization, homogeneity, and matching.

8. _____ is a threat to internal validity stemming from differential loss of subjects from groups.

9. In a(n) _____ design, data about causes are collected before data about effects.

10. Demonstrating the existence of a relationship between an independent variable and an outcome contributes to _____ conclusion validity.

11. The degree to which it can be inferred that the independent variable caused or influenced the outcome variable is _____ validity.

12. The type of validity referring to the generalizability of results is _____ validity.

13. Data are collected at a single point in time in a _____ study.

14. A(n) _____ is what would have happened to the same people simultaneously exposed and not exposed to a hypothesized causal factor.

15. A(n) _____ study is a nonexperimental design involving the comparison of a *case* and a matched counterpart.

49

16. A(n)_____ study involves the collection of data over an extended period of time.

17. _____ involves the deliberate pairing of participants in different groups with respect to key attributes as a method of controlling confounding variables.

18. Statistical _____ refers to the ability of the design to detect true relationships among variables.

19. A(n) _____ threat is an internal validity problem that concerns the effect of other things co-occurring with the independent variable.

20. In a delayed treatment design, control group members are _____-listed for the intervention.

21. In an intervention study, data collected before implementing the intervention are often called _____ data.

22. Intervention studies in which there is no randomization to treatment conditions are called _____.

23. Correlational studies examine _____ between variables but involve no intervention.

24. In _____ studies, researchers search for antecedent causes of an effect occurring in the present.

B. MATCHING EXERCISES

Match each research question from Set B with one (or more) of the phrases from Set A that indicates a potential reason for using a nonexperimental design. Indicate the letter(s) corresponding to your response next to each statement in Set B.

SET A

a. Independent variable cannot be manipulated

b. Possible ethical constraints on manipulation

c. Practical constraints on manipulation

d. No constraints on manipulation

SET B   **RESPONSES**

1. Does the use of certain tampons cause toxic shock syndrome?   _____

2. Does heroin addiction among mothers affect Apgar scores of infants?   _____

3. Is the age of a patient who is on hemodialysis related to the occurrence of the disequilibrium syndrome?   _____

4. What body positions aid respiratory function?   _____

5. Does the ingestion of saccharin cause cancer in humans?   _____

6. Does a nurse's attitude toward the elderly affect his or her choice of a clinical specialty?   _____

7. Does the use of touch by nursing staff affect patient morale?   _____

8. Does a nurse's gender affect his or her salary and rate of promotion? _____

9. Does extreme athletic exertion in young women cause amenorrhea? _____

10. Does assertiveness training affect a psychiatric nurse's job performance? _____

C. STUDY QUESTIONS

1. Suppose you wanted to study self-efficacy among successful dieters who lost 20 or more pounds and maintained their weight loss for at least 6 months. Specify at least two different types of comparison strategies that might provide a useful comparative context for this study. Do your strategies lend themselves to experimental manipulation? If not, why not?

2. Refer to the 10 hypotheses in Chapter 6 Exercises C.2 and C.3 on page 36. Indicate below whether these hypotheses could be tested using an experimental/quasi-experimental approach, a nonexperimental approach, or both.

Question Number	Experimental/Quasi-Experimental	Nonexperimental	Both
2a			
2b			
2c			
2d			
2e			
3a			
3b			
3c			
3d			
3e			

3. In the following study, the researchers used two comparison groups:
   - Hosseinabadi, R., Biranvand, S., Pournia, Y., & Anbari, K. (2015). The effect of acupressure on pain and anxiety caused by venipuncture. *Journal of Infusion Nursing, 38,* 397–405.
     a. Review the design for this study and comment on the appropriateness of having three groups.
     b. What biases were the researchers trying to avoid? Do you think they were successful?

4. Suppose that you were studying the effects of range-of-motion exercises on arm mobility among patients undergoing radical mastectomy. You start your experiment with 50 experimental subjects and 50 control subjects. Your intervention requires the experimental subjects to come for daily sessions over a 2-week period, while control subjects come only once at the end of 2 weeks.

Your final group sizes are 40 for the experimental group and 49 for the control group. The results of your study indicate that women in the experimental group did better in raising the arm of the affected side above head level than those in the control group. What effects, if any, do you think the attrition might have on the internal validity of your study?

5. Suppose that you were interested in testing the hypothesis that regular ingestion of aspirin reduced the risk of colon cancer. Describe how such a hypothesis could be tested using a retrospective case-control design. Now describe a prospective cohort design for the same study. Compare the strengths and weaknesses of the two approaches.

D. APPLICATION EXERCISES

Exercise D.1: Study in Appendix A

Read the Methods section of the report by Stephens and colleagues ("Smartphone technology and text messaging for weight loss in young adults") in Appendix A on pages 113–120 and then answer the following questions:

Questions of Fact

a. Was there an intervention in this study?

b. Is the design for this study experimental, quasi-experimental, or nonexperimental?

c. What were the independent and dependent variables?

d. Was randomization used? If yes, what specific method was used to assign subjects to groups?

e. In terms of the control group strategies described in the textbook, what approach did the researchers use?

f. What is the specific name of the research design used in this study?

g. Was any masking/blinding used in this study?

h. Would this study be described as longitudinal?

i. Which of the methods of research control described in this chapter were used to control confounding variables?

j. What confounding variables were controlled?

k. Was there any attrition in this study?

l. Was selection a threat to the internal validity of this study?

m. Was mortality a threat to the internal validity of this study?

Questions for Discussion

a. What was the intervention? Comment on how well the intervention was described, including a description of how it was developed and refined.

b. Comment on the researchers' control group strategy. Could a more powerful or effective strategy have been used?

c. Discuss ways in which this study achieved or failed to achieve the criteria for making causal inferences.

d. Comment on the researchers' use or nonuse of blinding.

e. Comment on the timing of postintervention data collection.

f. Is this study strong on external validity? What, if any, are the threats to the external validity of this study?

Exercise D.2: Study in Appendix D

Read the Methods section of the report by Eckhardt and colleagues ("Fatigue in the presence of coronary heart disease") in Appendix D on pages 139–150 and then answer the following questions:

Questions of Fact

a. Was there an intervention in this study?

b. Is the design for this study experimental, quasi-experimental, or nonexperimental?

c. Was this a cause-probing study?

d. What were the independent and dependent variables in this study?

e. Was the independent variable amenable to manipulation?

f. Was randomization used? If yes, what specific method was used to assign subjects to groups?

g. What is the specific name of the research design used in this study?

h. Was any blinding (masking) used in this study?

i. Would this study be described as longitudinal? Would it be described as prospective?

Questions for Discussion

a. Discuss ways in which this study achieved or failed to achieve the criteria for making causal inferences.

b. Comment on the timing of data collection. Would a different time perspective be useful?

10

Sampling and Data Collection in Quantitative Studies

A. FILL IN THE BLANKS

How many terms have you learned in this chapter? Fill in the blanks in the sentences below to find out. You can have fun with this section by doing it with a friend. Who is the first one to complete the sentence?

1. _____ sampling involves recruiting *every* eligible person over a specified period of time.

2. Specifications for a population are identified in the _____ criteria.

3. The total number of participants in a study is known as the study's sample _____.

4. An aggregate set of people/objects with specified characteristics is a(n) _____.

5. Subdivisions of a population are called _____.

6. _____ sampling involves sampling by convenience, but within specified subgroups of the population, to enhance representativeness.

7. The broad class of sampling in which every element of a population has an equal chance of being selected is _____ sampling.

8. In quantitative studies, the key criterion for evaluating a sample is its _____ of the population.

9. _____ sampling is the most widely used type of sampling in quantitative research.

10. Probability sampling involves the selection of sample members at _____.

11. Sampling _____ is the systematic overrepresentation or underrepresentation of some segment of the population.

12. In _____ sampling, the researcher samples every *k*th case, with the interval established by dividing the population size by the desired sample size.

13. In quantitative studies, researchers use _____ _____ to estimate how large a sample they need.

14. The most widely used method of data collection by nurse researchers is by _____-report.

15. The type of questions prevalent in mailed questionnaires are _____-ended questions.

16. The question, "What is it like to be a cancer survivor?" is a(n) _____-ended question.

17. A composite _____ with multiple items yields a score that places people on a continuum with regard to an attribute.

18. A(n) _____ scale is a type of summated rating scale used to measure agreement or disagreement with statements.

19. A scaling procedure to measure clinical symptoms is a(n) _____ analog scale.

20. The tendency to distort self-report information in characteristic ways is called a response _____ bias.

21. Methods of collecting data by watching behaviors and events are referred to as _____ methods.

22. In a structured observation, a(n) _____ is used with a category system to record frequencies of observed events or behaviors.

23. _____ sampling in observational studies is used to select periods when observations are made, either systematically or randomly.

24. _____ involves assigning numbers to attributes according to established rules.

25. _____ is the extent to which scores for people *who have not changed* are the same for repeated measurements.

26. An assessment of a composite scale's _____ _____ involves evaluating whether there is consistency across items designed to measure the same trait.

27. The method used to assess an instrument's stability is _____– _____ reliability.

28. _____ is the extent to which an instrument is actually measuring what it purports to measure.

29. _____ validity concerns the extent to which the scores on a measure are a good reflection of a "gold standard."

30. One means of assessing construct validity is through the known- _____ technique.

B. MATCHING EXERCISES

1. Match each statement relating to sampling for quantitative studies from Set B with one of the phrases from Set A. Indicate the letter corresponding to your response next to each of the statements in Set B.

SET A

a. Probability sampling

b. Nonprobability sampling

   c. Both probability and nonprobability sampling

   d. Neither probability nor nonprobability sampling

SET B   **RESPONSES**

   1. Includes systematic sampling   _____

   2. Allows an estimation of the magnitude of sampling error   _____

   3. Guarantees a representative sample   _____

   4. Includes quota sampling   _____

   5. Requires a sample size of at least 100 subjects   _____

   6. Elements are selected by nonrandom methods   _____

   7. Can be used with entire populations or with selected strata
   from the populations   _____

   8. Used to select populations   _____

   9. Elements have an equal chance of being selected   _____

   10. Is most widely used by nurse researchers   _____

   2. Match each descriptive statement regarding data collection methods from
   Set B with one (or more) of the statements from Set A. Indicate the letter(s)
   corresponding to your response next to each item in Set B.

SET A

   a. Self-reports

   b. Observations

   c. Biophysiologic measures

   d. None of the above

SET B   **RESPONSES**

   1. Cannot easily be gathered unobtrusively   _____

   2. Can be biased by the participants' desire to "look good"   _____

   3. Can be used to gather data from infants   _____

   4. Is a good way to obtain information about human behavior   _____

   5. Can be biased by the researcher's values and beliefs _____

   6. Can be combined with other data collection methods in a
   single study   _____

   7. Can yield quantitative information   _____

   8. Is the most widely used method of collecting data by
   nurse researchers   _____

   3. Match each descriptive statement regarding self-report methods from Set B
   with one of the statements from Set A. Indicate the letter corresponding to
   your response next to each item in Set B.

SET A

a. Interviews

b. Questionnaires

c. Both interviews and questionnaires

d. Neither interviews nor questionnaires

SET B   **RESPONSES**

1. Can provide participants the protection of anonymity   _____

2. Can be used with illiterate participants   _____

3. Can contain both open- and closed-ended questions   _____

4. Is the best way to measure human behavior   _____

5. Is generally an inexpensive method of data collection   _____

6. Can be distributed by mail   _____

C. STUDY QUESTIONS

1. Identify the type of quantitative sampling design used in the following examples:
   a. A sample of 250 members randomly selected from a roster of American Nurses Association members
   b. All the oncology nurses participating in a continuing education seminar
   c. Every 20th patient admitted to the emergency room
   d. Twenty male and 20 female patients admitted to the hospital with hypothermia
   e. Twenty-five internationally renowned critical care nurses selected for their expertise
   f. All patients receiving hospice services from Capital District Hospice in 2016

2. Suppose you have decided to use systematic sampling for a study. The population size is 5,000 and the desired sample size is 250. What is the sampling interval? If the first element selected is 23, what would be the second, third, and fourth elements selected?

3. Suppose you were interested in studying the attitude of nurse practitioners toward autonomy in work situations. Suggest a possible target and accessible population. What strata might be useful if quota sampling were used?

4. Below are several research problems. Indicate what methods of data collection (self-report, observation, biophysiologic measures, records) you might recommend using for each. Defend your response.
   a. What are the predictors of intravenous site symptoms?
   b. What are the health and mental health consequences of a sedentary lifestyle among community-dwelling elders?
   c. To what extent and in what manner do nurses interact differently with male and female patients?
   d. What are the effects of an HIV-prevention intervention on the risk-taking behavior of urban adolescents?

5. Identify five constructs of clinical relevance that would be appropriate for measurement using a visual analogue scale (VAS).

6. Which of the following measures could be assessed with respect to internal consistency?
   a. Infants' Apgar scores
   b. Blood pressure measurements
   c. A 10-item scale to measure resilience
   d. A visual analog scale measuring dyspnea

7. What types of groups might be useful for a known-groups approach to assessing construct validity for measures of the following:
   a. Fear of dying
   b. Children's aggressiveness
   c. Quality of life
   d. Compliance with a medication regimen
   e. Subjective pain

D. APPLICATION EXERCISES

Exercise D.1: Quantitative Appendix Studies

Which of the studies in Appendices A (by Stephens et al.) on pages 113–120, C (by Yackel et al.) on pages 131–138, and D (by Eckhardt et al.) on pages 139–150 used the following sampling methods?

a. Probability sampling
b. Convenience sampling
c. Consecutive sampling

Exercise D.2: Quantitative Appendix Studies

Which of the studies in Appendices A (by Stephens et al.) on pages 113–120, C (by Yackel et al.) on pages 131–138, and D (by Eckhardt et al.) on pages 139–150 used the following data collection methods?

a. Self-reports
b. Observational methods
c. Biophysiologic measures
d. Records

Exercise D.3: Study in Appendix D

Read the Methods and first part of the Results sections of the report by Eckhardt and colleagues ("Fatigue in the presence of coronary heart disease") in Appendix D on pages 139–150 and then answer the following questions:

Questions of Fact

a. What was the target population of this study? How would you describe the accessible population?

b. What were the eligibility criteria for the study?

c. Was the sampling method probability or nonprobability? What specific sampling method was used?

d. How were study participants recruited?

e. What efforts did the researchers make to ensure a diverse (and hence more representative) sample?

f. What was the sample size that the research team achieved?

g. Was a power analysis used to estimate sample size needs? If yes, what number of subjects did the power analysis estimate as the minimum needed number?

h. Were sample characteristics described? If yes, what were the main characteristics?

i. Did the researchers develop their own measures or did they use instruments or scales that had been developed by others?

j. What did the article say about the reliability and validity of key measures?

Questions for Discussion

a. Comment on the adequacy of the researchers' sampling plan and recruitment strategy. How representative was the sample of the target population? What types of sampling biases might be of special concern?

b. Do you think the sample size was adequate? Why or why not?

c. Comment on the adequacy of the data collection approaches used in this study. Did Eckhardt and her colleagues operationalize their outcome measures in the best possible manner?

d. Did the researchers' description of their measures inspire confidence in data quality in this study?

Qualitative Designs and Approaches

A. FILL IN THE BLANKS

How many terms have you learned in this chapter? Fill in the blanks in the sentences below to find out. You can have fun with this section by doing it with a friend. Who is the first one to complete the sentence?

1. Qualitative designs that are _____ require an ongoing analysis of data to suggest profitable new strategies.

2. _____ was Leininger's phrase for research at the interface between culture and nursing.

3. Ethnographers typically undertake _____ observation as a data collection strategy during their fieldwork.

4. Ethnographers rely on one or more key _____ to help them understand and interpret a culture.

5. An ethnography that studies small units in a group or culture is called a(n) _____ ethnography.

6. Phenomenologists study _____ experiences.

7. A phenomenological question is: What is the _____ of this phenomenon?

8. _____ phenomenology focuses on the *meaning* of experiences; another term used for this type of phenomenology is _____.

9. Descriptive phenomenologists use the strategy called _____ to hold in abeyance their presuppositions about a phenomenon.

10. Grounded theory researchers often identify a _____ social process (BSP) that explains how people resolve a problem.

11. The two originators of grounded theory were _____ and _____.

12. Grounded theorists use an analytic strategy called _____ comparison.

13. The systematic collection and analysis of materials relating to the past is known as _____ research.

14. In a(n) _____ study, a single person or group is at center stage.

15. In _____ analysis, the focus is on a *story*.

16. Research that seeks to be transformative is based on _____ theory.

17. _____ research focuses on gender domination.

18. Participatory _____ research is designed to be empowering for the group under study.

B. MATCHING EXERCISES

Match each descriptive statement from Set B with one of the research traditions from Set A. Indicate the letter corresponding to your response next to each item in Set B.

SET A

a. Ethnography

b. Phenomenology

c. Grounded theory

d. Ethnography, phenomenology, and grounded theory

SET B   RESPONSES

1. Is rooted in a philosophical tradition developed by Husserl and Heidegger   _____

2. Involves the study of both broadly defined cultures and more narrowly defined ones   _____

3. Uses qualitative data to address questions of interest   _____

4. Is an approach to the study of social processes and social structures   _____

5. Is concerned with the lived experiences of humans   _____

6. Strives to achieve an emic perspective on the members of a group   _____

7. Is closely related to a research tradition called hermeneutics   _____

8. Uses a procedure referred to as constant comparison   _____

9. Stems from a discipline other than nursing   _____

10. Developed by the sociologists Glaser and Strauss   _____

11. Is a tradition that is particularly well suited to a critical theory perspective   _____

12. Typically involves interviews with study participants   _____

C. STUDY QUESTIONS

1. For each of the research questions below, indicate what type of qualitative research tradition would likely guide the inquiry and why you think that would be the case.

   a. What is the social psychological process through which couples deal with the sudden loss of an infant through SIDS?

   b. How does the culture of suicide survivors' self-help group adapt to a successful suicide attempt by a former member?

   c. What is the lived experience of the spousal caretaker of a patient with Alzheimer's disease?

   d. What is the meaning of loneliness to childless widows with chronic health problems?

2. Skim the following two studies, which are examples of ethnographic and phenomenological studies that focused on alcohol/drinking. What were the central phenomena under investigation? Compare and contrast the methods used in these two studies (e.g., How were data collected? How many study participants were there? To what extent did the design unfold while the researchers were in the field?)

   • *Ethnographic Study:* Johnston, S., & Boyle, J. (2013). Northern British Columbian Aboriginal mothers: Raising adolescents with fetal alcohol spectrum disorder. *Journal of Transcultural Nursing, 24,* 60–67.

   • *Phenomenological Study:* Thurang, A. M., Palmstierna, T., & Tops, A. B. (2014). Experiences of everyday life in men with alcohol dependency—a qualitative study. *Issues in Mental Health Nursing, 35,* 588–596.

3. Skim the following open-access article about a participatory action research (PAR) study and comment on the roles of participants and researchers. How might the study have been different if a participatory approach had not been used?

   • *Loeb, S. J., Hollenbeak, C. S., Penrod, J., Smith, C. A., Kitt-Lewis, E., & Crouse, S. B. (2013). Care and companionship in an isolating environment: Inmates attending to dying peers. *Journal of Forensic Nursing, 9,* 35–44.

4. Read the following open-access article describing a case study and evaluate the extent to which a case study approach was appropriate. What were the drawbacks and benefits of using this approach?

   • *Harrison, T., Taylor, J., Fredland, N., Stuifbergen, A., Walker, J., & Choban, R. (2013). A qualitative analysis of life course adjustment to multiple morbidity and disability. *Research in Gerontological Nursing, 6,* 57–69.

5. Read the following open-access journal article about a grounded theory study and evaluate the extent to which the problem was amenable to the grounded theory tradition. Which school of grounded theory thought was followed in this study? Did the report explicitly discuss how the constant comparative method was used?

   • *Tseng, C. N., Huang, G., Yu, P., & Lou, M. (2015). A qualitative study of family caregiver experiences of managing incontinence in stroke survivors. *PLoS One, 10,* e0129540.

---

*A link to this open-access journal article is provided in the Internet Resources section on the textbook's thePoint website.

D. APPLICATION EXERCISES

Exercise D.1: Study in Appendix E

Read the Methodology section of the report by Byrne and colleagues ("Care transition experiences") in Appendix E on pages 151–168 and then answer the following questions:

Questions of Fact

a. In which tradition was this study based?

b. Which specific approach was used—that of Glaser and Strauss, Strauss and Corbin, or Charmaz?

c. What was the central phenomenon under study?

d. Was the study longitudinal?

e. What was the setting for this research?

f. Did the report indicate or suggest that constant comparison was used?

g. Was a core variable or basic social process identified? If yes, what was it?

h. Did the researchers use methods that were congruent with the chosen qualitative research tradition?

i. Did this study have an ideological perspective? If so, which one?

Questions for Discussion

a. How well is the research design described in the report? Were design decisions explained and justified?

b. Does it appear that the researchers made all design decisions up front, or did the design emerge during data collection, allowing them to capitalize on early information?

c. Were there any elements of the design or methods that appear to be more appropriate for a qualitative tradition other than the one the researchers identified as the underlying tradition?

Exercise D.2: Study in Appendix F

Read the Methods section of the report by Cummings ("Sharing a traumatic event") in Appendix F on pages 169–176 and then answer the following questions:

Questions of Fact

a. In which tradition was this study based? Within which specific school of inquiry was the study based?

b. What was the central phenomenon under study?

c. Was the study longitudinal?

d. What was the setting for this research?

e. Did the researcher make explicit comparisons?

f. Did the researchers use methods that were congruent with the chosen qualitative research tradition?

g. Did this study have an ideological perspective?

Questions for Discussion

a. How well is the research design described? Were design decisions explained and justified?

b. Does it appear that the researcher made all design decisions up front, or did the design emerge during data collection, allowing researchers to capitalize on early information?

c. Could this study have been undertaken within an ideological perspective? Why or why not?

d. Could the researcher have used narrative analysis in this study?

CHAPTER 12

Sampling and Data Collection in Qualitative Studies

A. FILL IN THE BLANKS

How many terms have you learned in this chapter? Fill in the blanks in the sentences below to find out. You can have fun with this section by doing it with a friend. Who is the first one to complete the sentence?

1. _____ sampling is a type of sampling based on referrals from early participants.

2. _____ sampling is preferred by grounded theory researchers.

3. A sampling approach in which participants are intentionally selected by the researchers to fulfill the needs of the study is known as _____ sampling.

4. A type of purposive sampling that involves deliberate attempts to draw from diverse groups is _____ sampling.

5. The principle used by qualitative researchers to determine when to stop sampling is called _____.

6. A(n) _____ guide is used in some qualitative studies to ensure that important question areas are covered in an interview.

7. An interview that is guided by an established list of topics or broad questions is _____ structured.

8. A completely unstructured interview typically begins with a(n) _____ question to begin an undirected conversation.

9. _____ is a technique wherein participants take pictures of their own environments and then explain the pictures to the researcher.

10. A technique for gathering in-depth information from 5 to 10 informants simultaneously is called a(n) _____ interview.

11. In ethnographic studies, researchers rely on _____ to provide insights about the culture and to provide guidance about activities and events to observe.

12. Participant observers record their observations, thoughts, and interpretations in _____ notes; they also maintain a daily _____ to record activities and events.

B. MATCHING EXERCISES

1. Match each type of sampling approach from Set B with one of the phrases from Set A. Indicate the letter corresponding to your response next to each of the statements in Set B.

SET A

a. Sampling approach for quantitative studies

b. Sampling approach for qualitative studies

c. Sampling approach for either quantitative or qualitative studies

d. Sampling approach for neither quantitative nor qualitative studies

SET B   RESPONSES

1. Typical case sampling   _____

2. Purposive sampling   _____

3. Systematic sampling   _____

4. Weighted sampling   _____

5. Consecutive sampling   _____

6. Extreme case sampling   _____

7. Stratified random sampling   _____

8. Quota sampling   _____

9. Theoretical sampling   _____

10. Power sampling   _____

2. Match each descriptive statement regarding data collection methods from Set B with one of the statements from Set A. Indicate the letter corresponding to your response next to each item in Set B.

SET A

a. Self-reports

b. Observations

c. Both self-reports and observations

d. Neither self-reports nor observations

SET B   RESPONSES

1. Is the primary source of data in phenomenological research   _____

2. Data are recorded in logs and field notes.   _____

3. Ethnographies rely on this as a data source.   _____

4. Photovoice is one approach.   _____

5. Mobile positioning is a strategy for collecting such data.   _____

6. Can be either structured for quantitative inquiries or unstructured for qualitative inquiries   _____

7. Usually relies on transcriptions in qualitative studies   _____

8. Can involve active participation of researchers   _____

9. Can be collected in focus groups   _____

10. Can rely on a topic guide   _____

C. STUDY QUESTIONS

1. Below are several research questions. Indicate which method of sampling you might recommend using for each and what you think the sample size might be. Defend your response.

   a. How does an elderly person manage the transition from a nursing home to a hospital and then back again?

   b. What is it like to be a patient undergoing in vitro fertilization and not get pregnant after many months of treatment?

   c. What is the process by which patients adjust to postdischarge life following a spinal cord injury?

   d. What arc the health beliefs and risk-taking behaviors of adolescent members of a vampire cult?

2. Suppose a qualitative researcher wanted to study the quality of life of cancer survivors. Suggest what the researcher might do to obtain a maximum variation sample and an extreme case sample.

3. The following open-access study relied primarily on a sample of convenience. Suggest ways in which the researchers might have improved the study by using a different sampling approach:

   • *Abedini, S., Morowatisharifabad, M. A., Enjezab, B., Barkhordari, A., & Fallahzadeh, H. (2014). Risk perception of nonspecific low back pain among nurses: A qualitative approach. *Health Promotion Perspectives*, 4, 221–229.

4. Below are several research questions. Indicate which type of unstructured self-report approach you might recommend using for each. Defend your response.

   a. How do parents of children with autism manage their frustration and fears?

   b. What are the barriers to preventive health care practices among the urban poor?

   c. What stresses does the spouse of a patient who is terminally ill experience?

   d. What are the coping mechanisms and perceived barriers to coping among patients with severely disfigured burn?

5. Suppose you were interested in studying patients' impatience and anxiety waiting for treatment in the waiting area of an emergency department. Develop a topic guide for a semistructured interview on this topic.

6. Suggest how you might collect data to address the following research question: *To what extent and in what manner do male and female nurses interact differently with male and female patients?* Would *participant* observation be appropriate? What are the possible advantages and drawbacks of such an approach?

---

*A link to this open-access journal article is provided in the Internet Resources section on the textbook's thePoint website.

7. Read one of the following open-access articles. Indicate how, if at all, you would augment the self-report data collected in the study with participant observation:

- *Lin, F. F., Foster, M., Chaboyer, W., & Marshall, A. (2016). Relocating an intensive care unit: An exploratory qualitative study. *Australian Critical Care, 29*, 55–60.

- *Ødbehr, L. S., Kvigne, K., Hauge, S., & Danbolt, L. J. (2015). Spiritual care to persons with dementia in nursing homes: A qualitative study of nurses and care workers experiences. *BMC Nursing, 14*, 70.

- *Woodgate, R. L., Edwards, M., Ripat, J. D., Borton, B., & Rempel, G. (2015). Intense parenting: A qualitative study detailing the experiences of parenting children with complex care needs. *BMC Pediatrics, 15*, 197.

D. APPLICATION EXERCISES

Exercise D.1: Study in Appendix B

Read the Methods sections of the report by Cricco-Lizza ("Rooting for the breast") in Appendix B on pages 121–130 and then answer the following questions:

Questions of Fact

a. What were the eligibility criteria for this study?

b. How were study participants recruited?

c. What type of sampling approach was used?

d. How many participants comprised the sample?

e. Was data saturation achieved?

f. Were sample characteristics described? If yes, what were those characteristics?

g. Did the researcher collect any self-report data? If no, could self-reports have been used? If yes, what concepts were captured by self-report?

h. What specific types of qualitative self-report methods were used?

i. Were examples of interview questions included in the report?

j. Did the report provide information about how long interviews took, on average?

k. How were the self-report data recorded?

l. Did this study collect any data through observation? If no, could observation have been used? If yes, what concepts were captured through observation?

m. If there were observations, how were observational data recorded?

n. Were any other types of data collected in this study?

o. Who collected the data in this study?

---

*A link to this open-access journal article is provided in the Internet Resources section on the textbook's thePoint website.

Questions for Discussion

a. Comment on the adequacy of the researcher's sampling plan and recruitment strategy for achieving the goals of this study.

b. Do you think Cricco-Lizza's sample size was adequate? Why or why not?

c. Cricco-Lizza used nurse experience as her key dimension of variability in selecting key informants. What other dimensions might have been used productively?

d. Comment on the adequacy of the researcher's description of her data collection methods.

e. Comment on the data collection approaches Cricco-Lizza used. Did she fully capture the concepts of interest in the best possible manner?

f. Comment on the procedures used to collect and record data in this study. Were adequate steps taken to ensure the highest possible quality data?

Exercise D.2: Study in Appendix E

Read the Method section of the article by Byrne and colleagues ("Care transition experiences") in Appendix E on pages 151–168 and then answer the following questions:

Questions of Fact

a. What were the eligibility criteria for this study?

b. How were study participants recruited?

c. What type of sampling approach was used?

d. How many study participants comprised the sample?

e. Was data saturation achieved?

f. Did the sampling strategy include confirming and disconfirming cases?

g. Were sample characteristics described? If yes, what were those characteristics?

h. Did the researcher collect any self-report data? If no, could self-reports have been used? If yes, what concepts were captured by self-report?

i. What specific types of qualitative self-report methods were used?

j. Were examples of interview questions included in the report?

k. Did the report provide information about how long interviews took on average?

l. How were the self-report data recorded?

m. Did this study collect any data through observation? If no, could observation have been used? If yes, what concepts were captured through observation?

Questions for Discussion

a. Comment on the adequacy of the researchers' sampling plan and recruitment strategy for achieving the goals of an in-depth study.

b. Assume that you had no resource constraints to address the research questions in this study. What sampling plan would you recommend?

c. Do you think the sample size in this study was adequate? Why or why not?

d. Comment on issues relating to the transferability of findings from this study.

Mixed Methods and Other Special Types of Research

A. FILL IN THE BLANKS

How many terms have you learned in this chapter? Fill in the blanks in the sentences below to find out. You can have fun with this section by doing it with a friend. Who is the first one to complete the sentence?

1. The type of research that integrates qualitative and quantitative data is _____ research.

2. Mixed methods designs can be characterized by decisions on _____ and _____.

3. In the notation QUAL + quan, the dominant strand is the _____ component.

4. The notation QUAL → quan signifies a design in which _____ data are collected first.

5. In mixed methods research, the design notation of an arrow (→) designates a design that is _____.

6. In mixed methods research, the design notation of a plus sign (+) designates a design that is _____.

7. The paradigm most often associated with mixed methods research is called _____.

8. A _____ _____ is a multiphase effort to refine and test the effectiveness of a clinical treatment.

9. Phase IV clinical trials are sometimes called _____ studies.

10. Phase III of a clinical trial is typically a(n) _____ controlled trial.

11. In nursing intervention research, the construct validity of a new intervention is enhanced by the development of a(n) _____.

12. An evaluation of how a new intervention gets implemented is called a(n) _____ analysis.

13. A(n) _____, which involves collecting self-report data about people's opinions, characteristics, and intentions, can be administered by telephone, mail, Internet, or in person.

14. _____ research involves efforts to understand the end results of health care practices.

15. In the Donabedian framework, the three key factors are process, outcomes, and _____.

16. A Plan-Do-Study-Act model is often used in _____ _____ projects.

17. A(n) _____ analysis involves undertaking a study using an existing data set to answer new questions.

18. The type of study that focuses on developing or improving research strategies is called a(n) _____ study.

B. MATCHING EXERCISES

1. Match each feature from Set B with one (or more) of the phrases from Set A that indicates a type of quantitative research. Indicate the letter(s) corresponding to your response next to each statement in Set B.

SET A

a. Clinical trial

b. Evaluation research

c. Survey research

d. Outcomes research

SET B   RESPONSES

1. Can involve an experimental design   _____

2. Examines the global effectiveness of nursing services _____

3. Data are always from self-reports.   _____

4. Often designed in a series of phases (typically four) _____

5. Includes process analyses   _____

6. Donabedian's framework is often used in this research. _____

7. May include an economic analysis   _____

8. Data can be used in a secondary analysis.   _____

C. STUDY QUESTIONS

1. Read one of the following open-access articles describing a study in which quantitative data were gathered and analyzed to address a research question. Suggest ways in which the collection of qualitative data might have enriched the study, strengthened its validity, or enhanced its interpretability:

   • *Pinar, R., & Afsar, F. (2015). Back massage to decrease state anxiety, cortisol level, blood pressure, heart rate and increase sleep quality in family caregivers

---

*A link to this open-access journal article is provided in the Internet Resources section on the textbook's thePoint website.

of patients with cancer: A randomised controlled trial. *Asian Pacific Journal of Cancer Prevention, 16*, 8127–8133.

- *Porter, L. S., Porter, B. O., McCoy, V., Bango-Sanchez, V., Kissel, B., Williams, M., & Nunnewar, S. (2015). Blended infant massage-parenting enhancement program on recovering substance-abusing mothers' parenting stress, self-esteem, depression, maternal attachment, and mother-infant interactions. *Asian Nursing Research, 9*, 318–327.

2. Read one of the following open-access articles describing a study in which qualitative data were gathered and analyzed to address a research question. Suggest ways that the findings could be validated or the emergent hypotheses could be tested in a quantitative study:

- *Adeola, M. T., Baird, C. L., Sands, L., Longoria, N., Henry, U., Nielsen, J., & Shields, C. G. (2015). Active despite pain: Patient experiences with guided imagery with relaxation compared to planned rest. *Clinical Journal of Oncology Nursing, 19*, 649–652.
- *Jervaeus, A., Nilsson, J., Eriksson, L. E., Lampic, C., Widmark, C., & Wettergren, L. (2016). Exploring childhood cancer survivors' views about sex and sexual experiences—findings from online focus group discussions. *European Journal of Oncology Nursing, 20*, 165–172.

3. Identify a nursing-sensitive outcome. Propose a research question that would use the outcome as the dependent variable. Would you consider the research to answer this question outcomes research?

4. Below is a brief description of a mixed methods study, followed by a critique. Do you agree with this critique? Can you add other comments regarding the study design?

FICTITIOUS STUDY

Aldrich conducted a study to examine the emotional well-being of women who had a mastectomy. Aldrich wanted to develop an in-depth understanding of the emotional experiences of women as they recovered from their surgery, including the process by which they handled their fears, their concerns about their sexuality, their levels of anxiety and depression, their methods of coping, and their social supports.

Aldrich's basic study design was a descriptive qualitative study. She gathered information from a sample of 26 women, primarily by means of in-depth interviews with the women on two occasions. The first interviews were scheduled within 1 month after the surgery. Follow-up interviews were conducted about 12 months later. Several women in the sample participated in a support group, and Aldrich attended and made observations at several meetings. Additionally, Aldrich decided to interview the "significant other" (usually the husbands) of most of the women, when it became clear that the women's emotional well-being was linked to the manner in which the significant other was reacting to the surgery.

In addition to the rich, in-depth information she gathered, Aldrich wanted to be able to better interpret the emotional status of the women. Therefore, at both the original and follow-up interview with the women, she administered a psychological scale known

---

*A link to this open-access journal article is provided in the Internet Resources section on the textbook's thePoint website.

as the Center for Epidemiological Studies Depression Scale (CES-D), a quantitative measure that has scores that can range from 0 to 60. This scale has been widely used in community populations and has cut-off scores designating when a person is at risk for clinical depression (i.e., a score of 16 and above).

Aldrich's qualitative analysis showed that the basic process underlying psychological recovery from the mastectomy was something she labeled "Gaining by Losing," a process that involved heightened self-awareness and self-respect after an initial period of despair and self-pity. The process also involved, for some, a strengthening of personal relationships with significant others, whereas for others, it resulted in the birth of awareness of fundamental deficiencies in their relationships. The quantitative findings confirmed that a very high percentage of women were at risk for being depressed at 1 month after the mastectomy, but at 12 months, the average level of depression was actually modestly lower than in the general population of women.

CRITIQUE OF THE FICTITIOUS STUDY

In her study, Aldrich embedded a quantitative measure into her field work in an interesting manner. The bulk of data were qualitative—in-depth interviews and in-depth observations. However, she also opted to include a well-known measure of depressive symptoms, which provided her with an important context for interpreting her data. A major advantage of using the CES-D is that this scale has known characteristics in the general population and therefore provided a built-in "comparison group."

Aldrich used a flexible design that allowed her to use her initial data to guide her inquiry. For example, she decided to conduct in-depth interviews with significant others when she learned their importance to the women's process of emotional recovery. Aldrich did do some advance planning, however, that provided general guidance. For example, although her questioning likely evolved while in the field, she had the foresight to realize that to capture a process as it evolved, she would need to collect data longitudinally. She also made the up-front decision to use the CES-D to supplement the in-depth interviews.

In this study, the findings from the qualitative and quantitative portions of the study were complementary. Both portions of the study confirmed that the women initially had emotional "losses," but eventually they recovered and "gained" in terms of their emotional well-being and their self-awareness. This example illustrates how the validity of study findings can be enhanced by the blending of qualitative and quantitative data. If the qualitative data alone had been gathered, Aldrich might not have gotten a good handle on the degree to which the women had actually "recovered" (vis-à-vis women who had never had a mastectomy). Conversely, if she had collected only the CES-D data, she would have had no insights into the process by which the recovery occurred.

D. APPLICATION EXERCISES

Exercise D.1: All Studies in the Appendices

Which of the studies in the appendices of this *Study Guide* (if any) could be considered:

a. A clinical trial?

b. An economic analysis?

c. Outcomes research?

d. Survey research?

e. A secondary analysis?

f. Methodologic research?

Exercise D.2: Study in Appendix D

Read the article by Eckhardt and colleagues ("Fatigue in the presence of coronary heart disease") in Appendix D on pages 139–150 and then answer the following questions:

Questions of Fact

a. Was this a mixed methods study? If yes, what was the purpose of the quantitative strand, and what was the purpose of the qualitative strand?

b. Which strand had priority in the study design?

c. Was the design sequential or concurrent?

d. Using the design names used in the textbook, what would the design be called?

e. How would the design be portrayed using the notation system described in the textbook? Did the researchers themselves use this notation?

f. What sampling design was used in this study?

g. What did the report say about integrating the two strands?

Questions for Discussion

a. Evaluate the use of a mixed methods approach in this study. Did the approach yield richer or more useful information than would have been achieved with a single-strand study?

b. Discuss the researchers' choice of a specific research design and the sampling design. Would an alternative mixed methods design have been preferable? If so, why?

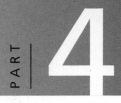

PART 4

Analysis and Interpretation in Quantitative and Qualitative Research

CHAPTER 14

Statistical Analysis of Quantitative Data

A. FILL IN THE BLANKS

How many terms have you learned in this chapter? Fill in the blanks in the sentences below to find out. You can have fun with this section by doing it with a friend. Who is the first one to complete the sentence?

1. The _____ level of measurement has order but provides no information about distance between values.

2. A(n) _____-level measurement has a rational zero point.

3. The lowest level of measurement is _____ measurement, which places objects into mutually exclusive categories.

4. Psychological scales yield _____-level measures.

5. A measure on an interval or ratio scale is often referred to as _____.

6. Distributions with a tail pointing to the left have a(n) _____ skew; those with a tail pointing to the right have a(n) _____ skew.

7. Distributions with a single high point are _____; those with two high points are _____.

8. A bell-shaped curve is a popular name for a(n) _____ distribution.

9. The most stable, and most frequently used, index of central tendency is known as the _____.

10. An index of central tendency that indicates the most "popular" value in a distribution is called _____.

11. The most widely used index of variability is the _____ deviation.

12. The distributions for two nominal-level variables can be displayed in a _____ table.

13. The _____ is a widely used risk index that summarizes the ratio of two probabilities—the likelihood of occurrence versus nonoccurrence.

14. _____ statistics is the broad class of statistics used to draw conclusions about a population.

15. _____ is the criterion used to establish the risk of a Type I error that is acceptable.

16. A _____ error occurs when a true null hypothesis is incorrectly rejected.

17. A _____ error is the error committed when a false null hypothesis is accepted.

18. A Type II error can occur when the analysis has insufficient _____, usually reflecting too small a sample.

19. The _____ of significance established the researcher's risk of making a Type I error.

20. The statistical test used to compare two group means is the _____.

21. Researchers establish a(n) _____ interval around a statistic to indicate the range within which a population parameter probably lies.

22. The statistical test used to compare means of three or more group means is _____.

23. An effect size index called _____ captures the magnitude of difference between two group means.

24. The index most often used as a correlation coefficient is called _____.

25. The statistic $r = .85$ indicates a strong, _____ relationship between two variables.

26. The _____ test is used to test hypotheses about differences in proportions.

27. Multiple _____ analysis could be used to predict body weight based on data about people's height, gender, and caloric intake.

28. In regression analysis, the independent variables are often called _____ variables.

29. The _____ of the multiple correlation coefficient (R) is an estimate of the proportion of variance in the outcome variable accounted for by the independent variables.

30. In ANCOVA, the confounding variable being statistically controlled is called a(n) _____.

31. _____ regression is a type of regression used to predict a nominal-level dependent variable from multiple predictors.

32. The index used to estimate internal consistency reliability is _____.

33. The preferred index for assessing test–retest reliability is the _____ coefficient.

34. Interrater reliability is evaluated using _____ when the ratings are dichotomous (e.g., presence vs. absence of a disease).

35. A measure's ability to identify a case correctly is its _____.

B. MATCHING EXERCISES

1. Match each variable in Set B with the level of measurement from Set A that captures the highest possible level for that variable. Indicate the letter corresponding to your response next to each variable in Set B.

SET A

a. Nominal scale

b. Ordinal scale

c. Interval scale

d. Ratio scale

SET B   RESPONSES

1. Hours spent in labor before childbirth   _____

2. Religious affiliation   _____

3. Time to first postoperative voiding   _____

4. Responses to a single Likert scale item   _____

5. Temperature on the centigrade scale   _____

6. Nursing specialty area   _____

7. Health status on the following scale: poor, fair, good, excellent   _____

8. Pulse rate   _____

9. Score on a 25-item Likert scale   _____

10. Highest academic degree attained (bachelor's, master's, doctorate)   _____

11. Apgar scores   _____

12. Marital status   _____

2. Match each statement or phrase from Set B with one of the phrases from Set A. Indicate the letter corresponding to your response next to each of the statements in Set B.

SET A

a. Index(es) of central tendency

b. Index(es) of variability

c. Index(es) of neither central tendency nor variability

d. Index(es) of both central tendency and variability

SET B   RESPONSES

1. The range   _____

2. In lay terms, an average   _____

3. A percentage   _____

4. Descriptor(s) of a distribution of scores   _____

5. Descriptor(s) of how heterogeneous a set of values is   _____

6. The standard deviation _____

7. The mode _____

8. The median _____

9. A normal distribution _____

10. The mean _____

C. STUDY QUESTIONS

1. Prepare a frequency distribution and frequency polygon for the set of scores below, which represent the ages of 30 women receiving a mammogram:

47 50 51 50 48 51 50 51 49 51

54 49 49 53 51 52 51 52 50 53

49 51 52 51 50 55 48 54 53 52

Describe the resulting distribution in terms of its symmetry and modality (i.e., whether it is unimodal or multimodal). What is the mode?

2. Calculate the mean, median, and mode for the following pulse rates:

78 84 69 98 102 72 87 75 79 84 88 84 83 71 73

Mean: _____   Median: _____   Mode: _____

3. Suppose a researcher has conducted a study concerning lactose intolerance in children. The data reveal that 12 boys and 16 girls have lactose intolerance, out of a sample of 60 children of each gender. Construct a crosstabs table and calculate the column percentages for each cell in the table, with gender listed in the columns (similar to Table 14.8 in the textbook). Discuss the meaning of these statistics. What test would we need to use to test the significance of group differences?

4. Below is a correlation matrix based on real data from a study of 997 low-income mothers. Answer the following questions with respect to this matrix:

   a. What is the correlation between body mass index (BMI) and scores on the physical health subscale?

   b. Is the correlation between physical health and mental health subscale scores significant at conventional levels?

   c. With which variable(s) is BMI correlated at the .01 level of significance?

   d. Explain what the correlation between the physical functioning scores and number of doctor visits means.

VARIABLE	1	2	3	4
1 Number of doctor visits	1.00			
2 Body mass index (BMI)	.13**	1.00		
3 Physical functioning	−.32**	−.13**	1.00	
4 Mental health score	−.13**	−.08*	.17**	1.00

*$p < .05$. **$p < .01$.

5. Indicate which statistical tests you would use to analyze data for the following variables:

   a. Variable 1 is psychiatric patients' gender; variable 2 is whether or not the patient has attempted suicide in the past 6 months.

   b. Variable 1 is the participation versus nonparticipation of patients with a pulmonary embolus in a special treatment group; variable 2 is the pH of the patients' arterial blood gases.

   c. Variable 1 is serum creatinine concentration levels; variable 2 is daily urine output.

   d. Variable 1 is patients' marital status (married vs. divorced/separated/widowed vs. never married); variable 2 is the patients' degree of self-reported depression (measured on a 20-item depression scale).

6. In the following examples, which multivariate procedure is most appropriate for analyzing the data?

   a. A researcher is testing the relationship between self-esteem, age, and the availability of family supports among a group of recently discharged psychiatric patients on the one hand and recidivism (i.e., whether they will be readmitted within 12 months after discharge) on the other.

   b. A researcher is comparing daily hours of sleep of recently widowed versus divorced individuals controlling for their age.

   c. A researcher wants to predict hospital staff absentee rates (number of days absent per year) based on salary, shift, number of years with the hospital, and number of children.

7. Below is a list of variables. Assume that you have data from 500 nurses on these variables. Develop two or three hypotheses regarding the relationships among these variables and indicate which statistical tests you would use to test your hypotheses.

   • Number of years of nursing experience
   • Type of employment setting (hospital, nursing home, public school system, other)
   • Annual salary
   • Marital status (married, never married, other)
   • Job satisfaction (as measured on a 10-item Likert-type scale)
   • Number of children younger than 18 years of age
   • Gender
   • Type of nursing preparation (diploma, associate's, bachelor's)

D. APPLICATION EXERCISES

Exercise D.1: Studies in Appendices A, C, and D

Which of the studies in Appendix A (Stephens et al.) on pages 113–120, Appendix C (Yackel et al.) on pages 131–138, and Appendix D (Eckhardt et al.) on pages 139–150 reported the following descriptive statistics:

a. Percentages?

b. Means and standard deviations?

c. Medians?

d. Mode?

Exercise D.2: Studies in Appendices A, C, and D

Which of the studies in Appendix A (Stephens et al.) on pages 113–120, Appendix C (Yackel et al.) on pages 131–138, and Appendix D (Eckhardt et al.) on pages 139–150 reported the following bivariate inferential statistics?

a. *t*-test

b. Chi-squared test

c. Pearson's *r*

Exercise D.3: Study in Appendix D

Read the Results section of the article by Eckhardt and colleagues ("Fatigue in the presence of coronary heart disease") in Appendix D on pages 139–150. Then answer the following questions:

Questions of Fact

a. Referring to Table 1, answer the following questions:
- Which variables described in the tables, if any, were measured as a nominal-level variable?
- Which variables described in the tables, if any, were measured as an ordinal-level variable?
- Which variables described in the tables, if any, were measured as an interval-level variable?
- Which variables described in the tables, if any, were measured as a ratio-level variable?
- State in one sentence what the "typical" participant was like demographically.
- What percentage of the *total* sample had a graduate degree?

b. Referring to Table 2, answer the following questions:
- With which variables were fatigue intensity scores significantly correlated at statistically significant levels?
- Were better educated people *more likely* or *less likely* to have high fatigue intensity?
- Were men or women more likely to have high scores on fatigue interference?

c. Which multivariate statistical analysis did the researchers use in this study?

d. Did the researchers report any values for R^2?

Questions for Discussion

a. Evaluate the statistical tests used in this research. Were the tests appropriate, given the level of measurement of the research variables? Should other statistics have been used as an alternative or as a supplement?

b. Some of the researchers' statistical results were nonsignificant. Is it possible that the study was underpowered (i.e., that a Type II error was committed)? Did the researchers undertake a power analysis?

c. Comment on the adequacy of the statistical tables. Were they easy to understand? Did they communicate important information effectively?

Interpretation and Clinical Significance in Quantitative Research

A. FILL IN THE BLANKS

How many terms have you learned in this chapter? Fill in the blanks in the sentences below to find out. You can have fun with this section by doing it with a friend. Who is the first one to complete the sentence?

1. Both researchers and consumers of quantitative research must develop a(n) _____ of the accuracy, meaning, and importance of the study results.

2. A famous research precept is that _____ does not prove that one variable caused another.

3. _____ size estimates such as *d* help to better understand the importance of the results.

4. The _____ guidelines for preparing research reports include a flow chart documenting participant flow in a study.

5. Researchers should take both the strengths and the _____ of their study into account when interpreting their findings.

6. A research _____ that is actually null is difficult to evaluate through standard statistical methods.

7. An important aspect of interpretation for clinical decision making is the degree of _____ of effects, usually communicated through confidence intervals (CIs).

8. Researchers' interpretations are presented in the _____ section of a report.

9. Results that are non _____ are especially difficult to interpret because of the possibility of a Type II error.

10. The _____ significance of research results is their practical importance to patients' daily lives or to health care decision making.

11. A widely used benchmark for clinical significance at the individual level is the _____ _____ _____.

12. Individuals' change scores in different groups can be classified as exceeding or not exceeding the MIC threshold and then compared in a(n) _____ analysis.

B. MATCHING EXERCISES

Match each statement or phrase from Set B with one or more of the phrases from Set A. Indicate the letter(s) corresponding to your response next to each of the statements in Set B.

SET A

a. Credibility of results

b. Precision of results

c. Magnitude of effects and importance

d. Generalizability of results

e. Implications of results

SET B   RESPONSES

1. Confidence intervals provide information about this.   _____

2. An analysis of threats to study validity is a way to
   address this.   _____

3. A consideration of how study limitations could be
   corrected in subsequent research is part of this.   _____

4. In assessing this, consideration is given to the characteristics
   of the study sample and the research setting.   _____

5. Effect size information can be especially useful for
   considering this.   _____

6. An analysis of the success of the researcher's "proxies" is an
   approach to this.   _____

7. Biases can reduce this.   _____

8. Statements about the utility of findings for clinical
   practice are part of this.   _____

C. STUDY QUESTIONS

1. Read one of the following studies and evaluate the extent to which the researchers assessed possible biases and commented on them in their discussions.
   - Azizan, A., & Justine, M. (2016). Effects of a behavioral and exercise program on depression and quality of life in community-dwelling older adults: A controlled, quasi-experimental study. *Journal of Gerontological Nursing, 42,* 45–54.

- Hadi, M. A., Alldred, D., Briggs, M., Marczewski, K., & Closs, S. J. (2016). Effectiveness of a community based nurse-pharmacist managed pain clinic: A mixed-methods study. *International Journal of Nursing Studies, 53*, 219–227.

2. In the following research article, a team of researchers reported that they obtained some nonsignificant results that were not consistent with expectations. Review and critique the researchers' interpretation of the findings and suggest some possible alternatives:

- McDonald, D. D., Martin, D., Foley, D., Baker, L., Hintz, D., Faure, L., . . . Price, S. (2010). Motivating people to learn cardiopulmonary resuscitation and use of automated external defibrillators. *Journal of Cardiovascular Nursing, 25*, 69–74.

3. In the following report, the researchers did not present a flow chart to track participant flow as recommended in the CONSORT guidelines. Use information in the report (see the section "Description of sample") to create one to the extent possible.

- Osterman, R. L., & Dyehouse, J. (2012). Effects of a motivational interviewing intervention to decrease prenatal alcohol use. *Western Journal of Nursing Research, 34*, 434–454.

4. Skim one of the following articles, the titles for which imply a causal connection between phenomena. Do you think a causal inference is warranted—why or why not?

- Goussé, V., Czernecki, V., Denis, P., Stilgenbauer, J. L., Deniau, E., & Hartmann, A. (2016). Impact of perceived stress, anxiety-depression and social support on coping strategies of parents having a child with Gilles de la Tourette syndrome. *Archives of Psychiatric Nursing, 30*, 109–113.
- Kramer, M., Brewer, B., & Maguire, P. (2013). Impact of healthy work environments on new graduate nurses' environmental reality shock. *Western Journal of Nursing Research, 35*, 348–383.
- *Theander, K., Hasselgren, M., Luhr, K., Eckerblad, J., Unosson, M., & Karlsson, I. (2014). Symptoms and impact of symptoms on function and health in patients with chronic obstructive pulmonary disease and chronic heart failure in primary health care. *International Journal of Chronic Obstructive Pulmonary Disease, 9*, 785–794.

5. Following is a fictitious research report and a critique of various aspects of it. This example is designed to highlight features about the form and content of both a written report and a written evaluation of the study's worth. To economize on space, the report is brief, but it incorporates essential elements for a meaningful appraisal. Read the report and critique and then determine whether you agree with the critique. Can you add other comments relevant to a critical appraisal of the study?

THE REPORT
The Role of Health Care Providers in Teenage Pregnancy by Phyllis Clinton

Background. Of the 20 million teenagers living in the United States, about one in four is sexually active by age 14 years; more than half have had sexual intercourse

---

*A link to this open-access journal article is provided in the Internet Resources section on the textbook's thePoint website.

by age 17 years (Kelman & Saner, 2009).[1] Despite increased availability of contraceptives, the number of teenage pregnancies has remained fairly stable over the past two decades. About 1 million girls under age 20 years become pregnant each year and, of these, about 500,000 become teenage mothers (U.S. Bureau of the Census, 2007).

Public concern regarding teenage pregnancy stems not only from the high rates but also from the extensive research that has documented the adverse consequences of early parenthood in the health arena. Pregnant teenagers have been found to receive less prenatal care (Tremain, 2000), to be more likely to develop toxemia (Schendley, 2002; Waters, 2004), to be more likely to experience prolonged labor (Curran, 1999), to be more likely to have low-birth-weight babies (Beach, 2004; Tremain, 2003), and to be more likely to have babies with low Apgar scores (Beach, 2004) than older mothers. The long-term consequences to the teenage mothers themselves are also bleak: Teenage mothers get less schooling, are more likely to be on public assistance, are likely to earn lower wages, and are more likely to get divorced if they marry than their peers who postpone parenthood (Jamail, 1999; North, 2002; Smithfield, 2008).

The 1 million teenagers who become pregnant each year have a difficult emotional decision—to carry the pregnancy to term and keep the baby, to have an abortion, or to deliver the baby and surrender it for adoption. Despite the widely reported adverse consequences of young parenthood cited earlier, most young women today are opting for delivery and child-rearing, often out of wedlock (Henderson, 2001; Jaffrey, 2007). Relatively few young mothers in recent years have been relinquishing their babies for adoption, forcing many couples with fertility problems to seek adoption options overseas (Smith, 2010).

The purpose of this study was to test the effect of a special intervention based on an outpatient clinic of a Chicago hospital on improving the health outcomes of a group of pregnant teenagers. Specifically, it was hypothesized that pregnant teenagers who were in the special program would receive more prenatal care, be less likely to develop toxemia, be less likely to have a low-birth-weight baby, spend fewer hours in labor, have babies with higher Apgar scores, and be more likely to use a contraceptive at 6 months postpartum than pregnant teenagers not enrolled in the program.

The theoretical model on which this research was based is an ecologic model of personal behavior (Brandenburg, 1984). A schematic diagram of the ecologic model is presented in Figure A. In this framework, the actions of the person are the focus of attention, but those actions are believed to be a function not only of the person's own characteristics, attitudes, and abilities but also of other influences in their environment. Environmental influences can be differentiated according to their proximal relationship with the target person. Health care workers and institutions are, according to the model, more distant influences than family, peers, and boyfriends. Yet it is assumed that these less immediate forces are real and can intervene to change the behaviors of the target person. Thus, it is hypothesized that pregnant teenagers can be influenced by increased exposure to a health care team providing a structured program of services designed to promote improved health outcomes.

Method. A special program of services for pregnant teenagers was implemented in the outpatient clinic of an inner-city public hospital in Chicago. The intervention involved 8 weeks of nutrition education and counseling, parenting education, instruction on prenatal health care, preparation for childbirth, and contraceptive counseling.

All teenagers with a confirmed pregnancy attending the clinic were asked if they wanted to participate in the special program. The goal was to enroll 150 pregnant

---

[1]All references in this example are fictitious.

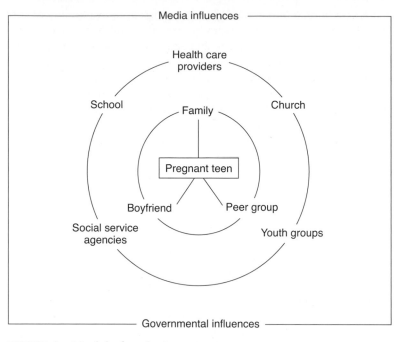

FIGURE A   Model of ecologic contexts.

teenagers during the program's first year of operation. A total of 276 teenagers attending the clinic were invited to participate; of these, 59 had an abortion or miscarriage and 108 declined to participate, yielding an experimental group sample of 109 girls.

To test the effectiveness of the special program, a comparison group of pregnant teenagers was needed. Another inner-city hospital agreed to cooperate in the study. Staff obtained information on the labor and delivery outcomes of the 120 teenagers who delivered at the comparison hospital, where no special teen–parent program was available. For both experimental group and comparison group subjects, a follow-up telephone interview was conducted at 6 months postpartum to determine if the teenagers were using birth control.

The outcome variables in this study were the teenagers' labor, delivery, and postpartum outcomes and their contraceptive behavior. Operational definitions of these variables are as follows:

Prenatal care: Number of visits made to a physician or nurse-midwife during the pregnancy, exclusive of the visit for the pregnancy test

Toxemia: Presence versus absence of preeclamptic toxemia as diagnosed by a physician or nurse-midwife

Labor time: Number of hours elapsed from the first contractions until birth of the baby to the nearest half hour

Low infant birth weight: Infant birth weights of less than 2,500 g versus those of 2,500 g or greater

Apgar score: The summary rating (from 0 to 10) of the health of the infant, taken at 1 minute after birth

Contraceptive use postpartum: Self-reported use of any form of birth control 6 months postpartum versus self-reported nonuse

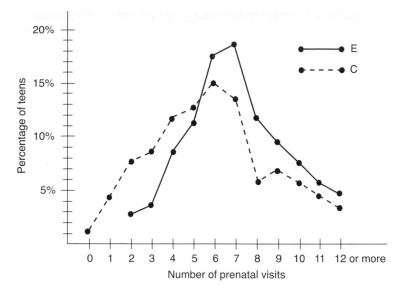

FIGURE B Frequency distribution of prenatal visits, by experimental versus comparison group. E, experimental group; C, comparison group.

The two groups were compared on these six outcome measures using *t*-tests and chi-squared tests.

Results. The teenagers in the sample were, on average, 17.6 years old at the time of delivery. The mean age was 17.0 years in the experimental group and 18.1 years in the comparison group (*p* < .05).

By definition, all the teenagers in the experimental group had received prenatal care. Two of the teenagers in the comparison group had no health care treatment before delivery. The distribution of visits for the two groups is presented in Figure B. The experimental group had a higher mean number of prenatal visits than the comparison group, as shown in Table A, but the difference was not statistically significant at the .05 level, using a *t*-test for independent groups.

In the sample as a whole, about 1 girl in 10 was diagnosed as having preeclamptic toxemia. The difference between the two groups was in the hypothesized direction, with 1.6% more of the comparison group teenagers developing this complication, but the difference was not significant using a chi-squared test.

The hours spent in labor ranged from 3.5 to 29.0 in the experimental group and from 4.5 to 33.5 in the comparison group. On average, teenagers in the experimental group spent 14.3 hours in labor, compared with 15.2 for the comparison group teenagers. The difference was not statistically significant.

Regarding low-birth-weight babies, a total of 43 girls out of 229 in the sample gave birth to babies who weighed less than 2,500 g (5.5 lb).[2] More of the comparison group teenagers (20.9%) than experimental group teenagers (16.5%) had low-birth-weight babies, but, once again, the group difference was not significant.

The 1-minute Apgar score in the two groups was quite similar—7.3 for the experimental group and 6.7 for the comparison group. This difference was nonsignificant.

---

[2]All mothers gave birth to live infants; however, there were two neonatal deaths within 24 hours of birth in the comparison group.

TABLE A   Summary of Experimental and Comparison Group Differences

| | Group | | | |
Outcome Variable	Experimental ($n = 109$)	Comparison ($n = 120$)	Difference	Test Statistic
Mean number of prenatal visits	7.1	5.9	1.2	$t = 1.83$, $df = 227$, NS
Percentage with toxemia	10.1	11.7	−1.6	$\chi^2 = 0.15$, $df = 1$, NS
Mean hours spent in labor	14.3	15.2	−.09	$t = 1.01$, $df = 227$, NS
Percentage with low-birth-weight baby	16.5	20.9	−4.4	$\chi^2 = 0.71$, $df = 1$, NS
Mean Apgar score	7.3	6.7	.6	$t = 0.98$, $df = 227$, NS
Percentage adopting contraception postpartum	81.7	62.5	19.2	$\chi^2 = 10.22$, $df = 1$, $p < .01$

Finally, the teenagers were compared with respect to their use of birth control 6 months after giving birth to their babies. For this variable, teenagers were coded as users of contraception if they were either using some method of birth control at the time of the follow-up interview or if they were nonusers but were sexually inactive (i.e., were using abstinence to prevent a repeat pregnancy). The results of the chi-squared test revealed that a significantly higher percentage of experimental group teenagers (81.7) than comparison group teenagers (62.5) reported using birth control after delivery. This difference was significant beyond the .01 level.

Discussion. The results of this evaluation were disappointing but not discouraging. There was only one outcome for which a significant difference was observed. The experimental program significantly increased the percentage of teenagers who used birth control after giving birth. Thus, one highly important result of participating in the program is that an early repeat pregnancy will be postponed. There is abundant research that has shown that repeat pregnancy among teenagers is especially damaging to their educational and occupational attainment and leads to particularly adverse labor and delivery outcomes in the higher order births (Jackson, 2007; Klugman, 2002).

The experimental group had more prenatal care but not significantly more. Perhaps part of the difficulty is that the program can only begin to deliver services once pregnancy has been diagnosed. If a teenager does not come in for a pregnancy test until her fourth or fifth month, this obviously puts an upper limit on the number of visits she will have; it also gives less time for her to eat properly, avoid smoking and drinking, and take other steps to enhance her health during pregnancy. Thus, one implication of this finding is that the program needs to do more to encourage early pregnancy screening. Perhaps a joint effort between the clinic personnel and school nurses in neighboring middle schools and high schools could be launched to publicize the need for a timely pregnancy test and to inform teenagers where such a test could be obtained. The two groups performed similarly with respect to the various labor and delivery outcomes chosen to evaluate the effectiveness of the new program. The issue of timeliness is again relevant here. The program may have been delivering services too late in the pregnancy for the instruction to have made much of an impact on the health of the mother and her child. This interpretation is supported, in part, by the fact that the one variable for which timeliness was *not* an issue (postpartum contraception) was, indeed, positively affected by program participation. Another possible implication is that the program itself should be made more powerful, for example, by lengthening or adding to instructional sessions.

Given that the experimental and comparison group differences were all in the hypothesized direction, it is also tempting to criticize the study's sample size. A larger sample (which was originally planned) might have yielded some significant differences.

In summary, the experimental intervention is not without promise. A particularly exciting finding is that participation in the program resulted in better contraceptive use, which will presumably lower the incidence of repeat pregnancy. It would be interesting to follow these teenagers 2 years after delivery to see if the groups differ in the rates of repeat pregnancy. It appears that more needs to be done to get these teenagers into the program early in their pregnancies. Perhaps then the true effectiveness of the program would be demonstrated.

CRITIQUE OF THE RESEARCH REPORT

In the following critique, we present some comments on various aspects of this research report. You are urged to read the report and form your own opinion about its strengths and weaknesses before reading our critique. An evaluation of a study is necessarily partly subjective. Therefore, you might disagree with some of the points made below, and you might have additional criticisms and comments. We believe, however, that most of the serious methodologic flaws of the study are highlighted in our critique.

Title. The title for the study is misleading. The research does *not* investigate the role of health care professionals in serving the needs of pregnant teenagers. A more appropriate title would be "Effects of an Intervention for Pregnant Teenagers on Health-Related Outcomes."

Background. The background section of this report consists of three distinct elements that can be analyzed separately: a literature review, statement of the problem, and a theoretical framework.

The literature review is relatively clearly written and well organized. It serves the function of establishing a need for an intervention by documenting the prevalence of teenage pregnancy and some of its adverse consequences. However, the literature review could be improved. First, an inspection of the citations suggests that the author is not as up-to-date on research relating to teenage pregnancy as she might have been. Most of the references date before 2010, so the review might be different if more recent studies were cited. Second, there is material in the literature review section that is not relevant and should be removed. For example, the paragraph on the options with which a pregnant teenager is faced (paragraph 3) is not germane to the research problem. A third and more critical flaw is what the review does *not* cover. Given the research problem, there are probably four main points that should be addressed in the review:

1. How widespread is teenage pregnancy and parenthood?

2. What are the social and health consequences of early childbearing?

3. What has been done by health care researchers to address the problems associated with teenage parenthood?

4. How successful have other interventions been?

The review adequately handles the first question: The need for concern is established. The second question is covered in the review, but perhaps more depth and more recent research is needed here. The new study is based on an assumption of negative health outcomes in teenage mothers. The author has strung together a series of references without giving the reader any clues about the reliability of the information. The author would have made her point more convincingly if she had added a sentence such as "For example, in a carefully executed prospective study involving nearly 4,000 pregnant women, Beach (2004) found that young maternal age was significantly associated with higher rates of prematurity and other negative neonatal outcomes." The third and fourth points that should have been covered are totally absent from the review. Surely, the author's intervention does not represent the first attempt to address the needs of pregnant teenagers. How is Clinton's intervention different from or better than other interventions? What reason does she have to believe that such an intervention might be successful? What was her intervention theory? Clinton has provided a rationale for addressing the problem but no rationale for the manner in which she has addressed it. If, in fact, there is little information about other interventions and their effectiveness in improving health outcomes, then the review should say so.

The problem statement and hypothesis were stated succinctly and clearly. The hypothesis is complex (there are multiple dependent variables) and directional (it predicts better outcomes among teenagers participating in the special program).

The third component of the Background section of the report is the theoretical framework. In our opinion, the theoretical framework chosen does little to enhance the research. The hypothesis is neither not generated on the basis of the model nor does the intervention itself grow out of the model. One gets the feeling that the model might have been slapped on as an afterthought to try to make the study seem more theoretical. Actually, if more thought had been given to this conceptual framework, it might have proved useful. According to this model, the most immediate and direct influences on a pregnant teenager are her family, friends, and sexual partner. One programmatic implication of this is that the intervention should involve one or more of these influences. For example, a workshop for the teenagers' parents could have been developed to reinforce the teenagers' need for adequate nutrition and prenatal care. A research hypothesis that could have been tested in the context of the model is that teenagers who are missing one of the direct influences would be especially susceptible to the influence of less proximal health care providers (i.e., the program). For example, it might be hypothesized that pregnant teenagers who do not live with both parents have to depend on alternative sources of social support (such as health care personnel) during the pregnancy. Thus, it is not that the theoretical context selected is far-fetched but rather that it was not convincingly linked to the actual research problem.

Method. The design used to test the research hypothesis was a widely used quasi-experimental design. Two groups, whose equivalence is assumed but not established, were compared on several outcome measures. The design is one that has serious problems because the preintervention comparability of the groups is unknown.

The most serious threat to the internal validity of the study is selection bias. Selection bias can work both ways—either to mask true treatment effects or to create the illusion of a program effect when none exists. This is because selection bias can be either positive (i.e., the experimental group can be initially advantaged in relation to the comparison group) or negative (i.e., the experimental group can have pretreatment disadvantages). In the present study, it is possible that the two hospitals served clients of different economic circumstances, for example. If the average income of the families of the experimental group teenagers was higher, then these teenagers would probably have a better opportunity for adequate prenatal nutrition than the comparison group teenagers. Or the comparison hospital might serve older teens, or a higher percentage of married teens, or a higher percentage of teens attending a special school-based program for pregnant students. None of these confounding variables, which could affect the mother's health, has been controlled.

Another way in which the design was vulnerable to selection bias is the high refusal rate in the experimental group. Of the 217 eligible teenagers, half declined to participate in the special program. We cannot assume that the 109 girls who participated were a random sample of the eligible girls. Again, biases could be either positive or negative. A positive selection bias would be created if, for example, the teenagers who were the most motivated to have a healthy pregnancy selected themselves into the experimental group. A negative selection bias would result if the teenagers from the most disadvantaged households or from families offering little support elected to participate in the program.

The researcher could have taken a number of steps to either control selection biases or, at the least, estimate their direction and magnitude. The following are among the most critical confounding variables: social class and family income, age, race and ethnicity, parity, participation in another pregnant teenager program, marital status, and prepregnancy experience with contraception (for the postpartum contraception outcome). The researcher should have attempted to gather information on these variables from experimental group and comparison group teenagers and from eligible teenagers in the experimental hospital who declined to participate in the program. To the extent that these groups were similar on these variables, the internal validity of the study, and thus the credibility of the results, would be enhanced. If sizable differences were observed, the researcher would at least know or suspect the direction of the biases and could factor that information into her interpretation and conclusions.

Had the researcher gathered information on the confounding variables, another possibility would have been to match experimental and comparison group subjects on one or two variables, such as family income and age. Matching is not an ideal method of controlling confounding variables; for one thing, matching on two variables would not equate the two groups in terms of the other confounding variables. However, matching is preferable to doing nothing to control extraneous variation.

So far we have focused our attention on the research design, but other aspects of the study are also problematic. Let us consider the decision the researcher made about the population. The target population is not explicitly defined by the researcher, but we can infer that the target population is pregnant young women younger than 20 years who carry their infants to delivery. The accessible population is pregnant teenagers from one area in Chicago. It cannot reasonably be assumed that the accessible population is representative of the target population. It is likely that the accessible population is quite different regarding health care, family intactness, and many other characteristics. The researcher should have more clearly discussed who the target population of this research was.

Clinton would have done well, in fact, to delimit the target population; had she done so, it might have been possible to control some of the confounding variables discussed previously. For example, Clinton could have established eligibility criteria that excluded multigravidas, very young teenagers (e.g., under age 15 years), or married teenagers. Such a specification would have limited the generalizability of the findings, but it would have enhanced the internal validity of the study because it probably would have increased the comparability of the experimental and comparison groups.

The sample was a sample of convenience, the least effective sampling design for a quantitative study. There is no way of knowing whether the sample represents the accessible and target populations. Although probability sampling likely was not feasible, the researcher might have improved her sampling design by using a quota sampling plan. For example, if the researcher knew that in the accessible population half of the families received public assistance, then it might have been possible to enhance the representativeness of the samples by using a quota system to ensure that half of the research subjects came from welfare-dependent families.

Sample size is a difficult issue. Many of the reported results were in the hypothesized direction but were nonsignificant. When this is the case, the adequacy of the sample size is always suspect, as Clinton pointed out. Each group had about 100 subjects. In many cases, this sample size would be considered adequate, but in the present case, it is not. One of the difficulties in testing the effectiveness of new interventions is that, generally, the experimental group is not being compared with a no-treatment group. Although the comparison group in this example was not getting the special program services, it cannot be assumed that this group was getting no services at all. Some comparison group members may have had ample prenatal care during which the health care staff may have provided much of the same information as they taught in the special program. The point is not that the new program was not needed but rather that unless an intervention is extremely powerful and innovative, the incremental improvement will typically be small. When relatively small effects are anticipated, the sample must be very large for differences to be statistically significant. Indeed, power analysis can be performed using the study findings. For example, a power analysis indicates that to detect a significant difference between the two groups with respect to one outcome—the incidence of toxemia—a sample of over 5,000 pregnant teenagers would have been needed. Had the researcher done a power analysis before conducting the study, she might have realized the insufficiency of her sample for some of the outcomes and might have developed a different sampling plan or identified different outcome variables.

The third major methodologic decision concerns the measurement of the research variables. For the most part, the researcher did a good job in selecting objective, reliable, and valid outcome measures. Also, her operational definitions were clearly worded and unambiguous. Two comments are in order, however. First, it might have been better to operationalize two of the variables differently. Infant birth weight might have been more sensitively measured as actual weight (a ratio-level measurement) instead of as a dichotomous variable. The contraceptive variable could also have been operationalized to yield a more sensitive (i.e., more discriminating) measure. For example, rather than measuring contraceptive use as a dichotomy, Clinton could have measured frequency of using contraception (e.g., never, sometimes, usually, or always), effectiveness of the *type* of birth control used, or a combination of these two.

A second consideration is whether the outcome variables adequately captured the effects of program activities. It would have been more directly relevant to the intervention to capture group differences in, say, dietary practices during pregnancy than in infant birth weight. None of the outcome variables measured the effects of parenting education. In other words, Clinton could have added more direct measures of the effectiveness of the intervention.

One other point about the methods should be made and that relates to ethical considerations. The article does not specifically say that subjects were asked for their informed consent, but that does not necessarily mean that no written consent was obtained. It is quite likely that the experimental group subjects, when asked to volunteer for the special program, were advised about their participation in the study and asked to sign a consent form. But what about the control group subjects? The article implies that comparison group members were given no opportunity to decline participation and were not aware of having their birth outcomes used as data in the research. In some cases, this procedure is acceptable. For example, a hospital or clinic might agree to release patient information without the patients' consent if the release of such information is done anonymously—that is, if it can be provided in such a way that even the researcher does not know the identity of the patients. In the present study, however, it is clear that the names of the comparison subjects were given to the researcher since she had to contact the comparison group at 6 months postpartum to determine their contraceptive practices. Thus, this study does not appear to have adequately safeguarded the rights of the comparison group subjects.

In summary, the researcher appears not to have given the new program a particularly fair test. Clinton should have taken a number of steps to control confounding variables and should have attempted to get a larger sample (even if this meant waiting for additional subjects to enroll in the program). In addition to concerns about the internal validity of the study, its generalizability is also questionable.

Results. Clinton did an adequate job of presenting the results of the study. The presentation was straightforward and succinct and was enhanced by the inclusion of a good table and figures. The style of this section was also appropriate: it was written objectively and was well organized.

The statistical analyses were also adequate. The descriptive statistics (means and percentages) were appropriate for the level of measurement of the variables. The two types of inferential statistics used (the *t*-test and chi-squared test) were also appropriate, given the levels of measurement of the outcome variables. The results of these tests were efficiently presented in a single table. Of course, more powerful statistics could have been used to control confounding variables (e.g., analysis of covariance). It appears, however, that the only confounding variable that could have been controlled statistically was the subjects' ages; no data were apparently collected on other confounding variables (social class, ethnicity, parity, and so on).

Discussion. Clinton's discussion section fails almost entirely to take the study's limitations into account in interpreting the data. The one exception is her acknowledgment that the sample size was too small. She seems unconcerned about the many threats to the internal or external validity of her research.

Clinton lays almost all the blame for the nonsignificant findings on the program rather than on the research methods. She feels that two aspects of the program should be changed: (1) recruitment of teenagers into the program earlier in their pregnancies and (2) strengthening program services. Both recommendations might be worth pursuing, but there is little in the data to suggest these modifications. With nonsignificant results such as those that predominated in this study, there are two possibilities to consider: (1) the results are accurate—that is, the program is not effective for those outcomes examined (although it might be effective for other measures), and (2) the results are false—that is, the existing program is effective for the outcomes examined, but the tests failed to demonstrate it. Clinton concluded that the first possibility was correct and therefore recommended that the program be changed. Equally plausible is the possibility that the study methods were too weak to demonstrate the program's true effects.

We do not have enough information about the characteristics of the sample to conclude with certainty that there were substantial selection biases. We do, however, have a clue that selection biases were operative in a direction that would make the program look less effective than it actually is. Clinton noted in the beginning of the results section that the average age of the teenagers in the experimental group was 17.0, compared with 18.1 in the comparison group—a difference that was significant. Age is inversely related to positive labor and delivery outcomes, indeed, that is the basis for having a special program for teenage mothers. Therefore, the experimental group's performance on the outcome measures was possibly depressed by the youth of that group. Had the two groups been equivalent in terms of age, group differences on the outcomes might have been larger and could have reached levels of statistical significance. Other uncontrolled pretreatment differences could also have masked true treatment effects.

For the one significant outcome, we cannot rule out the possibility that a Type I error was made—that is, that the null hypothesis was, in fact, true. Again, selection biases could have been operative. The experimental group might have contained many more girls who had preprogram experience with contraception; it might have contained more highly motivated teenagers, or more teenagers who already had multiple pregnancies than the comparison group. There simply is no way of knowing whether the significant outcome reflects true program effects or merely initial group differences.

Aside from Clinton's disregard for the problems of internal validity, she overstepped the bounds of scholarly speculation. She assumed that the program *caused* contraceptive improvements: "The experimental program significantly increased the percentage of teenagers who used birth control. . . . " Worse yet, she went on to conclude that repeat pregnancies will be postponed in the experimental group, although she does not know whether the teenagers used an effective contraception, whether they used it all the time, or whether they used it correctly.

As another example of going beyond the data, Clinton became overly invested in the notion that teenagers need greater and earlier exposure to the program. It is not that her hypothesis has no merit—the problem is that she builds an elaborate rationale for program changes with no apparent empirical support. She probably had information on when in the pregnancy the teenagers entered the program, but that information was not shared with readers. Her argument about the need for more publicity on early screening would have had more clout if she had reported that most teenagers entered the program during the fourth month of their pregnancies or later. Additionally, she could have marshaled more evidence in support of her proposal if she had been able to show that earlier entry into the program was associated with better health outcomes. For example, she could have compared the outcomes of teenagers entering the program in the first, second, and third trimesters of their pregnancies.

In conclusion, the study has several positive features. As Clinton noted, there is some reason to be cautiously optimistic that the program *could* have some beneficial effects. However, the existing study is too flawed to reach any conclusions, even tentatively. A replication with improved research methods is needed to solve the research problem.

D. APPLICATION EXERCISES

Exercise D.1: Study in Appendix A

Read the "Results" and "Discussion" sections of the report by Stephens and colleagues ("Smartphone technology and text messaging for weight loss in young adults") in Appendix A on pages 113–120 and then answer the following questions:

Questions of Fact

a. Was a CONSORT-type flow chart included in this report? If yes, what did it show?

b. Did the researchers provide evidence about the success of randomization—that is, whether those in the intervention and control groups were equivalent at the outset and thus, selection biases were absent?

c. Did the researchers report an analysis of attrition biases? Was attrition taken into account in the analysis of group differences on the outcomes?

d. Regarding the primary aim of the study, to compare intervention and control group outcomes on weight-related outcomes following the smartphone intervention, were hypotheses supported, nonsupported, or mixed?

e. Did the report provide information about the precision of results via confidence intervals?

f. Did the report provide information about magnitude of effects via calculation of effect sizes?

g. In the Discussion section, was there any explicit discussion about the study's internal validity?

h. In the Discussion section, was there any explicit discussion about the study's external validity (generalizability)?

i. In the Discussion section, was there any explicit discussion about the study's statistical conclusion validity?

j. Did the Discussion section link study findings to findings from prior research—that is, did the authors place their findings into a broader context?

k. Were any study limitations identified in the Discussion section?

l. Did the researchers explicitly comment on the clinical significance of the findings?

Questions for Discussion

a. Critique the analysis of biases in this report and possible resulting effects on the interpretation of the findings.

b. Do you agree with the researchers' interpretations of their results? Why or why not?

c. What is your assessment of the internal and external validity of the study?

d. To what extent do you think the researchers adequately described the study's limitations and strengths?

Exercise D.2: Study in Appendix D

Read the "Results" and "Discussion" sections of the report by Eckhardt and colleagues ("Fatigue in the presence of coronary heart disease") in Appendix D on pages 139–150 and then answer the following questions:

Questions of Fact

a. Were any biases discussed in this study? If yes, what did the researchers say?

b. Did the researchers state or imply any hypotheses? Were hypotheses supported or nonsupported?

c. Did the researchers make any unwarranted causal inferences about the relationship between variables in their study?

d. Did the report provide information about the precision of results via confidence intervals?

e. Did the report provide information about magnitude of effects via calculation of effect sizes?

f. In the Discussion section, was there any explicit discussion about the study's external validity (generalizability)?

g. Were any study limitations identified in the Discussion section?

h. Did the researchers explicitly comment on the clinical significance of any of the findings?

Questions for Discussion

a. Do you agree with the researchers' interpretations of their results? Why or why not?

b. Discuss the extent to which the Discussion included key results.

c. To what extent do you think the researchers adequately described the study's limitations and strengths?

d. How did the inclusion of qualitative data help in interpreting results?

Analysis of Qualitative Data

A. FILL IN THE BLANKS

How many terms have you learned in this chapter? Fill in the blanks in the sentences below to find out. You can have fun with this section by doing it with a friend. Who is the first one to complete the sentence?

1. After a category system is developed, the main task involves _____ the data.

2. Qualitative descriptive studies typically rely on _____ analysis to discover key themes and patterns.

3. In ethnographies, a broad unit of cultural knowledge is called a(n) _____.

4. The second level of analysis in Spradley's ethnographic method yielding an organizational structure for the data is called _____ analysis.

5. Colaizzi's approach is one method used in _____ phenomenological studies.

6. Van Manen's _____ approach involves analyzing every sentence.

7. A(n) _____ is a literary device sometimes used as part of an analytic strategy, especially by interpretive phenomenologists.

8. The hermeneutic _____ involves movement between parts and whole of a text being analyzed.

9. In Benner's hermeneutic approach, the presentation of _____ in reports allows readers to draw conclusions about the validity of the results.

10. _____ cases, in one approach to hermeneutic analysis, are strong examples of ways of being in the world.

11. The first stage of Glaserian grounded theory analysis involves _____ coding.

12. In Glaserian grounded theory, the type of coding focused on the core variable is _____ coding.

13. Grounded theorists document an idea in an analytic _____.

14. The concept of _____ fit in grounded theory involves comparing identified concepts with similar concepts from previous studies.

15. A recent approach to grounded theory analysis is called _____ grounded theory.

B. MATCHING EXERCISES

Match each descriptive statement from Set B with one or more types of qualitative analyses from Set A. Indicate the letter(s) corresponding to your response next to each item in Set B.

SET A

a. Grounded theory analysis

b. Phenomenologic/hermeneutic analysis

c. Ethnographic analysis

d. None of the above

SET B   RESPONSES

1. Involves the development of coding categories   _____
2. Begins with "open coding"   _____
3. One method of analysis was developed by Colaizzi.   _____
4. Data can be organized using computer software.   _____
5. One method of analysis was developed by Glaser and Strauss. _____
6. May involve the development of a taxonomy   _____
7. One analytic approach involves identifying paradigm cases. _____
8. Requires computer software   _____

C. STUDY QUESTIONS

1. What is wrong with the following statements?
   a. Perez conducted a grounded theory study about coping with a miscarriage in which she was able to identify four major themes.
   b. Marcolin's ethnographic analysis of Haitian clinics involved gleaning related thematic material from French poetry.
   c. Titterton's phenomenological study of the lived experience of Parkinson's disease focused on the domain of fatigue.
   d. Levine's grounded theory study of widowhood yielded a taxonomy of coping strategies.
   e. In her ethnographic study of the culture of a nursing home, Stimpfle used a rural nursing home as a paradigm case.

2. Use the category scheme presented in Box 16.1 on page 279 in the textbook to code the following segment from an actual interview:

   My first birth was horrendous. As soon as I became pregnant with my second child, I read absolutely everything I could possibly get my hands on about childbirth, from midwifery textbooks to independent research papers. I was determined that this next time was going to be very different. I would be very aware of the facts and I would have a better understanding of my own needs for privacy, control, and emotional support.

I then went about choosing an independent midwife. I interviewed two lovely women and asked them identical questions. I told them both that I had not dilated beyond 3 cm in my first birth and asked what they would do if I got to 3 cm then progress slowed. Midwife #1 said she would probably transfer me to the hospital. Midwife #2 said she would just wait until things changed. She talked about how much faith she had in the female body. I went with midwife #2.

During my pregnancy, I bought a copy of *Birthing from Within* and spent a lot of time painting my previous birth experience and how I envisioned birth #2. I truly nurtured myself. I swam, did yoga, walked, and spent lots of time outdoors and enjoyed being with my 2-year-old.

Over my pregnancy, I felt very supported by my midwife and I became able to trust her. My husband and I also hired a doula to make sure both he and I would be supported during this labor and delivery.

3. Suppose a researcher was studying people with hypertension who were struggling unsuccessfully for months to manage their weight. The researcher plans to interview 10 to 20 people for this study. Answer the following questions:

   a. What might be the research question that a phenomenologist would ask relating to this situation? And what might the research question be for a grounded theory researcher?

   b. Which do you think would take longer to do—the analysis of data for the phenomenological or the grounded theory? Why?

   c. What would the final "product" of the analyses be for the two different studies?

   d. Which study would have more appeal to you? Why?

4. Read the following open-access article and critique how well the researchers described the analytic process for this phenomenological study:

   - *Glenn, A. D. (2015). Using online health communication to manage chronic sorrow: Mothers of children with rare diseases speak. *Journal of Pediatric Nursing*, *30*, 17–24.

D. APPLICATION EXERCISES

Exercise D.1: Study in Appendix E

Read the "Design and Methods" and "Findings" sections of the report by Byrne and colleagues ("Care transition experiences") in Appendix E on pages 151–168 and then answer the following questions. (Note: The following questions supplement the critical thinking questions for Example 1 in the textbook on page 291):

Questions of Fact

a. Did the researchers audio-record and transcribe the interviews? If yes, who did the transcription? Did the report state how many pages of data comprised the data set?

---

*A link to this open-access journal article is provided in the Internet Resources section on the textbook's thePoint website.

b. Did data collection and data analysis occur concurrently?

c. Was a computer used to analyze the data? If yes, what software was used?

d. Were there any metaphors used to highlight key findings?

e. Did the researchers prepare any analytic memos?

f. Did the authors describe the coding process? If so, what did they say?

Questions for Discussion

a. Were data presented in a manner that allows you to be confident about the researchers' conclusions? Comment on the inclusion or noninclusion of figures that graphically represent the grounded theory.

b. Comment on the amount of verbatim quotes from study participants that were included in this report.

Exercise D.2: Study in Appendix F

Read the "Data Analysis" and "Results" sections of the article by Cummings ("Sharing a traumatic event") in Appendix F on pages 169–176 and then answer the following questions:

Questions of Fact

a. Did Cummings audiotape and transcribe the interviews?

b. Did Cummings organize her data manually or with the assistance of computer software? If the latter, what software was used?

c. Which phenomenologic analytic approach was adopted in this study?

d. Did Cummings prepare any reflecting memos or keep a reflective journal?

e. Did Cummings describe the coding process? If so, what did she say?

f. How many themes emerged in Cummings' analysis? What were they?

g. Did Cummings provide supporting evidence for her themes in the form of excerpts from the data?

Questions for Discussion

a. Discuss the thoroughness of Cummings' description of her data analysis efforts. Did the report present adequate information about the steps taken to analyze the data?

b. Discuss the effectiveness of Cummings' presentation of results. Does the analysis seem sensible, thoughtful, and thorough? Was sufficient evidence provided to support the findings? Were data presented in a manner that allows you to be confident about Cummings' conclusions?

CHAPTER 17

Trustworthiness and Integrity in Qualitative Research

A. FILL IN THE BLANKS

How many terms have you learned in this chapter? Fill in the blanks in the sentences below to find out. You can have fun with this section by doing it with a friend. Who is the first one to complete the sentence?

1. _____, which concerns confidence in the truth value of the findings, is a key criterion for assessing quality in qualitative studies.

2. Use of multiple means of converging on the truth is called _____.

3. The stability of data over time and conditions, analogous to reliability, is called _____.

4. The quality criterion concerning the extent to which qualitative findings can be applied to other settings is called _____.

5. The dependability of an inquiry can be enhanced by a(n) _____ trail that documents judgments and choices.

6. Transferability is enhanced through the researcher's use of _____ _____ in a research report.

7. The criterion of _____ refers to the potential for congruence between independent coders, analysts, or interpreters of qualitative data—its analog in quantitative studies is objectivity.

8. Credibility in qualitative inquiry has been described as analogous to _____ validity in quantitative inquiry.

9. Persistent _____ refers to a focus on the aspects of a situation that are relevant to the phenomena being studied.

10. A process by which researchers revise their interpretations by including cases that appear to disconfirm earlier hypotheses is a(n) _____ case analysis.

11. One method of enhancing credibility is to do _____ checks, which involve going back to participants to have them review preliminary findings.

12. _____ triangulation is achieved by having two or more researchers make key decisions and interpretations.

13. _____ is a quality criterion indicating the extent to which the researchers fairly and faithfully portray a range of different realities.

14. The strategy of _____ debriefing involves seeking the input from other researchers regarding the analysis of interpretation of qualitative data.

15. The strategy of _____ engagement involves a researcher's investment of sufficient time collecting and analyzing qualitative data.

B. MATCHING EXERCISES

Match each statement from Set B with one of the phrases from Set A. Indicate the letter corresponding to your response next to each of the statements in Set B.

SET A

a. Data source triangulation
b. Investigator triangulation
c. Method triangulation

SET B   RESPONSES

1. A researcher studying health beliefs of the rural elderly interviews old people and health care providers in the area.   _____

2. Two researchers independently interview 10 informants in a study of adjustment to a cancer diagnosis and debrief with each other to review what they have learned.   _____

3. A researcher studying embarrassment in school-based clinics observes interactions in the clinics and also conducts in-depth interviews with students.   _____

4. A researcher studying the process of resolving an infertility problem interviews husbands and wives separately.   _____

5. Themes emerging in the field notes of an observer on a psychiatric ward are categorized and labeled independently by the researcher and an assistant.   _____

C. STUDY QUESTIONS

1. Suppose you were conducting a grounded theory study of couples struggling to come to terms with a child's diagnosis of cancer. What might you do to incorporate various types of triangulation into your study?

2. What is your opinion about the value of member checking as a strategy to enhance credibility? Defend your position.

3. Read a research report in a recent issue of the journal *Qualitative Health Research*. Identify several examples of "thick description." Also, identify

areas of the report in which you feel additional thick description would have enhanced the transferability of the evidence.

4. Read the abstract, and then the Method section, of one of the following studies, published as open-access articles. Comment on the amount of information the researchers provided regarding the integrity and trustworthiness of the study:

- *Bragstad, L. K., Kirkevold, M., & Foss, C. (2014). The indispensable intermediaries: A qualitative study of informal caregivers' struggle to achieve influence at and after hospital discharge. *BMC Health Services Research*, *14*, 331.

- *de Valpine, M. G. (2014). Extreme nursing: A qualitative assessment of nurse retention in a remote setting. *Rural and Remote Health*, *14*, 2859.

- *Sebergsen, K., Norberg, A., & Talseth, A. (2016). Confirming mental health care in acute psychiatric wards, as narrated by persons experiencing psychotic illness: An interview study. *BMC Nursing*, *15*, 3.

D. APPLICATION EXERCISES

Exercise D.1: Study in Appendix E

Read the report by Byrne and colleagues ("Care transition experiences") in Appendix E on pages 151–168 and then answer the following questions:

Questions of Fact

a. Did the researchers devote a section of their report to describing their quality-enhancement strategies? If so, what was it labeled? If not, where was information about such strategies located?

b. What types of triangulation, if any, were used in this study?

c. Were any of the following methods used to enhance the credibility of the study?

- Prolonged engagement and/or persistent observation
- Member checks
- Search for disconfirming evidence
- Reflexivity
- Audit trail

Questions for Discussion

a. Discuss the thoroughness with which Byrne and colleagues described their efforts to enhance and evaluate the quality and integrity of their study.

---

*A link to this open-access journal article is provided in the Internet Resources section on the textbook's thePoint website.

b. How would you characterize the integrity and trustworthiness of this study based on the researchers' documentation? How would you describe the credibility, dependability, confirmability, authenticity, and transferability of this study?

Exercise D.2: Study in Appendix F

Read the report by Cummings ("Sharing a traumatic event") in Appendix F on pages 169–176 and then answer the following questions:

Questions of Fact

a. Did the researcher devote a section of the report to describing her quality-enhancement strategies? If so, what was it labeled? If not, where was information about such strategies located?

b. What types of triangulation, if any, were used in this study?

c. Were any of the following methods used to enhance the credibility of the study?

- Prolonged engagement and/or persistent observation
- Peer review and debriefing
- Member checks
- Search for disconfirming evidence
- Reflexivity
- Audit trail
- Researcher credibility

Questions for Discussion

a. Discuss the thoroughness with which Cummings described her efforts to enhance and evaluate the quality and integrity of her study.

b. How would you characterize the integrity and trustworthiness of this study based on the researchers' documentation? How would you describe the credibility, dependability, confirmability, authenticity, and transferability of this study?

c. Do you think that the researcher's maintenance of "an extensive audit trail" contributed to the integrity and trustworthiness of this study? Why or why not?

CHAPTER 18

Systematic Reviews: Meta-Analysis and Metasynthesis

A. FILL IN THE BLANKS

How many terms have you learned in this chapter? Fill in the blanks in the sentences below to find out. You can have fun with this section by doing it with a friend. Who is the first one to complete the sentence?

1. A systematic review that integrates study findings statistically is called a(n) _____.

2. A(n) _____ review is a preliminary exploration of the literature to clarify the evidence base.

3. Electronic searches can be supplemented by _____ searching journals known to publish relevant content.

4. The body of unpublished studies is sometimes referred to as _____ literature.

5. A concern in a systematic review is the _____ bias that stems from identifying only studies appearing in journals.

6. An appraisal of primary study _____ is undertaken in most systematic reviews, although approaches to using appraisal information vary.

7. In a meta-analysis, statistical _____ concerns dissimilarity among the effect size estimates of the various primary studies.

8. Another name for the effect index d for comparing two group means is *standardized mean* _____.

9. In a meta-analysis, a(n) _____ analysis involves examining the extent to which effects differ for different types of studies, people, or intervention elements.

10. A(n) _____ plot is a graphic display of the effect size (including CIs around them) of each primary study in a meta-analysis.

11. A systematic review that integrates qualitative study findings is most often called a(n) _____.

12. Noblit and Hare developed an approach to synthesizing qualitative findings called _____.

13. A(n) _____, which involves calculating manifest effect sizes, can lay the foundation for a metasynthesis.

14. In a meta-summary, a(n) _____ effect size is the percentage of reports that contain a given thematic finding.

15. In a meta-summary, a(n) _____ effect size is the percentage of all thematic findings that are contained in any given report.

B. MATCHING EXERCISES

Match each of the statements in Set B with the appropriate phrase in Set A. Indicate the letter(s) corresponding to your response next to each of the statements in Set B.

SET A

a. Meta-analysis

b. Metasynthesis

c. Neither meta-analysis nor metasynthesis

d. Both meta-analysis and metasynthesis

SET B   RESPONSES

1. Involves gathering data from human participants   _____

2. Focuses on synthesizing information from prior studies   _____

3. Relies on findings from qualitative studies   _____

4. May involve an assessment of publication bias   _____

5. Sandelowski developed important approaches for this   _____

6. Often involves calculating *d* or OR statistics   _____

7. CINAHL likely would be used for this in searching for
primary studies.   _____

8. Can involve the calculation of a frequency effect size   _____

C. STUDY QUESTIONS

1. Read one of the following meta-analysis reports published several years ago as open-access articles:
   - **Conn, V. S., Hafdahl, A. R., Brown, S. A., & Brown, L. M. (2008). Meta-analysis of patient education interventions to increase physical activity among chronically ill adults. *Patient Education and Counseling, 70*, 157–172.
   - **Dennis, C. L. (2005). Psychosocial and psychological interventions for prevention of postnatal depression: Systematic review. *BMJ, 331*, 15.
   - **DiCenso, A., Guyatt, G., Willan, A., & Griffith, L. (2002). Interventions to reduce unintended pregnancies among adolescents: Systematic review of randomised controlled trials. *BMJ, 324*, 1426.

---

*A link to this open-access journal article is provided in the Internet Resources section on the textbook's thePoint website.

Then search the literature for relevant quantitative primary studies published *after* this meta-analysis. Are new study results consistent with the conclusions drawn in the meta-analytic report? Are there enough new studies to warrant a new meta-analysis?

2. Read one of the following metasynthesis reports:

   - Beck, C. T. (2002). Postpartum depression: A metasynthesis. *Qualitative Health Research*, *12*, 453–472.
   - Lefler, L., & Bondy, K. N. (2004). Women's delay in seeking treatment with myocardial infarction: A meta-synthesis. *Journal of Cardiovascular Nursing*, *19*, 251–268.
   - Nelson, A. M. (2002). A metasynthesis: Mothering other-than-normal children. *Qualitative Health Research*, *12*, 515–530.

   Then, search the literature for related qualitative primary studies published *after* this metasynthesis. Are new study results consistent with the conclusions drawn in the metasynthesis report? Are there enough new studies to warrant a new metasynthesis?

3. Skim the following report, which involved a systematic review without a meta-analysis. Did the authors adequately justify their decision not to conduct a meta-analysis?

   - Hines, S., Ramsbotham, J., & Coyer, F. (2015). The effectiveness of interventions for improving the research literacy of nurses: A systematic review. *Worldviews on Evidence-Based Nursing*, *12*, 265–272.

D. APPLICATION EXERCISES

Exercise D.1: Study in Appendix G

Read the report on the meta-analysis by Chase and colleagues ("Effectiveness of medication adherence interventions") in Appendix G on pages 177–186 and then answer the following questions:

Questions of Fact

a. What was the stated purpose of this review? What were the independent and dependent variables in this review?

b. What inclusion criteria were stipulated? How many studies met all inclusion criteria?

c. What methods did the reviewers use to search for primary studies?

d. Did the authors present a flow chart showing the progression of potential studies through an identification and screening process? If no, was this information presented effectively in the text or in a table?

e. How many subjects were there in total, in all included studies combined?

f. What were the key demographic characteristics of subjects in the primary studies?

g. How many of the studies included in this meta-analysis used an experimental (randomized) design? How many were quasi-experimental?

h. Did the researchers rate each study in the data set for its quality? If yes, what aspects of the study were appraised? How many people evaluated the studies for quality? Was interrater agreement assessed?

i. Did the researchers set a threshold for study quality as part of their inclusion criteria? If yes, what was it?

j. What effect size measure was used in the analysis?

k. Did the researchers perform any tests for statistical heterogeneity? Was a fixed effects or random effects model used?

l. Were study-by-study effects presented in a forest plot?

m. Overall, what was the value of the effect size for the interventions? What was the confidence interval around the mean effect? Was the effect statistically significant?

n. Considering the information in Figure 1, answer the following questions:
   • In which study was the effect size the largest? Was this effect size statistically significant?
   • Were effect sizes nonsignificant in any studies?
   • Were there any studies where the effect size was in the opposite direction from what was anticipated?

o. Were subgroup analyses undertaken? If yes, what were the key findings?

Questions for Discussion

a. Was the size of the sample (studies and subjects) sufficiently large to draw conclusions about the overall intervention effects and about subgroup effects?

b. What other subgroups might have been interesting to examine (assume there was sufficient information in the original studies)?

c. How would you assess the overall rigor of this meta-analysis?

d. Based on this review, what is the evidence regarding interventions for medication adherence among patients with coronary artery disease?

e. Comment on the authors' discussion about study limitations.

f. Comment on the authors' discussion of the implications of this meta-analysis for clinical practice.

Exercise D.2: Study in Appendix H

Read the report on the metasynthesis by Beck ("A metaethnography of traumatic childbirth") in Appendix H on pages 187–198 and then answer the following questions:

Questions of Fact

a. In what way was this metasynthesis different from a typical metasynthesis?

b. What was Beck's position in the controversy regarding integration across different research traditions?

c. Were the data in the primary studies derived from interviews, observations, or both?

d. How many mothers participated in the six primary studies?

e. What approach was used to conduct this metasynthesis? Was the analytic process described?

f. Was a meta-summary performed?

g. How many shared themes were identified in this meta-synthesis? What were those themes?

h. Was Beck's analysis supported through the inclusion of raw data from the primary studies?

Questions for Discussion

a. Was the size of the sample (studies and subjects) sufficiently large to conduct a meaningful metasynthesis? Comment on the extent to which the diversity of the sample enhanced or weakened the metasynthesis.

b. Did the analysis and integration appear reasonable and thorough?

c. Were primary studies adequately described?

d. How would you assess the overall rigor of this metasynthesis? What would you recommend to improve its quality?

e. Based on this metasynthesis, what is the evidence regarding the experiences of birth trauma for mothers?

Journal of Cardiovascular Nursing. 2015 Dec 7. [Epub ahead of print]

Smartphone Technology and Text Messaging for Weight Loss in Young Adults
A Randomized Controlled Trial

Janna D. Stephens, PhD, RN; Allison M. Yager, BS; Jerilyn Allen, RN, ScD, FAAN

Background: Using smartphone technology and text messaging for health is a growing field. This type of technology is well integrated into the lives of young adults. However, few studies have tested the effect of this type of technology to promote weight loss in young adults **Objective:** The purpose of this study is to test the effectiveness of a behaviorally based smartphone application for weight loss combined with text messaging from a health coach on weight, body mass index (BMI), and waist circumference in young adults as compared with a control condition. **Methods:** Sixty-two young adults, aged 18 to 25 years, were randomized to receive (1) a smartphone application + health coach intervention and counseling sessions or (2) control condition with a counseling session. All outcome measures were tested at baseline and 3 months. These included weight, BMI, waist circumference, dietary habits, physical activity habits, and self-efficacy for healthy eating and physical activity. **Results:** The sample was 71% female and 39% white, with an average age of 20 years and average BMI of 28.5 kg/m^2. Participants in the smartphone + health coach group lost significantly more weight ($P = .026$) and had a significant reduction in both BMI ($P = .024$) and waist circumference ($P < .01$) compared with controls. **Conclusions:** The results of this weight loss trial support the use of smartphone technology and feedback from a health coach on improving weight in a group of diverse young adults.

KEY WORDS: self-efficacy, text messaging, weight loss, young adult

Overweight and obesity are major public health concerns in the United States. According to data published in 2014 by the National Health and Nutrition Examination Survey, more than one-half of US adults (60.3%) aged 20 to 39 years are overweight or obese with a body mass index (BMI) of 25 kg/m^2 or greater.[1] Weight gain is specifically a concern in college-aged individuals. Although the common theory that college freshman gain 15 lb has been disproven on

Janna D. Stephens, PhD, RN
Assistant Professor, College of Nursing, Ohio State University, Columbus
Allison M. Yager, BS
BSN Student, School of Nursing, Johns Hopkins University, Baltimore, Maryland.
Jerilyn Allen, RN, ScD, FAAN
Professor, School of Nursing, Johns Hopkins University, Baltimore, Maryland.

Research in this publication was supported by the National Institute of Nursing Research of the National Institute of Health under award numbers 1T32NR012704 (Cardiovascular Research Training Grant) and F31NR013811 (National Research Service Award). The content is solely the responsibility of the authors and does not necessarily represent the official views of the National Institutes of Health.

The authors have no conflicts of interest to disclose.

Correspondence
Janna D. Stephens, PhD, RN, 5910 Kyles Station Rd, Hamilton OH 45011 (Jsteph22@jhu.edu).

DOI: 10.1097/JCN.0000000000000307

most accounts,[2] studies have shown that many students do in fact gain weight.[3,4] A survey conducted in 2014 by the American College Health Association reported that more than 34% of undergraduate students are overweight or obese, and this number increases to 40% when surveying graduate students.[5] Being overweight greatly increases one's risk for stroke, heart disease, type 2 diabetes, and some forms of cancer.[6] Therefore, interventions to combat weight gain during these years are needed for healthy outcomes later in life.

The behaviors of college-aged individuals put them at risk for weight gain. Specifically, poor eating habits, decreased physical activity, decreased fruit and vegetable consumption, and increased alcohol consumption all contribute to weight gain.[7,8] The American College Health Association reports that 65% of students consume less than 2 servings of fruit/vegetables combined per day and that more than 50% of students report consuming alcohol in the past 9 days.[5] Of those consuming alcohol, 24% of students reported having 7 or more drinks the last time they drank.[5]

Technology is well integrated into the lives of young adults. Currently, 85% of young adults, aged 18 to 29 years, own a smartphone. Among those young adults owning a smartphone, 100% use their smartphone to send and receive text messages.[9] In addition, 77% of young adults have used their smartphone to look up health information.[9] A recent focus group study conducted by the first author identified that young adults are interested in using smartphone technology for weight loss; however, they know very little about the availability of different applications to assist with weight loss.[10]

Interventions for weight loss in this population have proven to be successful using various strategies. One study used technology and showed greater weight loss in a group that received a social networking site and text messages (−2.4 kg) compared with a social networking site alone (−0.63 kg).[11] Another study using the Internet reported increased fruit and vegetable consumption, although no differences in weight were noted.[12]

Smartphone technology can provide many tools to help one lose weight. However, there is limited knowledge on the use of smartphone technology for weight loss in young adults. Therefore, the purpose of this study is to test the effectiveness of a behaviorally based smartphone application combined with text messaging from a health coach on weight, BMI, and waist circumference in young adults as compared with a control condition.

Methods

The Young Adult Weight Loss Study was a randomized, controlled trial in which participants were randomly assigned to intervention or control. Assessments were completed at baseline and 3 months between 2014 and 2015. All participants provided informed written consent at baseline. The protocol was approved by the Johns Hopkins University Institutional Review Board. Study data were collected via paper/pencil questionnaires and a Web-based program for dietary recall. The Research Electronic Data Capture (REDCap), a secure, Web-based application, was used to store data.

Setting and Participants

Participants were recruited in and around the Johns Hopkins University campuses using many strategies including posters/flyers, Facebook, e-mail announcements, and word of mouth. Individuals between 18 and 25 years of age with a BMI between 25 and 40 kg/m^2 who owned an iPhone or Android phone were eligible to participate. Participants were not required to be a college undergraduate or graduate student. Interested individuals contacted the primary investigator to set up a telephone screening; if the individual qualified, they were asked to set up a baseline visit. Participants were excluded if they were currently participating in another structured weight loss program, were taking weight loss medications, were diagnosed with type I diabetes, or were currently pregnant or planning to become pregnant in the next 3 months. Individuals were also excluded if they currently exercised more than 150 min/wk at moderate intensity or have had symptoms of disordered eating in the previous 6 months. Symptoms of disordered eating were defined as answering yes to any question assessing binging/purging, laxative/diet pill use, and treatment for an eating disorder from the Eating Attitudes Test 26 (EAT-26) questionnaire.[13] Randomization to smartphone + health coach or control by blocks of 4 occurred after data were collected at the baseline visit. All participants received a $25 gift card for participation.

Outcome Measures

Data on the outcome measures were collected on all participants at baseline and 3 months. Body weight was measured using the Tanita BS-549 scale with the participant in light clothing. Height was measured using a wall stick measurement. Body mass index was then calculated using weight in kilograms/height in meters squared. Waist circumference was measured twice and then averaged according to the obesity guidelines.[14]

Physical activity was evaluated with the Godin Leisure-Time Exercise Questionnaire. The survey is self-administered and assesses strenuous, moderate, and mild activity over a 7-day period.[15] This survey method has been proven to be both valid and reliable in adults, with test-retest scores ranging from 0.74 to 0.81.[16] Nutrition data were collected using the National Cancer Institute's Automated Self-Administered 24-hour Recall (ASA-24). The ASA-24 is a Web-based, ASA 24-hour recall of foods and was filled out on the participant's computer. The ASA-24 provides analysis on calories, nutrients, and food group estimates.[17] It has been proven to be valid in an adult population, with the ASA-24 performing very close (87% matching) to standardized interviewer-administered 24-hour food recalls.[17] Information obtained from the ASA-24 included caloric intake, food pyramid equivalents, and nutrients from all foods reported according to the Food and Nutrient Database for Dietary Studies.[17]

Self-efficacy for healthy eating and exercise were evaluated with 2 questionnaires. Both of the self-efficacy scales were self-administered by the participant. The Self-Efficacy for Healthy Eating is a 13-item questionnaire that explores a person's belief in their ability to make better food choices in given situations. A reliability coefficient of 0.87 indicated high internal consistency on the scale tested in a group of adults, ages 19 to 64 years.[18] Self-efficacy for physical activity was assessed using a 14-item questionnaire called the Self-Efficacy for Exercise Scale. This questionnaire assesses individuals' belief in their ability to exercise in given situations. This scale was determined to be reliable and valid in a population of adults, with an internal consistency of 0.90 and a test-retest correlation of 0.67.[19]

Interventions

The behavioral intervention was based on self-efficacy theory, a construct of social cognitive theory, which was used in our previous pilot study that focused on smartphone applications for weight loss in adults.[20] The self-efficacy theory states that there are 4 ways to increase one's self-efficacy: mastery experience, social modeling, social support, and verbal persuasion.[21] These 4 mechanisms were built into the intervention, which focused on increasing the participant's self-efficacy to achieve better health outcomes related to weight loss. The goals for both groups were to lose 1 to 2 lb per week and increase participation in physical activity. Participants were encouraged to exercise at least 150 minutes per week at moderate intensity, which would meet the Physical Activity Guidelines for Americans.[22] Both groups received a 1-time counseling session before randomization. This was a 20-minute session that discussed healthy eating, limiting alcohol and sugar-sweetened beverages, and increasing physical activity. After this session, participants were randomized to 1 of 2 groups, control or smartphone + health coach (intervention) for the 3-month study period.

Smartphone + Health Coach Group

Participants in this group were given an additional 30- to 40-minute counseling session on energy balance, nutrient density of foods, sugar-sweetened beverage consumption, and physical activity; therefore, they had 2 sessions total during their baseline visit. Participants were encouraged to identify specific goals that their health coach could help them achieve.

Participants were also guided to download and use the Lose it! application. This application is a free, commercially available smartphone application that is focused on nutrition and physical activity self-monitoring. Participants were encouraged to log all food and exercise into the daily log in the application. They were instructed to follow the caloric budget set by the application using the Mifflin equation. The application also offered social networking through a "friend" feature, which allowed individuals to view peer weight loss and physical activity participation and also allowed the interaction between peers. Participants were encouraged to use this feature.

Individualized text messages were delivered to the participant's smartphone from a health coach. The participants were asked to not text their health coach back. Based on data from a focus group study conducted by the first author, the participants could choose any frequency of messages they wanted to receive from a health coach, anywhere from 1 time per week up to 3 times per day.[9] The smartphone application provided the health coach with the ability to monitor and track all participant progress on a real-time basis and text messages focused on current diet or physical activity status (see Table 1). Texts were sent from the health coach's cell phone at the specified time and frequency of the participant.

TABLE 1 Example Text Messages	
Nutrition/Exercise Focus	Example Text Message
Physical activity guidelines for Americans	I noticed you came very close to meeting your goal of 150 minutes of exercise last week. Great job! Let's work hard to meet that 150-minute goal this week
Physical activity social support	Working out with a group can be fun and motivating! Reach out to friends today and do something you all enjoy!
Breakfast consumption	Did you know that people who skip breakfast tend to snack more during the day? Try eating a balanced breakfast each morning!
Nutrient density/sugar-sweetened beverages	Drinking your calories does not provide a nutrient-rich diet! Keep up the good work of drinking zero-calorie beverages!

Control Group

The control group was asked to not use any smartphone applications focused on weight loss for the duration of the study. They received the Lose It! application with a training session at their 3-month visit.

Statistical Analysis

The study was powered to detect statistically significant differences in weight loss between the 2 groups. Using an effect size of 0.8, calculated from a similar study,[10] an α of 0.05, and a power of 80%, the sample size was determined to be 51. The sample size was increased by 15% to allow for attrition, to give a total sample size of 60, or 30 per group. Group differences in baseline sociodemographic and anthropometric characteristics were examined using Wilcoxon rank-sum tests and χ^2 or Fisher exact tests. The primary outcomes were changes from baseline to 3 months in weight in kilograms, BMI, and waist circumference in centimeters. Secondary outcomes were changes in diet, physical activity, and self-efficacy for diet and physical activity. A completers analysis was performed using generalized linear models, which were used to test for group differences, time effects, and interactions between group*time. All statistical analyses were done using Statistical Analysis System (SAS).

Results

Baseline Characteristics

Baseline characteristics of participants by group are shown in Table 2. Of the 62 participants enrolled, 71% were female, 33.8% were Asian, and 12.9% were African American. The overall median age was 20.0

TABLE 2	Baseline Sample Characteristics by Treatment Group			
Characteristics	Total	Control	Smartphone + Health Coach	P
n	62	31	31	
Age, median (range), y	20.0 (18.0–25.0)	20.0 (18.0–24.0)	20.0 (18.0–25.0)	1
Race, n (%)				.7917
White	24 (38.7)	12 (38.7)	12 (38.7)	
Black	8 (12.9)	5 (16.1)	3 (9.7)	
Asian	21 (33.8)	9 (29.0)	12 (38.7)	
Other	9 (14.5)	5 (16.1)	4 (12.9)	
Sex, n (%)				.6322
Male	18 (29.0)	8 (25.8)	10 (32.3)	
Female	44 (71.0)	22 (71.0)	21 (67.7)	
BMI, median (range), kg/m^2	28.5 (25.0–40.4)	26.6 (25.0–39.7)	29.0 (25.2–40.4)	.0898
Waist circumference, median (range), cm	93.8 (81.0–120.0)	93.5 (81.0–120.0)	95.8 (82.5–120.0)	.294
Type of smartphone				.3493
iPhone	49 (79.0)	23 (74.2)	26 (83.9)	
Android phone	13 (21.0)	8 (25.8)	5 (16.1)	

Abbreviation: BMI, body mass index.

(18.0–25.0) years and median BMI was 28.5 (25.0–40.4) kg/m^2. Although the sample included both non–college and college students, only 10% of study participants were not current undergraduate or graduate students. There were no significant differences in baseline characteristics between the 2 groups.

Recruitment and Retention

The Figure is the CONSORT diagram reporting the participant flow through the study. We assessed 87 individuals for eligibility.

A total of 66 individuals met the criteria to participate. Of those, 4 (6%) declined to participate. The primary reason for refusal was lack of interest in participating in a study for 3 months. A total of 62 individuals were randomized to 1 of the 2 groups, which represented 71% of those who originally expressed interest in participating.

Fifty-nine (95%) returned at 3 months for follow-up measurements. Retention rates were similar in the 2 groups, 97% in the control group and 94% in the intervention group.

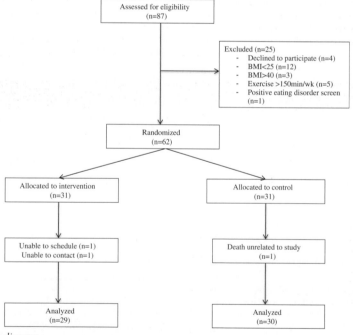

FIGURE. *Study flow diagram.*

Weight, Body Mass Index, and Wait Circumference

Changes from baseline to 3 months can be found in Table 3. The control group gained a slight amount of weight (0.3 kg) from baseline to 3 months, whereas participants in the smartphone + health coach group lost a significant amount (-1.8 kg, $P < .01$); the difference in weight change between groups was statistically significant ($P = .026$). The smartphone group also had a significant decrease in BMI ($P < .01$) and waist circumference ($P < .01$). The differences in BMI and waist circumference changes between groups were also statistically significant ($P = .024$ for BMI, $P < .01$ for waist circumference). Seven (24%) participants in the smartphone group who completed the study lost enough weight to change their weight status; 5 (17%) moved into the normal weight category and 2 (7%) went from the obese category to overweight.

Self-reported Behaviors

Changes in self-reported behaviors can also be found in Table 3. The smartphone + health coach group improved significantly in healthy eating self-efficacy ($P = .032$). They also improved in overall physical activity performed ($P < .01$); however, the differences were not significant when compared with the control group. Although both groups showed improvement in self efficacy for physical activity, neither change was statistically significant. A comparison of degree of change between groups was also performed (group × time interaction with all subjects) adjusting for self-efficacy for healthy eating and exercise. When adjusting for self-efficacy for healthy eating, the data show

that it is a slight mediator for change in weight with a P value shifting from $P = .026$ for nonadjusted to $P = .052$ when adjusted. Tests were also run for BMI and waist circumference, but there was no shift in P value, suggesting that self-efficacy for healthy eating does not entirely account for the treatment group effect.

A total of 37 (63%) participants completed the diet questionnaire at follow-up, 22 (73%) control and 15 (52%) smartphone + health coach. Table 4 displays the results from the ASA-24. The smartphone group consumed significantly more fiber than the control group did at follow-up ($P = .049$). There were no additional significant differences between the 2 groups at follow-up. However, participants in the smartphone group consumed slightly more protein, more vegetables, more fruit, fewer total carbohydrates, and fewer added sugars than did participants in the control arm.

Application Use and Text Messaging

The number of text messages sent varied from 1 per day to 3 times per day. No participants requested less than 1 message per day. Overall, 22 (71%) participants requested 3 messages per day, 4 (13%) requested 2 per day, and 5 (16%) requested 1 per day. All text messages were delivered to participants successfully; no error messages were received and all messages were labeled as delivered. Also, no issues were reported by participants.

All participants assigned to the smartphone group logged exercise and diet. Over the 3-month period, 6 (21%) participants logged exercise on more than 50% of days and 18 (62%) logged diet on more than 50% of days. Of those participants who logged on

TABLE 3 Preintervention and Postintervention Measurements of Body Size and Self-reported Behaviors

	Control			Smartphone + Health Coach			
	Pre	Post	P^a	Pre	Post	P^b	P^c
Body size							
Weight, median (range), kg	75.8 (63.0–103.7)	77.3 (66.0–106.2)	.764	82.8 (61–117.5)	80.1 (57.1–120.7)	<.01	.026
BMI, median (range), kg/m²	27.9 (25.0–39.7)	27.6 (25.1–37.7)	.811	29.8 (25.5–40.2)	28.4 (24.7–41.3)	<.01	.024
Waist circumference, median (range), cm	93.3 (81–120)	92.3 (81–117)	.964	95.8 (82.5–120)	92.3 (77–122)	<.01	<.01
Self-reported behaviors							
Self-efficacy (healthy eating), raw score (range)	102 (60–130)	109 (77–130)	.273	100 (66–120)	106 (73–128)	.032	.190
Self-efficacy (exercise), raw score (range)	87.5 (54–131)	92 (42–124)	.258	86 (25–127)	97 (30–140)	.151	.541
Physical activity, 7-day recall, raw score (range)	34 (3–108.5)	36 (6.0–92)	.099	32 (0–72)	43 (15–81)	<.01	.503

Variables summarized as median (range) and compared from pre-post using Wilcoxon rank-sum test; between-group interaction tested using repeated-measures analysis of variance.
Abbreviation: BMI, body mass index.
[a]Comparison of post versus pre in the control group (group effect in generalized linear model for control only).
[b]Comparison of post versus pre in the smartphone group (group effect in generalized linear model for treated only).
[c]Comparison of degree of change between groups (group × time interaction with all subjects).

TABLE 4	Diet Quality of Study Participants During Follow-Up			
Diet Parameter, Median (Range)	Total Study Population (N = 37)	Control (n = 22)	Smartphone + Health Coach (n = 15)	P
Calories	1356.7 (586–3288)	1282.2 (831–3288)	1670.5 (586–2689)	.221
Protein	61.1 (24.2–137.5)	58.7 (24.2–110.3)	78.5 (28.3–137.5)	.080
Total fat	47.7 (14.0–129.9)	44.8 (22.2–129.9)	53.7 (14.0–111.5)	.394
Total carbs	175.9 (73.3–453.7)	176.7 (73.3–453.7)	170.0 (85.9–312.0)	.816
Total sugar	61.8 (10.7–180.7)	60.5 (14.8–180.7)	65.0 (10.7–163.3)	.378
Total fiber	14.6 (2.1–61.7)	13.0 (2.1–61.7)	18.4 (7.2–31.7)	.049
Water	1638.8 (717–4277)	1541.3 (851–4277)	1684.1 (717–3869)	.816
Total sodium	2781.4 (1223–4784)	2720.3 (1272–4542)	2792.9 (1223–4784)	.631
Saturated fat	14.6 (2.6–43.9)	13.3 (6.6–43.9)	18.2 (2.6–41.2)	.506
Total vegetables	1.1 (0.0–6.1)	1.0 (0.0–6.1)	1.2 (0.5 4.2)	.193
Total fruit	0.7 (0.0–5.0)	0.5 (0.0–5.0)	0.9 (0.0–4.0)	.219
Total dairy	1.1 (0.0–5.2)	0.9 (0.0–5.2)	1.4 (0.0–2.9)	.768
Added sugars	7.1 (0.0–28.6)	8.2 (0.7–28.6)	5.6 (0.0–23.6)	.077

Continuous variables summarized as median (range) and compared between groups using Wilcoxon rank-sum test.

more than 50% of days, 3 (50%) logged physical activity on more than 75% of days and 7 (38%) logged diet on more than 75% of days. Table 5 displays the significant relationship between number of physical activity days logged and weight loss (0.03 kg weight loss per additional day of physical activity [PA] logging; $P = .026$). The 6 participants who logged PA more than 50% of the time lost 1.57 kg more than those who did not. When the threshold was reduced to 25% days logged, the 9 participants logging PA 25% or more of the time lost 1.43 kg more than those logging PA less than 25% of the time. The same directional trends were observed with increased logging frequency for food as well, but these were not significant ($P = .226$), possibly because of overall good compliance with food logging.

Discussion

To date, to the authors' knowledge, this is the first trial focused on young adults that used both individualized text messages and a smartphone application for weight loss. This trial showed that the use of a smartphone application combined with individualized text messages is successful in helping individuals to lose weight. Individuals in the smartphone group lost significantly more weight, had a significant decrease in BMI, and significantly decreased their waist circumference compared with the control group. However,

many individuals did not meet the recommended goal in the study to lose 1 to 2 lb per week. The mean weight loss in the smartphone + health coach group was 4 lb over the 3-month trial. These results are promising when examining other similar research. Although studies using technology or text messaging have seen improvements in weight, many did not report any significant improvements when compared with a control condition.[23,24] It is possible that the combination of a smartphone application with text messaging led to significant improvements in body weight in this group of young adults.

It is noteworthy that self-efficacy increased significantly for healthy eating ($P = .03$) in the smartphone + health coach group and both groups experienced an increase in self-efficacy for exercise, although this was not significant. It is possible that there were differences in self-efficacy between men and women or based on racial category in this study; however, these differences were not tested. Recent studies conducted in college-aged individuals reported implications for testing the differences in self-efficacy between men and women and also indicate possible racial differences in self-efficacy for improving certain health behaviors. A study published in 2015 by Bruce et al[25] reported significantly lower self-efficacy for changing sugar-sweetened beverage consumption in African American college men compared with white college men. In addition, a study examining

TABLE 5	Relationships Between Logging Consistency and Weight Change			
	n/N	B	95% CI	P
No. days logged (PA)	—	−0.03[a]	−0.05 to −0.01	.026
Logging >50% PA	6/29	−1.57[b]	−3.31 to 0.17	.089
No. days logged (food)	—	−0.02[a]	−0.04 to 0.01	.226
Logging >50% food	18/29	−0.70[b]	−2.24 to 0.74	.375

Abbreviation: CI, confidence interval.
[a]Expected weight change per additional day of logging.
[b]Expected weight change for more than 50% logging versus less than 50% logging.

What's New and Important

- This is the first study to examine use of smartphone technology and text messaging for weight loss in young adults.
- This study shows that using smartphone technology and text messaging can help young adults lose weight.
- Increased logging of physical activity on a smartphone led to increases in weight loss.

Korean college students reported that self-efficacy for physical activity is a significant predictor of physical activity in Korean men but not in Korean women.[26] Future studies should include analyses on differences in self-efficacy but should also examine other components of social cognitive theory, such as social support or outcome expectations, which are known predictors of behaviors.[21]

An increase in logging into the smartphone application for both physical activity and diet led to better outcomes with weight loss. It is therefore important that accountability be a focus in future interventions. Accountability in this study was exhibited through the behavior of logging into an application; however, accountability could be achieved many different ways in upcoming trials. In trials that use technology, increasing compliance and accountability with smartphone logging could be achieved through a counselor stressing the importance of logging during a session or more frequent reminders could be sent to participant phones.

There are several strengths to note in this study. Strengths of the study include the randomized design powered to detect significant differences between groups, use of a commercially available smartphone application, and an attrition rate of only 5%. In addition, the study population was diverse: 38 (62%) participants were from a minority group and 21 (33%) identified as Asian and 8 (13%) identified as African American.

Study limitations include the small sample size and limited generalizability of the study population in that most were attending college at a single university on the east coast. Also, the study was of short duration (3 months) with no extended follow-up. Finally, it cannot be determined whether differences between groups were a result of the health coach text messaging or the smartphone application.

Conclusion

This randomized controlled trial using a smartphone application for weight loss combined with individualized text messages has provided valuable information that the combination of self-monitoring via an application and feedback from a health coach is successful in helping young adults lose weight. The study had a meaningful impact on weight, BMI, and waist circumference. In future trials, a sample that includes equal amounts of individuals attending college and those not attending college could strengthen the generalizability of the results. Smartphone technology seems to be an appropriate resource to use when working with the young adult population and it has the potential to greatly impact the serious public health problem of obesity.

REFERENCES

1. Ogden CL, Carroll MD, Kit BK, Flegal KM. Prevalence of childhood and adult obesity in the United States, 2011–2012. *JAMA*. 2014;311(8):806–814.
2. Holm-Denoma JM, Joiner TE, Vohs KD, Heatherton TF. The "freshman fifteen" (the "freshman five" actually): predictors and possible explanations. *Health Psychol*. 2008; 27(supplement 1):S3–S9.
3. Economos CD, Hildebrandt ML, Hyatt RR. College freshman stress and weight change: differences by gender. *Am J Health Behav*. 2008;32(1):16–25.
4. Gropper SS, Newton A, Harrington P, Simmons KP, Connell LJ, Ulrich P. Body composition changes during the first two years of university. *Prev Med*. 2011;52(1):20–22.
5. American College Health Association. *American College Health Association- National College Health Assessment II: Undergraduate Students Reference Group Executive Summary Spring 2014*. Hanover, MD: American College Health Association; 2014.
6. Burton BT, Foster WR, Hirsch J, Van Itallie TB. Health implications of obesity: an NIH consensus development conference. *Int J Obes*. 1985;9:155–169.
7. Kasparek DG, Corwin SJ, Valois RF, Sargent RG, Morris RL. Selected health behaviors that influence college freshman weight change. *J Am Coll Health*. 2008;56(4):437–444.
8. Lloyd-Richardson EE, Lucero ML, DiBello JR, Jacobson AE, Wing RR. The relationship between alcohol use, eating habits and weight change in college freshmen. *Eat Behav*. 2008; 9(4):504–508.
9. Smith A. U.S. smartphone use in 2015. April 1, 2015. http://www.pewinternet.org/2015/04/01/us-smartphone-use-in-2015/. Accessed April 20, 2015.
10. Stephens J, Moscou-Jackson G, Allen JK. Young adults, technology, and weight loss: a focus group study. *J Obes*. 2015;2015:379769.
11. Napolitano MA, Hayes S, Bennett GG, Ives AK, Foster GD. Using Facebook and text messaging to deliver a weight loss program to college students. *Obesity (Silver Spring)*. 2013; 21(1):25–31.
12. Lachausse RG. My student body: effects of an internet-based prevention program to decrease obesity among college students. *J Am Coll Health*. 2012;60(4):324–330. doi:10.1080/07448481 .2011.623333.
13. Garner DM, Olmsted MP, Bohr Y, Garfinkel PE. The eating attitudes test: psychometric features and clinical correlates. *Psychol Med*. 1982;12(4):871–878.
14. National Heart, Lung and Blood Institute. *Guidelines on Overweight and Obesity: Electronic Textbook*. Bethesda, MD: National Institutes of Health.
15. Godin G, Shephard RJ. Godin Leisure-Time Exercise Questionnaire. *Med Sci Sports Exerc*. 1997;26(suppl 6):S36–S38.
16. Jacobs DR Jr, Ainsworth BE, Hartman TJ, Leon AS. A simultaneous evaluation of 10 commonly used physical activity questionnaires. *Med Sci Sports Exerc*. 1993;25(1): 81–91.

17. Kirkpatrick SI, Subar AF, Douglass D, et al. Performance of the Automated Self-Administered 24-hour Recall relative to a measure of true intakes and to an interviewer-administered 24-h recall. *Am J Clin Nutr.* 2014;100(1):233–240.

18. Schouwstra SJ. The Nutrition Efficacy Scale: development and construct validation using the deductive design. *UvA-Dare.* 2014;78–117.

19. Wilson M, Allen DD, Li JC. Improving measurement in health education and health behavior research using item response modeling: comparison with the classical test theory approach. *Health Educ Res.* 2006;21(suppl 1):i19–i32.

20. US Department of Health and Human Services. Physical activity guidelines for Americans, 2008. http://health.gov/paguidelines. Accessed April 20, 2015.

21. Glanz K, Rimer BK, Viswanath K. *Health Behavior and Health Education.* 4th ed. San Francisco, CA: Jossey-Bass; 2008.

22. Allen JK, Stephens J, Dennison Himmelfarb CR, Stewart KJ, Hauck S. Randomized controlled pilot study testing use of smartphone technology for obesity treatment. In: *J Obes,* vol. 2013;2013:151597.

23. Zuercher JL. *Developing Strategies for Helping Women Improve Weight-Related Health Behaviors.* Chapel Hill, NC: University of North Carolina at Chapel Hill; 2009.

24. Hebden L, Cook A, van der Ploeg HP, King L, Bauman A, Allman-Farinelli M. A mobile health intervention for weight management among young adults: a pilot randomized controlled trial. *J Hum Nutr Diet.* 2014;27(4):322–332.

25. Bruce MA, Beech BM, Thorpe RJ Jr, Griffith DM. Racial disparities in sugar-sweetened beverage consumption change efficacy among male first-year college students [published online ahead of print August 15, 2015]. In: *Am J Mens Health.* pii:1557988315599825.

26. Choi JY, Chang AK, Choi EJ. Sex differences in social cognitive factors and physical activity in Korean college students. *J Phys Ther Sci.* 2015;27(6):1659–1664.

MCN American Journal of Maternal Child Nursing. 2009 Nov–Dec; 34(6): 356–64

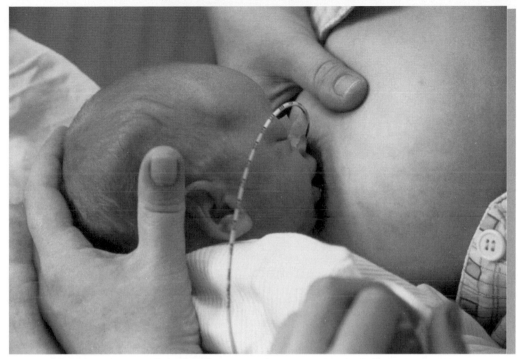

Rooting for the Breast:
Breastfeeding Promotion in the
NICU

Roberta Cricco-Lizza, PhD, MPH, RN

This study explored the structure and process of breastfeeding promotion in the neonatal intensive care unit (NICU). Mother's milk is particularly important for the health of premature and high-risk infants (American Academy of Pediatrics, 2005; Ip et al., 2007). Ingestion of breast milk in the NICU by low birth weight infants has been linked to beneficial health outcomes and enhanced cognitive development (Vohr et al., 2006). Breast milk provides protection against infections, sepsis, necrotizing enterocolitis, and retinopathy of prematurity (Furman, Taylor, Minich, & Hack, 2003; Hylander, Strobino, Pezzullo, & Dhannireddy, 2001; Schanler, Lau, Hurst, & Smith, 2005). The American Academy of Pediatrics recommends direct breastfeeding and/or use of mother's own pumped milk for high-risk infants; however, these reported rates are low for NICU babies (Espy & Senn, 2003). In addition to

121

Abstract

Purpose: This study explored the structure and process of breastfeeding promotion in the NICU.

Methods: An ethnographic approach was used with the techniques of participant observation, interviewing, and artifact assessment. This 14-month study took place in a level IV NICU in a Northeastern US children's hospital. General informants consisted of 114 purposively selected NICU nurses. From this group, 18 nurses served as key informants. There was an average of 13 interactions with each key informant and 3.5 for each general informant. Audiotaped interviews, feeding artifacts, and observational notes were gathered for descriptions of breastfeeding promotion. Data were coded and analyzed for recurring patterns. NUD*IST-aided data management and analysis.

Findings: There were three main findings: (1) organizational and human resources were developed to create a web of support to promote breastfeeding in the NICU; (2) variations in breastfeeding knowledge and experience within the nursing staff, marketing practices of formula companies, and insufficient support from other health professionals served as sources of inconsistent breastfeeding messages; and (3) promotion of breastfeeding in this NICU is evolving over time from a current breast milk feeding focus to the goal for a future breastfeeding process orientation.

Clinical Implications: NICU nurses should advocate for organizational and human resources to promote breastfeeding in the unit. To decrease inconsistent messages, staff development should be expanded to all professionals, and formula marketing practices should be curtailed.

Keywords: Breastfeeding; NICU; Nurses; Promotion.

maternal and neonatal issues, staff and hospital factors also influence NICU breastfeeding rates (Lessen & Crivelli-Kovach, 2007; Merewood, Philipp, Chawla, & Cimo, 2003).

Maternity practices in the United States are often not evidence based and have been shown to impede breastfeeding (Centers for Disease Control and Prevention, 2008; DiGirolamo, Grummer-Strawn, & Fein, 2001). The World Health Organization (WHO) and the United Nations Children's Fund (UNICEF) (1992) launched the Baby-Friendly Hospital Initiative (BFHI) to protect, promote, and support breastfeeding in birth environments. The recommended practices in this Initiative have been linked to improved breastfeeding rates, but they generally pertain to routine births in hospitals and birthing centers (Kramer et al., 2001). Mothers of high-risk infants face unique challenges to the initiation and continuation of breastfeeding (Meier, 2001; Spatz, 2006). Hospitals must address these challenges to prepare the NICU staff to support breastfeeding families. However, mothers have reported problems with hospital routines and inadequate support for breastfeeding from nurses and physicians in the NICU (Cricco-Lizza, 2006). Hospitals with NICU breastfeeding promotion programs have positively influenced breastfeeding rates (Dall'Oglio et al., 2007; do Nascimento & Issler, 2005).

More research is needed about effective ways to promote breastfeeding in the NICU. Structures and processes in an organization can advance or can hamper the implementation of health promotion strategies, and much can be gained by exploring the context of everyday practices (Yano, 2008). This report is part of a larger qualitative study of NICU nurses and infant feeding. In a previous publication from this study, nurses' personal contexts of infant feeding outside of the NICU were examined. The nurses identified a formula feeding norm during their own childhoods and described limited exposure to breastfeeding in nursing school (Cricco-Lizza, 2009). The current article examines the structures and processes that were developed to promote breastfeeding in the NICU.

Methods

An ethnographic approach was used with the techniques of participant observation, interviewing, and artifact analysis. By combining these three techniques, multiple sources of information were obtained for a comprehensive view of breastfeeding promotion in the NICU. The sample consisted of 114 nurses who were considered "general informants," purposefully selected to provide a wide angle view of breastfeeding promotion, and 18 "key informants" chosen from that group who were followed more intensively for an in-depth view. Both key and general informants were selected for maximal variety of infant feeding and NICU clinical experiences. The 14-month study was conducted in a level IV NICU in a freestanding children's hospital in the Northeastern United States. This study was approved by the Human Subjects' Committees and study information was provided to the nurses through the intranet, staff meetings, and individual encounters in the NICU. Nurses who served as key informants for the study signed informed consent before formal interviews.

Sample

From 250 nurses employed in this NICU, 114 served as the general informants; 96 of these were White, 9 African American, 8 Asian, and 1 Hispanic. Only one was a male. About 30% of the general informants had taken a hospital breastfeeding course developed before this study was initiated. The age of the 18 key informants ranged from 22 to 51 (mean = 33). Of these, 17 were female; 16 were White and 2 were African American. Two had diplomas in nursing, 1 had an associate degree, 14 had a BSN, and 1 had a master's degree. The key informants were almost evenly divided among all four expertise levels of the clinical ladder, from novices to clinical experts. About half of these key informants had taken the hospital breastfeeding course and almost one-fourth were on the breastfeeding committee.

Data Collection
Participant Observation

Unobtrusive observations focused on the nurses' behaviors during interactions with babies, families, nurses, and other healthcare professionals throughout everyday NICU activities. Included in these observations were feedings and routine care, shift reports, breastfeeding committee meetings, nutrition meetings, psychosocial rounds, and nurse-run breastfeeding support groups for parents. There were 128 observation sessions, which took place for 1 to 2 hours

> Nurses who had taken the breastfeeding course said that it helped them feel "comfortable," "competent," and "prepared" to teach breastfeeding to families.

during varying days and times of the week. The investigator introduced herself as a nurse researcher who was interested in learning about NICU nurses' perspectives about infant feeding. The researcher role evolved from observation to informal interviews over time. The nurses were asked about breastfeeding promotion within the context of everyday nursing care in the NICU. The general informants were observed/informally interviewed an average of 3.5 times each (range 1-24) over the study period. All observational data and informal interview data were documented immediately after each session.

Artifact Analysis

Documents can serve as a resource for investigating social meaning and practice (Miller & Alvarado, 2005). Breastfeeding standards of care, teaching plans, and policies and procedures were purposefully gathered and reviewed early in the study. These documents provided insight into officially recognized standards of care for infant feeding in this NICU. They also served as a springboard for lines of inquiry that were further developed during observations and interviews. In addition, parent education materials, posters on the unit, and signs placed at the bedside provided other sources of data about breastfeeding promotion in this NICU.

Formal Interviewing

Each of the 18 key informants engaged in a formal, 1-hour, tape-recorded interview in a private room near the NICU. Open-ended interview questions probed nursing perspectives about breastfeeding promotion in the NICU. In addition to the formal interview, they were also informally interviewed and/or observed a total of 3 to 43 times each (mean of 13.1) over the entire study. The formal interviews were transcribed verbatim and the transcriptions and tapes were reviewed for accuracy.

Data Analysis and Verification

The data from formal and informal interviews, observations, NICU artifacts, and ongoing memos were analyzed concurrently with data collection. QSR NUD*IST was used to facilitate data management, retrieval, and analysis. The data were examined line-by-line in an iterative fashion and codes were inductively derived for meaning. These codes were restructured into categories and then analyzed for patterns. Ongoing contact with general and key informants facilitated pattern identification and verification. The findings were continuously verified through triangulation of interviewing, participant observation, and artifact assessment and this helped to decrease bias. A peer-review group of pre- and postdoctoral nurse researchers also provided oral and written critique throughout the course of the study.

Findings

Organizational and Human Resources Were Developed To Create a Web of Support To Promote Breastfeeding in the NICU
Organizational Resources

There was consistent evidence that organizational resources had been developed in the NICU to encourage breastfeeding. A general informant described how multidisciplinary NICU representatives had reviewed the state of the science on breastfeeding. She said that they used these findings to conceptualize *"a continuum from informed decision making, pump access with establishment and maintenance of milk supply, breast milk feeding, skin-to-skin care, nonnutritive sucking, transition to breast, to preparation for discharge."*

A review of unit documents demonstrated that breastfeeding standards of care and policies and procedures clearly communicated unit-approved statements supporting the use of human milk and breastfeeding in the NICU. Breastfeeding teaching plans and educational materials were observed to be readily available on the unit and examination of the content showed that these documents focused on the specific needs of families with high-risk infants. The general and key informants referred to these documents and discussed how they were used during interactions with parents. One nurse said, *"We try to give them information. We have booklets, printouts, whatever about breastfeeding."*

Another stated, *"We present them with breastfeeding information as soon as they come in the door."* The admission packet for parents described breastfeeding as a *"wonderful"* decision for the health of the baby.

Discussion with general and key informants revealed an understanding of the breast milk management system in this NICU. These breast milk handling procedures were generally followed by the nurses, although discussion between the nurses and mothers about milk supply was sometimes overlooked, and occasionally this information did not get transmitted in shift reports. Observations in the unit showed that pump rooms were easily accessible and used by NICU mothers. These spaces had high visibility and accessibility in a central location. Rolling breast pumps were also on hand for bedside pumping and a rental station was available to support breast pumping away from the NICU. Observations also revealed that current literature about medications and breast milk was on reserve in the NICU. All of these structures and processes provided a foundation to promote breastfeeding.

Interviews of general and key informants demonstrated that these organizational resources were initiated by the NICU lactation and nursing professionals in this NICU, and further developed through the combined actions of the NICU breastfeeding committee members. NICU nurses, along with the lactation staff, served on this committee and they met on a monthly basis to discuss any ongoing issues related to breastfeeding on the unit. Observations demonstrated that the nurses who served on this committee were the leaders in all phases of breastfeeding promotion on the unit. Specific activities observed during this study included conference planning, quality improvement studies, World Breastfeeding Week events, and skin-to-skin care promotion. These activities had ripple effects throughout the unit. For example, one key informant stated, *"We had posters all around for World Breastfeeding Week, and a mother read… about all the benefits… and said, 'you know because of that I'm breastfeeding my baby.'"* Observations also demonstrated that there was an increase in mothers asking about doing skin-to-skin care after the breastfeeding committee members placed skin-to-skin posters in the NICU.

Efforts were also expended beyond the NICU to strengthen intra- and extra-hospital support for breastfeeding promotion. The breastfeeding committee successfully lobbied the hospital foundation to remove a public display panel within the hospital corridors that promoted bottle feeding. This committee also designated annual awards to staff nurses who were most active in breastfeeding promotion. Furthermore, the committee members conducted an annual breastfeeding conference and they were observed sharing the latest research-based feeding practices with NICU nurses from the varied hospitals in this perinatal catchment area. In addition, they used conference gatherings as opportunities to encourage staff nurses to become politically active in support of statewide breastfeeding legislation.

Human Resources

Staff development factors were also important for breastfeeding promotion in the unit. The NICU had lactation consultants and a nursing clinical specialist who provided weekday support for mothers who wanted to breastfeed their NICU babies. Bedside staff nurse support was important for initial referral and continuing assistance of these mothers. All nurses in the NICU were required to complete a Web-based module about the handling, storage, and management of breast milk. General and key informants also talked about the additional 16-hour breastfeeding course that had been developed before this study took place, and had been offered over the past few years at this hospital. They said that this course included information about breastfeeding benefits, anatomy and physiology of lactation, and specific NICU issues of pumping, lactoengineering, skin-to-skin care, transition to the breast, test weights, and concerns related to the transfer of viruses and drugs. They stated that they also received clinical experience with assessment of positioning, latch, and breastfeeding. The nurses who completed this course identified that they learned important information for their NICU nursing practice. Some nurses said: *"A lot of the things were new to me"* and *"It was excellent, very informative."* Other nurses said that this course helped them feel *"comfortable,"* *"competent,"* and *"prepared"* to teach breastfeeding to families. One new graduate nurse stated, *"I don't hesitate to…help the baby latch on…try different holds…try different techniques."* There was also evidence that the benefits of this course extended to personal experiences outside of the NICU setting. For example, one nurse said that this course was the biggest influence on her decision to breastfeed her own child. She stated, *"From working here and becoming educated [and] knowing all the benefits it has for the baby and for the mom… I just thought that it would be a good thing to do."*

The nurses who completed this breastfeeding course were expected to act as bedside breastfeeding supporters and some of them served on the breastfeeding committee or helped to coordinate the parents' breastfeeding support group. Observations in the NICU demonstrated that the nurses who had taken this course were very positive about breastfeeding promotion. In varied situations these nurses were observed encouraging mothers who had low supplies and educating them about steps to take to increase yield. In one particular situation on the night shift, a new graduate nurse worked closely supporting and teaching new parents how to assess intake. She said that she felt pleased with her ability to facilitate their infant feeding. Another nurse was heard telling parents *"We want to help you"* when the mother was discouraged with pumping.

Variations in Breastfeeding Knowledge and Experience Within the Nursing Staff, Marketing Practices of Formula Companies and Insufficient Support From Other Health Professionals Served as Sources of Inconsistent Messages for Breastfeeding

Breastfeeding Knowledge and Experience of the NICU Nurses

There were considerable variations in the breastfeeding knowledge and experience of the NICU nurses. The 16-hour breastfeeding course was a requirement for all orientees, but for the rest of the NICU staff, it was optional. One of the key informants said, *"There's no requirement"* for existing NICU staff members to take the breastfeeding classes. During the study there were about 45 nurses out of 250 who had completed these classes and all had been paid for their time in class. Another key informant stated that nurses who had not taken this course were *"not practicing based on evidence right now; they are practicing based on their beliefs."* The NICU nurses freely spoke about their education for infant feeding and whether or not they had taken the breastfeeding course. One of the NICU nurses who had chosen not to take the course stated, *"I feel like for me if there's certain stuff I need to know, I'd rather know how to give a kid a bolus and do different stuff like that than breastfeed. I'd rather grab somebody else you know, a resource nurse or lactation consultant."* Another nurse voiced similar reasons why she had decided not to take the breastfeeding course. She asserted, *"If you give me a list of 10 different things to pursue interest-wise, breastfeeding would be somewhere towards the bottom. It's not something that I have ever gone out of my way to get involved in."* She said, *"If I have to go to an in-service I will, but I don't go out of my way to pursue* [breastfeeding] *conferences."*

The nurses who had not completed the breastfeeding course were generally more detached from breastfeeding promotion activities. Observations throughout the study demonstrated that these nurses were more likely to miss opportunities for breastfeeding promotion during the work day. Nurses who had not taken this course sometimes treated breast milk and formula as equivalent or did not promote direct breastfeeding to pumping mothers. For example, a mother who was committed to breastfeeding expressed concern to her nurse over her baby's difficulty eating. She asked the nurse what the goal was for her child. This nurse said that she had to take a certain amount of *"p.o. feeds"* or the rest would be given by tube. When the mother asked the meaning of the term *"p.o. feeds,"* the nurse replied, *"all of the feeds by bottle."* This general informant seemed unaware that she had dismissed breastfeeding.

Formula Company Marketing

The marketing practices of formula companies also presented challenges for breastfeeding promotion. The nurses frequently identified formula companies when they talked about infant feeding information that was perceived as educational. One key informant said, *"Formula reps come in and do a little lunch and do a little slideshow."* Many of the informants said that they attended these formula company-sponsored in-services and they talked confidently about the messages learned there. One nurse said that she was told that a certain formula *"is better for eye and brain development."* Another nurse stated that a particular formula company publishes *"a calendar every year with kids that have been on some of their different formulas, very specialized formulas, just to show you... how these kids have progressed* [and] *grown."* She said, *"They help them because they have these special formulas available."* One other nurse also went to these in-services and said that it helped in, *"finding ... what formulas* [were] *most like breast milk and really helped the baby with digestion."* Another nurse stated that the formula companies have an annual conference and the *"topics are non formula related so you can get a big audience of nurses to go, but in between the speakers it's almost commercial breaks for the product."* She said that they offer *"good topics and it's really reasonable and you get really good food... and you get contact hours for certification."* This nurse declared that the formula companies were *"trying to push the science of 'this is such a superior product' and that may catch the nurses."* One of the nurses who supported breastfeeding also sarcastically referred to *"the cutest lunch bags"* that the formula representative was giving to the staff.

Insufficient Support from other Healthcare Professionals

Other challenges for breastfeeding promotion included the varied feeding approaches of other professionals. Some of the nurses did not feel that the physicians promoted breastfeeding. One key informant said, *"The doctors here are more totally focused on the disease process, getting the baby better... getting the baby out of here. I don't think I've EVER heard... a doctor here question the mom about how she was planning to feed the baby. I think they're too busy. And it's just the LAST thing on their list of priorities."*

Observations at the bedside established that the lactation staff and nurses were the most likely to promote breastfeeding with the parents. Nurses' interactions with mothers and members of other disciplines were frequently observed. The physicians rarely mentioned breastfeeding. The speech/infant feeding therapists focused on bottle feeding and in one case, one of them made deprecating comments to the nurse and parents about the pumping advice of the lactation staff. Infant feeding instructions posted at the bedside by these therapists consistently described procedures for the use of pacifiers and bottles.

Promotion of Breastfeeding in This NICU Is Evolving Over Time From a Current Breast Milk Feeding Focus To the Goal for a Future Breastfeeding Process Orientation

The general and key informants identified that there had been significant changes in breastfeeding promotion in the NICU over the past 5 years. The NICU had not documented rates of breastfeeding or breast milk feeding prior to instituting their efforts to promote breastfeeding. However, one key informant repeated a common refrain when she said, *"We really have grown."* Another nurse described her individual growth and the changes that had occurred in the unit since she took the breastfeeding course. She said: *"I feel since I started here we have come a long way as far [as] educating nurses and I think people are a lot more comfortable now, educating families and mothers about breastfeeding. Although I was a new nurse and really hadn't been exposed that much to breastfeeding, I didn't know much about it. You know it was a little uncomfortable for me...because people asked me questions and I didn't know what to tell them or how to help them. But now that we've been educated, I think that it's a lot easier."*

> *"I feel since I started here we have come a long way as far [as] educating nurses and I think people are a lot more comfortable now, educating families and mothers about breastfeeding."*

There was general acknowledgement that support for breastfeeding still varied in the NICU. One nurse said, *"I think that more [nurses] are understanding the importance of breast milk but I don't think that 100% of them are."* This nurse felt that some nurses' *"lack of information"* and *"lack of awareness of its importance"* interfered with breastfeeding promotion. Another nurse said, *"I would say some nurses do a better job at trying to steer them [mothers] towards breastfeeding or pumping than other nurses."*

There were variations in the breastfeeding measures currently collected by the staff on the unit. During the study, monthly rates for percent of NICU babies ever receiving any human milk varied from 53% to 95% with an average of 71%. The nurses did not gather measures about any differences in the percentage of feeds of breast milk consumed or rates of transition to actual breastfeeding. In general, the nurses were more oriented to breast milk feeding than actual breastfeeding. Frequently, the nurses mentioned the scientific advantages of breast milk when they engaged in breastfeeding promotion. During the parents' breastfeeding support meetings, the nurses often used cards that listed varying science-based statements about the properties of breast milk. Likewise one of the breastfeeding promotion signs on the unit was worded, *"Breast milk is more than nutrition. It is protection."* The focus was usually on breast milk as a scientific product rather than breastfeeding as human process between mother and baby.

Interviews and observations demonstrated that breast milk feeding was more widespread than actual breastfeeding. Overall one of the key informants said, *"We've come a long way here. More [babies] receive breast milk at this point than ever in our past."* Another key informant further clarified this. She said, *"We are trying to work on the notion that baby can go to breast for the first oral feed. It doesn't need to be the bottle. That's a hard notion."* Other nurses concurred that it was the *"transition to the breast"* that was the area most in need of improvement. During observations some of the nurses could be seen handing a defrosted bottle of breast milk to a mother instead of helping her to breastfeed. When one key informant was asked about this practice, she stated, *"It does get overlooked sometimes definitely...I know that plenty of time we feed the kid the bottle."* Another key informant spoke for many when she attributed this practice to: *"Doctors and nurses being uncomfortable with the breastfeeding, extra work for the nurses, getting the test weight scale, and making sure that the screens are up and appropriate. And just, you know, it IS a lot of extra work."*

There was also evidence that attempts to make the NICU more breastfeeding supportive occasionally took its toll on the staff. One general informant who was a member of the breastfeeding committee said that it was discouraging because one nurse helps with breastfeeding and the next one does not. A key informant described the continuing struggle to promote breastfeeding in the NICU. She said: *"But the difficult thing is trying to change culture and practice in this unit. It's very difficult...For instance with breastfeeding, we've made such headway in the last couple of years, but sometimes we have to stop and look back and say we are making headway because on a daily basis, at times, it doesn't feel that way because you are constantly struggling or you feel like that somebody is always trying to undo something that you've done."*

Nevertheless, the breastfeeding committee members remained committed to breastfeeding promotion and to changing the NICU culture to support high-risk families with this process. One of them reflected a common sentiment when she stated: *"I think we send the message that it's important…That we've made such a change in our culture and it's not 100% across the board, but there are enough of us that we are making a change happen. And [it is one] that moms really value."* These nurses had a long term view of the change process in the NICU and decided to work together over time to overcome the hurdles. Another breastfeeding committee member said: *"It's really up to us. It's not fair if we don't provide the adequate education and be able to give the parents the proper information to make an informed decision…. And WE CAN, as NICU nurses, we can get there.*

> "It's really up to us. It's not fair if we don't provide the adequate education and … give the parents the proper information to make an informed decision….and WE CAN, as NICU nurses, we can get there."

Discussion/Clinical Nursing Implications

The BFHI has provided clear guidelines to promote breastfeeding in birth settings; however, high-risk infants require special care to safeguard their need for breastfeeding. These infants face distinctive challenges related to their compromised physical states and their separation from their mothers, and many questions exist about how NICUs can support these vulnerable families. This study used an ethnographic approach to examine the organizational and human resource support for breastfeeding promotion in the NICU and detailed the multifaceted elements that should be considered in a high-risk setting.

The staff in this particular NICU had limited experience and exposure to breastfeeding during their formative years and in their nursing school education (Cricco-Lizza, 2009). This greatly increased the demand on the institution to develop resources to meet the needs for breastfeeding promotion. Leaders in lactation and nursing spearheaded the changes that initiated this still evolving process. They started a breastfeeding committee that actively involved the staff nurses in this evidence-based change process. As a group

they developed systems of support and material resources for pumping and breast milk management, and constructed wide ranging policy, procedure, and teaching materials as staff resources. This infrastructural support was highly visible for the staff and parents and clearly communicated the value of breastfeeding within the daily activities of the unit. The group also took these changes outside of the NICU into the hospital itself, the multiple hospitals in this perinatal catchment area and on to legislators in this state. In such a manner they built a multifaceted web of support. This web could be further enhanced by efforts to gather more detailed data about breast milk and breastfeeding rates. These rates could guide breastfeeding promotion efforts within the unit.

Development of human resources met with mixed success. The breastfeeding course was specifically geared for breastfeeding promotion in an acute care setting. The staff members who completed this 2-day session served as extensions of the lactation staff and as bedside sources of breastfeeding expertise. Siddell, Marinelli, Froman, and Burke (2003) demonstrated that a breastfeeding educational intervention significantly increased NICU nurses' breastfeeding knowledge and altered some attitudes about breastfeeding. The findings of this ethnographic study support this and showed that these nurses not only served as leaders on the unit, but some also took this knowledge back into their personal lives outside of the NICU. Jones, Shapiro, and Roshon (2007) determined that an organized team of experts coupled with training and continued troubleshooting could affect culture change in an acute care setting. During the time of the study, about 45 NICU nurses had fulfilled the course requirements to serve as these bedside supporters. These nurses promoted breastfeeding and acted as change agents in this NICU. Those nurses who did not take the course maintained a more detached stance in breastfeeding activities. In the demanding setting of the NICU, nurses without the breastfeeding training missed opportunities to promote and support breastfeeding. This uneven knowledge and skill with breastfeeding could serve as a source of inconsistent messages for families. This finding suggests that the time is right to implement the breastfeeding course for the entire staff. Breastfeeding training for all staff members is a requirement for birth hospitals for BFHI and is probably even more important for the vulnerable babies in non-birth hospital NICUs.

Nurses were also exposed to formula marketing messages in educational forums for NICU staff. Many of these nurses had not attended the breastfeeding course and identified these formula programs as sources for infant feeding

CLINICAL IMPLICATIONS

NICU nurses should:

❖ Develop organizational and human resources for breastfeeding promotion

❖ Provide breastfeeding education for all NICU staff

❖ Encourage multidisciplinary representation for breastfeeding committees and projects

❖ Limit formula marketing practices in the NICU to avoid inconsistent feeding messages

❖ Utilize in-house experts to provide staff education about infant feeding

❖ Gather specific breastfeeding and breast milk feeding rates to guide promotion efforts

education. Bernaix (2000) found that knowledge about breastfeeding was predictive of maternal child nurses' supportive behaviors for breastfeeding, and emphasized the need for accurate knowledge. The NICU nurses in this current study repeated some of the non-evidence-based formula company claims, and some accepted small gifts and lunches from the sales representatives. The American Academy of Pediatrics (2005) has identified formula marketing as an obstacle to breastfeeding. This study suggests that direct infant formula marketing to professionals by formula representatives also compromises clear messages about breastfeeding promotion in the NICU. Sponsored educational offerings, gifts, and meals can create conflicts of interest and serve as threats to professional integrity (Erlen, 2008; Hagen, Pijl-Zieber, Souveny, & Lacroix, 2008; Stokamer, 2003).

The nurses also perceived a lack of support for breastfeeding from other NICU healthcare professionals. The study findings demonstrated that there were inconsistent recommendations from health professionals in this NICU. Mothers have previously reported conflicting breastfeeding advice from professionals (McInnes & Chambers, 2008). do Nascimento and Issler (2005) found that a trained interdisciplinary team provided consistent information and attained a 94.6% rate for breast milk consumption at discharge from a Brazilian NICU. Multidisciplinary commitment is crucial for successful implementation of evidence-based practice in critical care units (Weinert & Mann, 2008).

This study also indicated that inconsistent messages can contribute to decreased morale and frustration for the nurses who do promote breastfeeding. The findings revealed that breastfeeding promotion in the NICU was not without its difficulties and that implementation occurred over time. Nevertheless, infrastructural and human resource development set the foundation for breastfeeding promotion and helped to buffer some of the inconsistent messages generated by formula marketing and the lack of breastfeeding education among some nurses and health professionals. To ensure that messages are clear and consistent, education about breastfeeding should be required for all staff members who interact with NICU parents. In addition, NICUs should reconsider whether outside corporations should be allowed access to the unit to market their products to the hospital staff. NICU babies should receive care based on scientific evidence that is not conflicting with commercial interests. Feeding education could be easily provided by experts in nutrition from within the NICU.

This article focused on structure and processes of breastfeeding promotion. Future manuscripts will shed further light on the nurses' infant feeding beliefs and experiences and how these get expressed in the everyday demands of nursing in the NICU setting. ❖

Acknowledgments

The author acknowledges funding from the National Institute of Nursing Research/National Institutes of Health Grant to the University of Pennsylvania School of Nursing, Research on Vulnerable Women, Children and Families (T32-NR-07100) and the Xi Chapter of Sigma Theta Tau International Honor Society of Nursing. The author also thanks Drs. Janet Deatrick, Sandra Founds, Diane Spatz, and Frances Ward for support during this study.

Roberta Cricco-Lizza, PhD, MPH, RN, is associated with Center for Health Disparities Research, University of Pennsylvania School of Nursing, Philadelphia, PA. She can be reached via e-mail at rcricco@nursing.upenn.edu

The author has disclosed that there are no financial relationships related to this article.

References

American Academy of Pediatrics. (2005). Breastfeeding and the use of human milk. *Pediatrics, 115,* 496-506.

Bernaix, L. W. (2000). Nurses' attitudes, subjective norms, and behavioral intentions toward support of breastfeeding mothers. *Journal of Human Lactation, 16,* 201-209.

Centers for Disease Control and Prevention. (2008). Breastfeeding-related maternity practices at hospitals and birth centers—United States, 2007. *Morbidity and Mortality Weekly Review, 57,* 521-525.

Cricco-Lizza, R. (2006). Black non-Hispanic mothers' perceptions about the promotion of infant feeding methods by nurses and physicians. *Journal of Obstetric, Gynecologic and Neonatal Nursing, 35,* 173-180.

Cricco-Lizza, R. (2009). Formative infant feeding experiences and education of NICU nurses. *MCN The American Journal of Maternal Child Nursing.*

Dall'Oglio, I., Salvatori, G., Bonci, E., Nantini, B., D'Agostino, G., & Dotta, A. (2007). Breastfeeding promotion in neonatal intensive care unit: Impact of a new program toward a BFHI for high-risk infants. *Acta Paediatric 96,* 1626-1631.

DiGirolamo, A. M., Grummer-Strawn, L. M., & Fein, S. (2001). Maternity care practices: Implications for breastfeeding. *Birth, 28,* 94-100.

do Nascimento, M. B., & Issler, H. (2005). Breastfeeding the premature infant: Experience of a baby-friendly hospital in Brazil. *Journal of Human Lactation, 21*, 47-52.

Erlen, J. A. (2008). Conflict of interest: Nurses at risk! *Orthopedic Nursing, 27*, 135-139.

Espy, K. A., & Senn, T. E. (2003). Incidence and correlates of breast milk feeding in hospitalized preterm infants. *Social Science and Medicine, 57*, 1421-1428.

Furman, L., Taylor, G., Minich, N., & Hack, M. (2003). The effect of maternal milk on neonatal morbidity of very low-birth-weight infants. *Archives of Pediatrics Adolescent Medicine, 157*, 66-71.

Hagen, B., Pijl-Zieber, E. M., Souveny, K., & Lacroix, A. (2008). Let's do lunch? The ethics of accepting gifts from the pharmaceutical industry. *Canadian Nurse, 104*, (4), 30-35.

Hylander, M. A., Strobino, D., Pezzullo, J. C., & Dhanireddy, R. (2001). Association of human milk feedings in retinopathy of prematurity among very low birth weight infants. *Journal of Perinatology, 21*, 356-362.

Ip, S., Chung, M., Raman, G., Magula, N., DeVine, D., Trikalinos, T., et al. (2007). *Breastfeeding and maternal and infant health outcomes in developed countries* (Evidence Report/Technology Assessment No. 153). AHRQ Publication No. 07-E007. Rockville, MD: Agency for Healthcare Research and Quality.

Jones, A. E., Shapiro, N. I., & Roshon, M. (2007). Implementing early goal-directed therapy in the emergency setting: The challenges and experiences of translating research innovations into clinical reality in academic and community settings. *Academic Emergency Medicine, 14*, 1072-1078.

Kramer, M. S., Chalmers, B., Hodnett, E. D., Sevkovskaya, Z., Dzikovick, I., Shapiro, S., et al. (2001). Promotion of breastfeeding intervention trial (PROBIT): A randomized trial in the Republic of Belarus. *Journal of the American Medical Association, 285*, 413-420.

Lessen, R., & Crivelli-Kovach, A. (2007). Prediction of initiation and duration of breastfeeding for neonates admitted to the neonatal intensive care unit. *Journal of Perinatal Nursing, 21*, 256-266.

McInnes, R. J., & Chambers, J. A. (2008). Supporting breastfeeding mothers: Qualitative synthesis. *Journal of Advanced Nursing, 62*, 407-427.

Meier, P. P. (2001). Breastfeeding in the special care nursery: Prematures and infants with medical problems. *Pediatric Clinics of North America, 48* (2), 425-442.

Merewood, A., Philipp, B. L., Chawla, N., & Cimo, S. (2003). The baby-friendly hospital initiative increases breastfeeding rates in a US neonatal intensive care unit. *Journal of Human Lactation, 19*, 166-171.

Miller, F. A., & Alvarado, K. (2005). Incorporating documents into qualitative nursing research. *Journal of Nursing Scholarship, 37*, 348-353.

Schanler, R. J., Lau, C., Hurst, N. M., & Smith, E. O. (2005). Randomized trial of donor human milk versus preterm formula as substitutes for mothers' own milk in the feeding of extremely premature infants. *Pediatrics, 116*, 400-406.

Siddell, E., Marinelli, K., Froman, R. D., & Burke, G. (2003). Evaluation of an educational intervention on breastfeeding for NICU nurses. *Journal of Human Lactation, 19*, 293-302.

Spatz, D. L. (2006). State of the science: Use of human milk and breastfeeding for vulnerable infants. *Journal of Perinatal and Neonatal Nursing, 20*, 51-55.

Stokamer, C. L. (2003). Pharmaceutical gift giving: Analysis of an ethical dilemma. *Journal of Nursing Administration, 33*, 48-51.

Vohr, B. W., Poindexter, B. B., Dusick, A. M., McKinley, L. T., Wright, L. L., Langer, J. C., et al. (2006). Beneficial effects of breast milk in the neonatal intensive care unit on the developmental outcome of extremely low birth weight infants at 18 months of age. *Pediatrics, 118*(1), pp. e115-e123. Retrieved June 1, 2009, from http://pediatrics.aappublications.org/cgi/content/full/118/1/e115

Weinert, C. R., & Mann, H. J. (2008). The science of implementation: Changing the practice of critical care. *Current Opinion in Critical Care, 14*, 460-465.

World Health Organization and United Nations Children's Fund. (1992). Baby Friendly Hospital Initiative. Geneva: WHO/UNICEF.

Yano, E. (2008). The role of organizational research in implementing evidence-based practice: QUERI series. *Implementation Science, 3*, 29. Retrieved June 1, 2009, from http://www.pubmedcentral.nih.gov/ articlerender.fcgi?tool=pubmed&pubmedid=18510749

Nursing Research • January/February 2010 • Vol 59, No 1S, S58–S65

A Nurse-Facilitated Depression Screening Program in an Army Primary Care Clinic

An Evidence-Based Project

Edward E. Yackel ▼ Madelyn S. McKennan ▼ Adrianna Fox-Deise

▶ **Background:** Depression, sometimes with suicidal manifestations, is a medical condition commonly seen in primary care clinics. Routine screening for depression and suicidal ideation is recommended of all adult patients in the primary care setting because it offers depressed patients a greater chance of recovery and response to treatment, yet such screening often is overlooked or omitted.

▶ **Objective:** The purpose of this study was to develop, to implement, and to test the efficacy of a systematic depression screening process to increase the identification of depression in family members of active duty soldiers older than 18 years at a military family practice clinic located on an Army infantry post in the Pacific.

▶ **Methods:** The Iowa Model of Evidence-Based Practice to Promote Quality Care was used to develop a practice guideline incorporating a decision algorithm for nurses to screen for depression. A pilot project to institute this change in practice was conducted, and outcomes were measured.

▶ **Results:** Before implementation, approximately 100 patients were diagnosed with depression in each of the 3 months preceding the practice change. Approximately 130 patients a month were assigned a 311.0 Code 3 months after the practice change, and 140 patients per month received screenings and were assigned the correct International Classification of Diseases, Ninth Revision Code 311.0 at 1 year. The improved screening and coding for depression and suicidality added approximately 3 minutes to the patient screening process. The education of staff in the process of screening for depression and correct coding coupled with monitoring and staff feedback improved compliance with the identification and the documentation of patients with depression. Nurses were more likely than primary care providers to agree strongly that screening for depression enhances quality of care.

▶ **Discussion:** Data gathered during this project support the integration of military and civilian nurse-facilitated screening for depression in the military primary care setting. The decision algorithm should be adapted and tested in other primary care environments.

▶ **Key Words:** decision algorithm · depression screening · evidence-based practice · military primary care clinic

Mental illness ranks first among morbidities that cause disability in the United States, Canada, and Western Europe, with the associated healthcare cost in the United States estimated at $150 billion in 2003 (Centers for Disease Control and Prevention [CDC], 2003). A psychometric comparison of military and civilian populations in primary care settings revealed no statistical difference in the prevalence of mood disorders (Jackson, O'Malley, & Kroenke, 1999). However, Waldrep, Cozza, and Chun (2004) found that the deployment of a spouse or parent can challenge the ability of a military family member to cope with a preexisting medical or mental health illness. These authors recommended that clinicians identify those family members who require additional services and suggested actions that might mitigate the impact of deployment on the family unit.

Depression is a common medical condition seen frequently in primary care clinics. Patients with depression who present to primary care clinics have a greater chance of responding to treatment and recovery if primary care providers screen for depression using a short self-administered questionnaire as part of a comprehensive disease management program (DMP). The role of nurses in the process of screening for depression has yet to be delineated, so this evidence-based practice (EBP) project was designed to develop, to implement, and to evaluate a standardized nursing procedure to improve the screening of family members for depression at a military family practice clinic located on a U.S. Army infantry post in Hawaii. This EBP project was based on the Veterans Administration/Department of Defense Behavioral Health Clinical Practice Guideline (VA/DoD BHCPG, 2002) for screening and treatment of depression as the DMP to guide practice change.

The absence in this clinic of a systematic method to screen family members of deployed soldiers for depression and the inability to estimate rates of depression in this clinical population were the problem-focused triggers for this project. National standards and guidelines that call for the

Edward E. Yackel, MSN, RN, FNP-BC, is Lieutenant Colonel, U.S. Army Nurse Corps, McDonald Army Health Center, Fort Eustis, Virginia.

Madelyn S. McKennan, MSN, RN, FNP-BC, is Lieutenant Colonel, U.S. Army Nurse Corps, Schofield Barracks Army Health Clinic, Honolulu, Hawaii.

Adrianna Fox-Deise, RN, FNP, is Instructor, School of Nursing and Dental Hygiene, University of Hawaii at Manoa.

131

screening of all adults for depression in primary care settings, such as the VA/DoD BHCPG (2002) and the recommendations and rationale published by the U.S. Preventive Services Task Force (USPSTF, 2002), were the knowledge-focused triggers that guided practice change in this primary care clinic.

A multidisciplinary panel of stakeholders—advanced practice registered nurses (APRNs), physicians, certified nurse assistants (CNAs), registered nurses (RNs), psychologist, and clinic administrators—formed the EBP team. This team was led by a change champion (an APRN) and an opinion leader (a physician). The change champion was an expert clinician who had positive working relationships with other healthcare professionals and who was passionate and committed about screening for depression in primary care. Similarly, the opinion leader was viewed as an important and respected source of influence among his peer group, demonstrated technical competence, and excelled as a teacher and mentor on the subject of depression. The EBP team met to review both problem- and knowledge-focused triggers and determined that screening for depression was a priority for the organization. The EBP project received enthusiastic support throughout the organization and at the highest levels of nursing leadership.

Because of the relevance to the outpatient setting in taking into account clinical decision making, the clinician, and organizational perspectives (Titler et al., 2001), the Iowa Model of Evidence-Based Practice to Promote Quality Care (see the Titler and Moore editorial in this supplement) was chosen to guide an EBP improvement systematically in a military primary practice clinic.

Literature Review

The published medical and nursing literature was reviewed to identify studies evaluating the efficacy of screening for depression in primary care and methodological approaches to such screening. The MEDLINE, the Cochrane, and the Cumulative Index to Nursing and Allied Health Literature databases were searched for English-language articles using eight subject headings (primary care, clinical practice guidelines, mental health, depression instruments, depression screening, suicide screening, military healthcare, and deployment). In addition, bibliographies of the articles obtained were searched for relevant articles to generate additional references. Editorials were rejected, as were articles with data targeting pediatric populations exclusively. Two guidelines (graded as Level I), 3 Level I articles, 17 Level II articles, and 10 Level III articles were critiqued using USPSTF criteria by two APRNs, a physician, and a nurse researcher for inclusion in a literature synthesis. Level I articles included evidence obtained from at least one randomized controlled trial. Level II articles included evidence from well-designed controlled trials without randomization (classified as Level II-1), evidence from cohort or case–control analytic studies (Level II-2), and evidence from multiple time series with or without intervention (Level II-3). Level III articles included opinions of respected authorities that were based on clinical experience or descriptive studies and case reports (Harris et al., 2001). The literature synthesis (Table 1) facilitated the categorization of articles into three focus areas: (a) prevalence of depression in primary care populations; (b) depression management programs and evaluation of suicidal risk; and (c) depression screening instruments and their use in primary care settings.

Prevalence of Depression   Depression is a common medical condition associated with high direct and indirect healthcare costs (Badamgarav et al., 2003; Valenstein, Vijan, Zeber, Boehm, & Buttar, 2001). Dickey and Blumberg (2002) analyzed data from the 1999 National Health Interview Survey and found that 6.3% or 12.5 million noninstitutionalized U.S. adults suffer from major depression. The prevalence of major depression in primary care settings is 5% to 9% among adults, with half of these unrecognized and untreated (Hirschfeld et al., 1997; Hunter, Hunter, West, Kinder, & Carroll, 2002; Simon & VonKorff, 1995). Depressive illness in primary care is less severe than in mental health settings; thus, the short-term prognosis, the chance of recovery, and the response to treatment are greater in primary care settings (Dickey & Blumberg, 2002; Pignone et al., 2002; Simon & VonKorff, 1995).

Within the next 20 years, depression is projected to be the second highest cause of disability in the world and to have a lifetime prevalence of 15% to 25% (Badamgarav et al., 2003). Depression has been shown to increase the morbidity and mortality associated with other chronic diseases, such as diabetes and cardiovascular disorders (Hunter et al., 2002; Pignone et al., 2002). Furthermore, family members of patients with depression have increased physical morbidity and psychopathology (Sobieraj, Williams, Marley, & Ryan, 1998). A majority of adult patients with mental health concerns such as depression will seek and receive care in primary care settings (Dickey & Blumberg, 2002; Pignone et al., 2002).

The lifetime suicide risk for all patients diagnosed with major depressive disorder has been estimated as 3.5% (Blair-West, Mellsop, & Eyeson-Annan, 1997). Harris and Barraclough (1997) found a 12- to 20-fold risk for suicide associated with depressive disorder using the general population for comparison. Suicide is the second-leading cause of death among those aged 25 to 34 years, accounting for 12.9% of all deaths annually (CDC, 2007). Luoma, Martin, and Pearson (2002) reviewed 40 studies examining rates of contact with primary care providers before suicide and found that approximately 45% of patients who committed suicide had contact with a primary care provider within 1 month of taking their lives, suggesting that screening for risk of suicide in patients with depression is important in primary care settings. Although the literature supports the efficacy of DMPs that include screening for depression, the USPSTF (2004) found insufficient evidence to recommend for or against screening for risk of suicide by primary care clinicians. Focusing on the detection and care of patients with depression who are at higher risk for self-harm and improving the ability of primary care providers to identify and to treat those at risk for suicide are suggested strategies for suicide prevention efforts (Luoma et al., 2002; Schulberg et al., 2005).

Depression Screening Instruments

A variety of self-administered questionnaires are available for assessing the severity of depression and risk of suicide in primary care. The Patient Health Questionnaire depression module (PHQ-9) and a two-item version of the PHQ depression module, the PHQ-2, provide primary care providers with valid and reliable measures to assess patients with depression in busy primary care settings (Kroenke, Spitzer, & Williams, 2001, 2003). The PHQ-9 is the self-administered

TABLE I. Selected Literature Synthesis

Focus area	Journal or source	Year	Description	Level of evidence
Prevalence of depression	General Hospital Psychiatry	1995	Literature review	Literature synthesis
	JAMA	2006	Population-based descriptive study	Level II-3
	Military Medicine	1999	Psychometric comparison: military vs. civilian	Level II-3
	Archives of Family Medicine	1995	Epidemiological study with 1- year follow-up	Level II-2
	Journal of the American Board Family Practice	2005	Descriptive study	Level III
	Military Medicine	2002	Comparative study: PHQ vs. progress notes	Level II-3
	Iraq War Clinicians Guide	2004	Opinion by respected authority	Level III
	American Journal of Psychiatry	2003	Meta-analysis	Level I
	National Mental Health Information Center	1999	Survey report	Level III
	JAMA	1997	Consensus statement	Level III
Depression management programs and evaluation of suicide risk	Annals of Internal Medicine	2002	Systematic literature review	Guideline/Level I
	General Hospital Psychiatry	1992	Abstract	Level III
	American Journal of Psychiatry	2002	Meta-analysis of descriptive studies/reports	Level III
	Journal of General Internal Medicine	1996	Structured interviews, comparison of three studies	Level II-1
	Annals of Family Medicine	2005	Randomized controlled trial	Level I
	British Journal of Psychiatry	1997	Meta-analysis	Level II-1
	Centers for Disease Control and Prevention	2007	Report/literature review	Level III
Depression screening instruments	American Journal of Managed Care	2004	Psychometric comparison of one-item depression screen versus PHQ	Level II-3
	Journal of General Internal Medicine	1997	Comparing validity of PHQ-2 to validity of other known measures	Level II-2
	Medical Care	2003	Survey, nonrandomized	Level II-2
	Psychotherapy and Psychosomatics	2004	Descriptive comparison of three questionnaires	Level II-3
	Journal of General Internal Medicine	2001	PHQ-9 compared with other measures/nonrandomized	Level II-2
	Department of Veterans Affairs	2000	Clinical practice guideline	Guideline/level I
	JAMA	1999	Criterion standard study: PRIME MD	Level I
	American Journal of Obstetrics and Gynecology	2000	Validity study of PHQ in obstetrician-gynecologist patients	Level II-2

Note. Level I articles included evidence obtained from at least one randomized controlled trial. Level II articles included evidence from well-designed controlled trials without randomization (classified as Level II-1), evidence from cohort or case–control analytic studies (Level II-2), and evidence from multiple time series with or without intervention (Level II-3). Level III articles included opinions of respected authorities that were based on clinical experience or descriptive studies and case reports (Harris et al., 2001).

depression module of the Primary Care Evaluation of Mental Disorders (a diagnostic instrument for common mental disorders designed for primary care providers to assess the cognitive and physical symptoms of depressive disorders; Hunter et al., 2002). Kroenke et al. (2001) examined the validity of the PHQ-9 by analyzing data from 6,000 patients aged 18 years or older who had completed the PHQ-9 in eight primary care clinics and seven obstetrics-gynecology clinics. Recent data show that the PHQ-9 has a sensitivity of 88% and a specificity of 88% for major depression, with excellent internal reliability ($\alpha = .89$) and validity in measuring the severity of depression (Corson, Gerrity, & Dobscha, 2004; Kroenke et al., 2001). Lowe et al. (2004) compared the criterion validity of the PHQ-9 for diagnosing depressive episodes with two other well-established instruments and concluded that the PHQ-9 demonstrated a diagnostic advantage and had superior criterion validity when compared with the other instruments. The last item of the PHQ-9 assesses patients for suicidal risk, which is one of the diagnostic criteria for depressive disorders. Feeling suicidal predicts plans to attempt suicide with 83% sensitivity, 98% specificity, and 30% positive predictive value when asked as a single self-report item (Olfson, Weissman, Leon, Sheehan, & Farber, 1996). Corson et al. (2004) reported that use of the PHQ-9 death or suicide item identified one third (7%) of patients in a VA primary care clinic with active suicidal ideation who would not have been treated otherwise.

Shorter screening tests with questions about depressed mood and anhedonia (inability to have pleasurable feelings) appear to detect a majority of depressed patients (Pignone et al., 2002). The PHQ-2 is a self-administered questionnaire used to ascertain the frequency of depressed mood and anhedonia over the past 2 weeks. Kroenke et al. (2003) established the criterion validity of the PHQ-2 by comparing its operating characteristics with an interview by an independent mental health provider and reported a sensitivity of 83% and a specificity of 92%. Corson et al. and Kroenke et al. reported 97% sensitivity and 91% specificity for depression when using the PHQ-2 to screen for this disorder in a VA primary care setting. Thus, the literature provides strong evidence for the validity of the PHQ-2 as a brief screening measure that facilitates the diagnosis of major depression. However, it is recognized as an initial step in a DMP that requires further assessment and implementation to care for patients with major depression (Corson et al., 2004; Kroenke et al., 2003; USPSTF, 2002).

The VA/DoD BHCPG (2002) for screening and treatment of depression is an example of a DMP that includes screening for depression and suicide. The guideline is designed for use by providers who care for patients with depression in military primary care clinics. The VA/DoD BHCPG DMP describes (a) the screening and recognition of depression and suicidal ideation; (b) the assessment of physical and mental status; (c) the diagnostic criteria and assessment of risk factors; (d) a treatment plan that includes suggestions for managing medications, counseling, and referral criteria; (e) patient and family education; and (f) the monitoring and documentation of follow-up. The VA/DoD BHCPG is designed for the primary care setting and describes the role of primary care providers, but it does not explicate the role of nursing staff in implementing the process.

Evidence has been found that screening improves the identification of depressed patients and that effective follow-up and treatment of depressed adults decrease clinical morbidity in primary care settings (USPSTF, 2002). Evidence-based guidelines, patient education, collaborative and multidisciplinary care, and monitoring are used in DMPs to provide comprehensive care for patients with chronic diseases such as depression (Badamgarav et al., 2003). The DMPs that include screening for depression are more effective than the programs that are focused on depression screening alone (Bijl,

van Marwijk, de Haan, van Tilburg, & Beekman, 2004; Pignone et al., 2002). Badamgarav et al. (2003) systematically reviewed the published medical literature evaluating the effectiveness of DMPs for chronic conditions such as depression and found that disease management improves the detection and care of patients with depression. Similarly, a systematic review and a meta-analysis of randomized controlled trials of DMPs for depression concluded that the costs of depression programs are within the cost range of other public health improvements and that enhanced quality of care is possible (Neumeyer-Gromen, Lampert, Stark, & Kallischnigg, 2004). Primary care providers play a vital role in DMPs to improve the detection and care of patients with depression. Notably absent from the literature are descriptors of nursing processes that facilitate screening for depression and the role that nurses play in the DMPs. The purpose of this EBP project was to implement and to evaluate the change process methodology involved in screening family members of military active duty soldiers for depression.

Setting

The setting for this EBP project was a military family practice clinic with an enrollment of 14,322 family members and approximately 175 daily patient visits. Before implementation of the project, only female family members were screened routinely for depression (at well-woman visits), and nurses did not participate in screening for depression. This process resulted in 100 cases of depression being captured a month. Family members of military active duty soldiers older than 18 years who could read, write, and communicate in English were screened. Patient care was documented in a hard-copy medical record or in the military's electronic medical record, the Armed Forces Health Longitudinal Technology Application (AHLTA). The selection of the screening process for the EBP project was based on the VA/DoD BHCPG for screening and treatment of depression and similar patient populations studied by other investigators (Kroenke et al., 2003; Olfson et al., 1996). All military family members have open access to mental health services. Patients who require inpatient psychiatric care are referred by their primary care provider or mental health provider to a regional military medical center.

Implementation: Decision Algorithm

Two questions from the PHQ-2 ("During the past month, have you often been bothered by feeling down, depressed or hopeless?" and "During the past month, have you often been bothered by little interest or pleasure in doing things?") and one question from the PHQ-9 ("Do you have thoughts that you would be better off dead or hurting yourself in some way?") were selected for use in the project. The decision algorithm for nurses (Figure 1) integrates the PHQ-2 and the PHQ-9 questions as steps in the depression screening process. The first step of the depression screening process prompts nursing staff to ask the PHQ-2 questions in an effort to determine the presence of depressed mood or anhedonia. A negative response to the PHQ-2 questions concludes the depression screening process, and the primary care provider addresses the patient's primary complaint. The second step of the screening process directs nurses to ask the PHQ-9 question (suicidal ideation) when a positive response is given to

Copyright © 2018. Wolters Kluwer.

Reprinted with permission.   Study Guide for Essentials of Nursing Research: Appraising Evidence for Nursing Practice, 9e

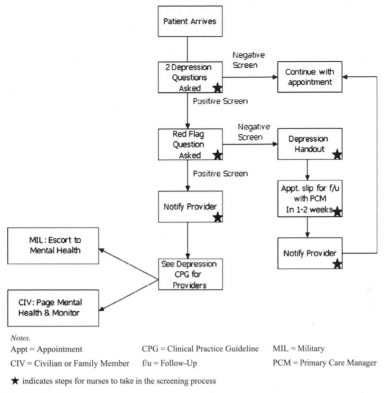

Notes.

Appt = Appointment   CPG = Clinical Practice Guideline   MIL = Military

CIV = Civilian or Family Member   f/u = Follow-Up   PCM = Primary Care Manager

★ indicates steps for nurses to take in the screening process

FIGURE 1. A decision algorithm for nurses.

either of the PHQ-2 questions. A patient who denies suicidal ideation is given a depression handout listing behavioral health support services, locations of clinics, and contact numbers. Subsequently, the patient is offered a follow-up appointment in 1 or 2 weeks with the primary care provider to discuss assessment and treatment of depression. The patient's appointment continues after the nurse reports the results of the depression screening to the primary care provider. A patient who responds positively to the PHQ-9 (*red flag*) question is referred immediately to a mental health professional for further evaluation. Documentation of the depression screening process is completed by nurses in the AHLTA system. Primary care providers are encouraged to use the VA/DoD BHCPG to assess and to treat patients with depression.

Piloting the Change

Creating an environment for a practice change to occur is an important element in the EBP process; therefore, a pilot project was undertaken to identify barriers in implementing the decision algorithm. A physician, a CNA, and two RNs (a nurse researcher and a research assistant) from the EBP team were selected to model the change in clinical practice over a 3-day period. The experienced nurse researcher instructed the CNA on depression, depression screening, and integra-

tion of the EBP decision algorithm into existing screening practices by providing verbal education and written materials. The CNA was required to verbalize and to demonstrate the use of the decision algorithm before starting the pilot. All patients meeting the inclusion criteria were screened for depression using the decision algorithm. The experienced nurse researcher and research assistant observed screening practices during the pilot to evaluate the process and outcomes and to make recommendations aimed at improving the process.

Instituting the Change in Practice

Feedback from all participants in the pilot project was used to formulate six recommendations aimed at minimizing barriers in implementing the decision algorithm and in instituting the change in practice: (a) integrate the PHQ-2 and the PHQ-9 depression screening questions into both the hard-copy medical record and the AHLTA system to add continuity during unscheduled computer downtime; (b) educate staff (providers and nurses) on the decision algorithm and the documentation process for both hard-copy and electronic medical records; (c) provide depression awareness education by a mental health professional to increase the nursing staff's comfort when asking questions about depression; (d) post the decision algorithm at the nursing team center to foster recognition and comprehension; (e) display depression posters prominently in patient care areas to sensitize the patient population to this common mental health condition; and (f) educate providers (physicians, APRNs, and physician assistants) on the need to document and use the International Classification of Diseases, Ninth Revision (ICD-9) Code 311.0 (depressive disorder, not otherwise specified) consistently to simplify data retrieval from military medical databases. Forty staff members (RNs, LPNs, CNAs, APRNs, PAs, and MDs) were educated in using the decision algorithm and the documentation process for both the hard-copy and the electronic medical record by the family practice clinic head nurse (EBP team member). A psychologist provided depression education to 17 nurses (RN, LPN, or CNA). This included the definition of depression, how to approach asking questions on depression, and role playing the depression screening process. Thirteen of the family practice clinic providers (100%) were educated by the opinion leader on the use of Code 311.0 to document the diagnosis of depression. Depression posters were displayed in patient care areas, the decision algorithm was displayed at the nursing team center, and the PHQ-2 and the PHQ-9 questions were integrated into the hard-copy and the AHLTA medical record.

Results

Outcome Measures

Four measures were used to assess the success of implementing the EBP decision algorithm in the family practice clinic: (a) number of patients diagnosed with depression; (b) satisfaction of providers and nurses; (c) compliance in documentation (measured via random chart audits); and (d) time–motion evaluation of the patient screening process. Data collection began 3 months after implementation of the decision algorithm by the RN researcher.

An assessment of the numbers of patients diagnosed with depression was based on data gathered from a military medical database to establish the number of family members diagnosed with depression in the family practice clinic using the ICD-9 Code 311.0 before and after the practice change. With nurses administering the depression screening to all adult patients (not just females) and providers using Code 311.0 to identify those with depression, approximately 130 patients a month were assigned a Code 311.0 3 months into the practice change and 140 patients a month at 1 year after the practice change (Figure 2). A possible correlation between deployment of soldiers to Iraq and increase in the number of family members presenting for treatment of depression was not examined.

The satisfaction of providers and nursing staff was measured at 3 and 12 months after the change in practice using one question answered on a 4-point Likert scale: "Implementing depression screening enhances the quality of care in the family practice clinic." Participants rated their level of agreement from 1 (*strongly disagree*) to 4 (*strongly agree*). Three months after implementation, 64% of the nurses and 45% of the providers strongly agreed that screening for depression enhanced the quality of care in the clinic. At 1 year after the implementation of the decision algorithm, 95% of nurses and 54% of providers strongly agreed that screening for depression enhanced the quality of care.

The nurse researcher evaluated staff compliance in documenting the process of screening for depression using a standardized audit form to review systematically selected (every fourth record from 11 providers) electronic medical records. Thirty records that met selection criteria were audited at 3 months, and 30 different records were audited at 6 months after the practice change was implemented. The number of records to audit was determined on the basis of patient visits per day and the rate of major depression in primary care (5–9%) obtained from the literature review. Three months into the practice change, 26 (87%) of 30 reviewed charts showed evidence of documentation for depression screening; 7 (27%) of 26 charts verified that patients screened for depression were positive for depressed mood or anhedonia without suicidal ideation. Six months after the practice change, evidence of documentation for depression screening was shown in 29 (97%) of the 30 charts, and patients who were screened for depression were positive for depressed mood or anhedonia without suicidal ideation in 10 (33%) charts. The

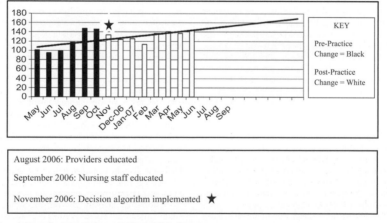

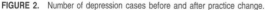

August 2006: Providers educated

September 2006: Nursing staff educated

November 2006: Decision algorithm implemented ★

FIGURE 2.   Number of depression cases before and after practice change.

nurse researcher was unable to determine the compliance of nursing staff in documenting notification of a mental health provider, given that no cases of suicidal ideation were identified in the audited charts. An important facet of compliance with documentation throughout the institutionalization of the decision algorithm was continual education and feedback to both providers and nurses on requirements.

Time–motion data were collected for the length of time it took to screen patients. The screening process included greeting the patient, obtaining weight and vital signs, escorting the patient into an examination room, reviewing demographic data, reviewing the screening questions on depression and suicide, and entering data into the AHLTA system. Variability among the nurses in the process for screening patients during the first month of the project initially resulted in a time variance of 11 minutes, with a range of 5 to 30 minutes for each screening. The clinic head nurse standardized the screening process by asking the nurses to enter data into the AHLTA in the examination rooms instead of returning to the team center. This resulted in a mean time reduction of 4 minutes, 58 seconds after the practice change. The mean time added per patient encounter after the practice change was 2 minutes, 53 seconds.

Discussion

Data gathered during the EBP project support the relevance of a nurse-facilitated program to screen for depression in a primary care setting. The VA/DoD BHCPG is designed for primary care and describes the role of primary care providers in the DMP but it does not describe the role of nurses in the depression screening process. The decision algorithm was a valuable tool defining the steps to be followed by nurses when screening patients for depression. More important, incorporating nurses into the depression screening process accomplished the first step of the VA/DoD BHCPG in a multidisciplinary effort consistent with recommendations found in the literature.

Nurses can be instrumental in depression screening in the primary care setting, leading to appropriate referral for further care. The prevalence, the morbidity, and the mortality associated with depression necessitate that nurses be involved integrally in this process as part of the healthcare team. In this pilot project, one provider, a CNA, and two RNs identified barriers in implementing the decision algorithm into the business practices of the family practice clinic. Although procedural barriers to the implementation of the decision algorithm were addressed, incorporating the process of screening for depression into existing screening practices was not clearly defined. The wide range seen in screening times during the first month of the project was most likely related to procedural differences in whether nursing staff entered vital signs and questionnaire data into the electronic medical record (the AHLTA) during or after seeing the patient. Standardization of the time of data entry improved screening times. A mandatory program for reconciling medications was implemented during the EBP project and may have affected the outcome of the time–motion study because the effects of implementing both screening for depression and medication reconciliation might have been measured.

A majority of staff members strongly agreed that screening for depression is a quality component of clinical practice, despite both providers and nurses acknowledging an increased workload because of the EBP project. The decision algorithm was designed to allow primary care providers the option of implementing the VA/DoD BHCPG upon notification of screening results by nurses. The hope was that if the nursing staff followed the procedural steps outlined in the decision algorithm, the need for providers to intercede in the process of screening for depression would be mitigated. However, clinical assessment of the presenting illness and trends in patients' healthcare utilization may have affected how providers responded to the screening results. Some providers were not comfortable with the process of screening for depression, which may have played a role also in how they responded to patients who reported anhedonia or depressed mood. Conversely, nurses who were comfortable with screening for depression were more likely to respond that such screening enhanced the quality of patient care. The difference between nurse and provider levels of comfort may have been the result of the difference in the educational offerings presented to each group. Nurses were offered depression awareness training and repeated education on the decision algorithm and documentation requirements, whereas providers were educated only on the management of depression in primary care and implementation of the decision algorithm. Standardization of educational offerings for all members of the healthcare team is recommended to provide consistent information and continuity of care and to foster trust in the depression screening process.

Both providers and nurses considered depression screening beneficial to family members of deployed soldiers. One year after the practice change, 10 providers were asked to reflect on how many patients had a positive screening for suicidal ideation that required immediate referral to a behavioral health specialist. These providers estimated that approximately 36 patients reported suicidal ideation who would not otherwise have been detected. Although no data were obtained on the relationship between the deployment of soldiers and reports of depression and suicidal ideation by family members, further study on the relationship between these variables is recommended.

Implications for Practice and Research

The integration of a nurse-facilitated depression screening program into the business practices of a busy military family practice clinic was viewed by providers, nursing staff, and nursing leadership as a quality component of clinical practice that benefited the population served. The Iowa Model of Evidence-Based Practice to Promote Quality Care (Titler et al., 2001) and the decision algorithm for nurses were essential tools in implementing practice change and appear to have great utility in the primary care setting. The use of an EBP model provides a systematic method for nurses to evaluate critically, to define, and to implement changes in practice. The decision algorithm for nurses was a valuable tool in the depression screening process and should be tested in other primary care settings. In addition, further study is warranted to determine whether having nurses screen for depression influences the practice patterns of primary care providers when implementing a DMP such as the VA/DoD BHCPG. ▼

Accepted for publication September 30, 2009.

This project was funded by an award from the TriService Nursing Research Program, grant no. N03-P18. The Uniformed Services University of the Health Sciences (USUHS), 4301 Jones Bridge Rd., Bethesda, MD 20814-4799, is the awarding and administering office.

This project was sponsored by the TriService Nursing Research Program, Uniformed Services University of the Health Sciences; however, the information or content and conclusions do not necessarily represent the official position or policy of, nor should any official endorsement be inferred by, the TriService Nursing Research Program, Uniformed Services University of the Health Sciences, the Department of Defense, or the U.S. Government.

The following people contributed to the study: Nathan DeWeese, MD; Ms. Renee Latimer, RN, MPH; Mrs. Charlotte Grant, NA; Mr. Wesley Grant, NA; Richard Schobitz, PhD; and Mr. Adrian Santos, RN, BSN.

The authors thank LTC Debra Mark and LTC Mary Hardy, who were responsible for implementation of the Evidence-Based Practice Training Program at Tripler Army Medical Center, and CAPT Patricia Kelley, without whom we could not have conducted this project.

The views and opinions expressed in this article are solely those of the authors and do not reflect the policy or position of the Department of the Army, the Department of Defense, or the U.S. Government.

Corresponding author: Edward E. Yackel, MSN, RN, FNP-BC, U.S. Army Nurse Corps, McDonald Army Health Center, Fort Eustis, VA 23604 (e-mail: Ed.yackel@us.army.mil).

References

Badamgarav, E., Weingarten, S. R., Henning, J. M., Knight, K., Hasselbald, V., Gano, A. Jr., et al. (2003). Effectiveness of disease management programs in depression: A systematic review. *American Journal of Psychiatry, 160*(12), 2080–2090.

Bijl, D., van Marwijk, H. W., de Haan, M., van Tilburg, W., & Beekman, A. J. (2004). Effectiveness of disease management programmes for recognition, diagnosis and treatment of depression in primary care. *European Journal of General Practice, 10*(1), 6–12.

Blair-West, G. W., Mellsop, G. W., & Eyeson-Annan, M. L. (1997). Down-rating lifetime suicide risk in major depression. *Acta Psychiatrica Scandinavica, 95*(3), 259–263.

Centers for Disease Control and Prevention. (2003). *Healthy people 2010: Progress review focus area 18.* Retrieved July 5, 2006, from http://www.cdc.gov/nchs/about/otheract/hpdata2010/focusareas/fa18-mentalhealth.htm

Centers for Disease Control and Prevention. (2007). *Suicide: Facts at a glance.* Retrieved July 22, 2007, from http://www.cdc.gov/injury

Corson, K., Gerrity, M. S., & Dobscha, S. K. (2004). Screening for depression and suicidality in a VA primary care setting: 2 items are better than 1 item. *American Journal of Managed Care, 10*(11 Pt. 2), 839–845.

Dickey, W. C., & Blumberg, S. J. (2002). *Prevalence of mental disorders and contact with mental health professionals among adults in the United States, National Health Interview Survey, 1999.* Retrieved July 5, 2006, from http://mentalhealth.samhsa.gov/publications/allpubs/SMA04-3938/Chapter08.asp

Harris, E. C., & Barraclough, B. (1997). Suicide as an outcome for mental disorders. A meta-analysis. *British Journal of Psychiatry, 170,* 205–228.

Harris, R. P., Helfan, M., Woolf, S. H., Lohr, K. N., Mulrow, C. D., Teutsch, S. M., et al. (2001). Current methods of the US Preventive Services Task Force: A review of the process. *American Journal of Preventive Medicine, 20*(Suppl. 3), 21–35.

Hirschfeld, R. M., Keller, M. B., Panico, S., Arons, B. S., Barlow, D., Davidoff, F., et al. (1997). The National Depressive and Manic-Depressive Association consensus statement on the undertreatment of depression. *JAMA, 277*(4), 333–340.

Hunter, C. L., Hunter, C. M., West, E. T., Kinder, M. H., & Carroll, D. W. (2002). Recognition of depressive disorders by pri-

mary care providers in a military medical setting. *Military Medicine, 167*(4), 308–311.

Jackson, J. L., O'Malley, P. G., & Kroenke, K. (1999). A psychometric comparison of military and civilian medical practices. *Military Medicine, 164*(2), 112–115.

Kroenke, K., Spitzer, R. L., & Williams, J. B. (2001). The PHQ-9: Validity of a brief depression severity measure. *Journal of General Internal Medicine, 16*(9), 606–613.

Kroenke, K., Spitzer, R. L., & Williams, J. B. (2003). The Patient Health Questionnaire-2: Validity of a two-item depression screener. *Medical Care, 41*(11), 1284–1292.

Lowe, B., Grafe, K., Zipfel, S., Witte, S., Loerch, B., & Herzog, W. (2004). Diagnosing ICD-10 depressive episodes: Superior criterion validity of the Patient Health Questionnaire. *Psychotherapy and Psychosomatics, 73*(6), 386–390.

Luoma, J. B., Martin, C. E., & Pearson, J. L. (2002). Contact with mental health and primary care providers before suicide: A review of the evidence. *American Journal of Psychiatry, 159*(6), 909–916.

Neumeyer-Gromen, A., Lampert, T., Stark, K., & Kallischnigg, G. (2004). Disease management programs for depression: A systematic review and meta-analysis of randomized controlled trials. *Medical Care, 42*(12), 1211–1221.

Olfson, M., Weissman, M. M., Leon, A. C., Sheehan, D. V., & Farber, L. (1996). Suicidal ideation in primary care. *Journal of General Internal Medicine, 11*(8), 447–453.

Pignone, M., Gaynes, B. N., Rushton, J. L., Mulrow, C. D., Orleans, C. T., Whitener, B. L., et al. (2002). *Screening for depression: Systematic evidence review no. 6.* Prepared by the Research Triangle Institute, University of North Carolina Evidence-Based Practice Center under Contract No. 290-97-0011. Rockville, MD: Agency for Healthcare Research and Quality.

Schulberg, H. C., Lee, P. W., Bruce, M. L., Raue, P. J., Lefever, J. J., Williams, J. W. Jr., et al. (2005). Suicidal ideation and risk levels among primary care patients with uncomplicated depression. *Annals of Family Medicine, 3*(6), 523–528.

Simon, G. E., & VonKorff, M. (1995). Recognition, management and outcomes of depression in primary care. *Archives of Family Medicine, 4*(2), 99–105.

Sobieraj, M., Williams, J., Marley, J., & Ryan, P. (1998). The impact of depression on the physical health of family members. *British Journal of General Practice, 48*(435), 1653–1655.

Titler, M. G., Kleiber, C., Steelman, V. J., Rakel, B. A., Budreau, G., Everett, L. Q., et al. (2001). The Iowa Model of Evidence-Based Practice to Promote Quality Care. *Critical Care Nursing Clinics of North America, 13*(4), 497–509.

United States Preventive Services Task Force. (2002). Screening for depression: Recommendations and rationale. *Annals of Internal Medicine, 136*(10), 760–764.

United States Preventive Services Task Force. (2004). Screening for suicide risk: Recommendation and rationale. *Annals of Internal Medicine, 140*(10), 820–821.

Valenstein, M., Vijan, S., Zeber, J. E., Boehm, K., & Buttar, A. (2001). The cost-utility of screening for depression in primary care. *Annals of Internal Medicine, 134*(5), 345–360.

Veterans Administration/Department of Defense. (2002). *Management of major depressive disorder (MDD) in adults in the primary care setting, initial assessment and treatment.* Retrieved January 25, 2006, from http://oqp.med.va.gov/cpg/cpg.htm

Waldrep, D. A., Cozza, S. J., & Chun, R. S. (2004). XIII. The impact of deployment on the military family. From the National Center for Post-Traumatic Stress Disorder. *Iraq War Clinician Guide.* Retrieved August 29, 2006, from http://www.ptsd.va.gov/professional/manuals/manual-pdf/iwcg/iraq_clinician_guide_ch_13.pdf

Nursing Research. 2014 Mar–Apr; 63(2): 83–93

Fatigue in the Presence of Coronary Heart Disease

Ann L. Eckhardt ▼ Holli A. DeVon ▼ Mariann R. Piano ▼ Catherine J. Ryan ▼ Julie J. Zerwic

Background: Fatigue is a prevalent and disabling symptom associated with many acute and chronic conditions, including acute myocardial infarction and chronic heart failure. Fatigue has not been explored in patients with stable coronary heart disease (CHD).

Objectives: The purpose of this partially mixed sequential dominant status study was to (a) describe fatigue in patients with stable CHD; (b) determine if specific demographic (gender, age, education, income), physiological (hypertension, hyperlipidemia), or psychological (depressive symptoms) variables were correlated with fatigue; and (c) determine if fatigue was associated with health-related quality of life. The theory of unpleasant symptoms was used as a conceptual framework.

Methods: Patients ($N = 102$) attending two cardiology clinics completed the Fatigue Symptom Inventory, Patient Health Questionnaire-9, and Medical Outcomes Study Short Form-36 to measure fatigue, depressive symptoms, and health-related quality of life. Thirteen patients whose interference from fatigue was low, moderate, or high participated in qualitative interviews.

Results: Forty percent of the sample reported fatigue more than 3 days of the week lasting more than one half of the day. Lower interference from fatigue was reported on standardized measures compared with qualitative interviews. Compared with men, women reported a higher fatigue intensity ($p = .003$) and more interference from fatigue ($p = .007$). In regression analyses, depressive symptoms were the sole predictor of fatigue intensity and interference.

Discussion: Patients with stable CHD reported clinically relevant levels of fatigue. Patients with stable CHD may discount fatigue as they adapt to their symptoms. Relying solely on standardized measures may provide an incomplete picture of fatigue burden in patients with stable CHD.

Key Words: coronary heart disease & fatigue & mixed methods

Fatigue is often defined as the subjective sensation of extreme and persistent exhaustion, tiredness, and lack of energy (Aaronson et al., 1999; Dittner, Wessely, & Brown, 2004; Ream & Richardson, 1996). Similar to other symptoms such as pain, fatigue is multidimensional, is influenced by physical and psychosocial factors, and shares common features with some mood and anxiety disorders (Aaronson et al., 1999; American Psychiatric Association, 2013). In patients with coronary heart disease (CHD), fatigue is a prevalent and debilitating symptom associated with poor quality of life and reduced physical activity (Pragodopol & Ryan, 2013).

CHD, also referred to as ischemic heart disease and acute coronary syndrome (ACS), encompasses conditions that arise because of atherosclerosis and a reduction in coronary artery blood flow (American Heart Association, 2013). Emerging evidence indicates that new onset or elevated levels of fatigue may be associated with an impending ACS event or may indi-

cate worsening or progressive CHD. Among patients ($N = 256$, mean age = 67 years) presenting to the emergency department for ACS, patients reported that "unusual fatigue" was one of the three most prevalent symptoms that propelled them to seek care (DeVon, Ryan, Ochs, & Shapiro, 2008). In a large prospective longitudinal study enrolling only men ($N = 5,216$, mean age = 59 years), Ekmann, Osler, and Avlund (2012) found that fatigue was associated with first hospitalization for nonfatal ischemic heart disease (hazard ratio [HR] = 1.98, 95% CI [1.09, 3.61]) and all-cause mortality (HR = 3.99, 95% CI [2.27, 7.02]). After adjusting for smoking and alcohol consumption, fatigue remained the only significant predictor of first hospitalization for nonfatal ischemic heart disease in men. In a large study enrolling women and men ($N = 11,795$, mean age = 57 years), Lindeberg, Rosvall, and Östergren (2012) found that exhaustion predicted cardiac events in both men (HR = 1.49, 95% CI [1.06, 2.11]) and women (HR = 1.78, 95% CI [1.23, 2.58]). After adjusting for depression and anxiety, the association between exhaustion and CHD was strengthened in men (HR = 1.62, 95% CI [1.05, 2.50]) but was no longer statistically significant in women.

Fennessy et al. (2010) found that both men and women reported moderate-to-high levels of fatigue at the time of acute myocardial infarction (AMI). Women reported significantly less fatigue 30 days after AMI, whereas men did not report

Ann L. Eckhardt, PhD, RN, is Assistant Professor, School of Nursing, Illinois Wesleyan University, Bloomington.

Holli A. DeVon, PhD, RN, is Associate Professor; Mariann R. Piano, PhD, RN, is Professor and Department Head; Catherine J. Ryan, PhD, RN, is Clinical Assistant Professor; and Julie J. Zerwic, PhD, RN, is Professor and Executive Associate Dean, Department of Biobehavioral Health Science, College of Nursing, University of Illinois at Chicago.

DOI: 10.1097/NNR.0000000000000019

139

a change. Using quantitative coronary artery angiography, Zimmerman-Viehoff and colleagues (2013) examined the relationship between vital exhaustion (Maastricht questionnaire) and progression of coronary artery atherosclerosis in women ($N = 103$, mean age = 55 years) who had experienced an acute coronary event. Vital exhaustion significantly correlated with coronary artery diameter, with women having the highest vital exhaustion scores (46-57) showing the most pronounced coronary artery diameter narrowing ($M = 0.21$ mm, 95% CI [0.15, 0.27]) compared with intermediate vital exhaustion scores (43-45; coronary artery diameter, $M = 0.11$ mm, 95% CI [0.05, 0.17]). Women with vital exhaustion scores in low (score: 20-34) and lower intermediate (score: 35-42) range had no significant change in coronary artery diameter. These findings indicate that women with the highest level of vital exhaustion had the fastest coronary artery atherosclerosis progression.

Considering that fatigue may be an indicator of new onset or progressive CHD, it is important to determine the severity and characteristics of fatigue in a stable CHD population. Stable CHD is defined as patients who have been diagnosed with CHD but have not experienced a worsening of symptoms, symptoms at rest, or an episode of ACS for at least 60 days (Goblirsch et al., 2013). Therefore, the purpose of this partially mixed sequential dominant status study was to

1. describe fatigue (intensity, distress, timing, and quality) in patients with stable CHD;

2. determine if specific demographic (gender, age, education, income), physiological (hypertension, hyperlipidemia), or psychological (depressive symptoms) variables were correlated with fatigue; and

3. determine if fatigue was associated with health-related quality of life (HRQoL).

ORGANIZING FRAMEWORK

The organizing framework for this study was derived from the theory of unpleasant symptoms, which includes physiological, psychological, and situational factors that influence the symptom experience and describes symptoms in terms of intensity, distress, timing, and quality (Lenz, Pugh, Milligan, Gift, & Suppe, 1997). Although not consistent across all CHD studies, others have reported that fatigue is associated with gender, age, HRQoL, medication type, smoking status, pain, and depressed mood (DeVon et al., 2008; Ekmann et al., 2012; Fink et al., 2012; Fink, Sullivan, Zerwic, & Piano, 2009; Hägglund, Boman, Stenlund, Lundman, & Brulin, 2008; McSweeney & Crane, 2000; Shaffer et al., 2012). Figure 1 depicts the conceptualization of the theory of unpleasant symptoms for the current study as adapted by the authors.

In the theory of unpleasant symptoms, gender and age are considered situational factors, whereas depressed mood is categorized as a psychological factor. The symptom experience was examined using the Fatigue Symptom Inventory (FSI; Hann et al., 1998). The average of the first three FSI questions was used to evaluate symptom (fatigue) intensity.

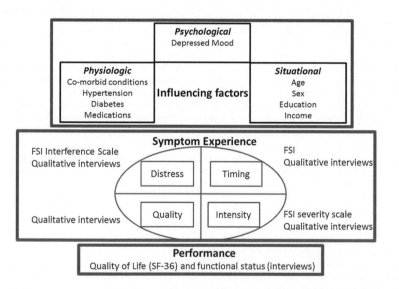

FIGURE 1 Organizing framework based on the theory of unpleasant symptoms used to understand fatigue in the presence of coronary heart disease.

The FSI-Interference Scale was used to determine symptom (fatigue) distress. The distress dimension within the theory of unpleasant symptoms refers to the degree to which a person is bothered by the symptom and the symptom interferes with activities of daily living. The FSI has several items, which corresponded to the timing of fatigue (time of day, number of days per week fatigue occurs, and pattern of fatigue). The Short Form-36 (McHorney, Ware, & Raczek, 1993), a measure of HRQoL, was used as a reflection of performance. Qualitative interviews were completed to obtain a comprehensive description of fatigue and add descriptive depth to each of the dimensions within the theory of unpleasant symptoms.

METHODS

Research Design

The study was conducted using a partially mixed sequential dominant status design, whereby the main study design was quantitative (QUAN) followed by a qualitative (qual) component (QUAN → qual). In a partially mixed sequential dominant status design, the qualitative and quantitative elements are deployed one after the other with one method being emphasized over the other (Leech & Onwuegbuzie, 2009). This mixed-methods design was chosen to achieve complementarity, which seeks to achieve convergence between quantitative and qualitative findings and to provide descriptive depth through qualitative interviews (Greene, 2007). The cross-sectional quantitative data were collected first, and participants for the qualitative component were recruited from this sample. Integration of qualitative and quantitative data occurred at the data analysis and discussion stages.

Sample and Setting

One hundred and two participants with stable CHD were recruited from two cardiology clinics during routine cardiovascular appointments. One clinic served primarily minority, urban patients ($n = 51$), and one served predominantly Caucasian patients from a small city in a rural setting ($n = 51$). Eligibility was determined by review of medical records. Inclusion criteria included a diagnosis of stable CHD, the ability to speak and read English and living independently. Exclusion criteria included heart failure with reduced ejection fraction (ejection fraction < 40%), terminal illness with prediction of less than 6 months to live, myocardial infarction or coronary artery bypass grafting in the past 2 months, unstable angina, symptoms due to worsening or exacerbation of cardiac disease, and hemodialysis. These exclusion criteria were chosen to eliminate patients with a recent acute event, those with new or worsening symptoms of CHD, and those with comorbid conditions known to be associated with significant fatigue. The institutional review boards at both sites approved the study. All participants provided written informed consent.

Quantitative Measurement

Fatigue Fatigue was measured using the FSI, a 14-item self-report instrument measuring fatigue intensity, duration, and interference with activities of daily living over the past week (Hann et al., 1998). The FSI has been used to measure fatigue in patients with AMI (Fennessy et al., 2010; Fink et al., 2010) and patients with heart failure (Fink et al., 2009). Similar to others, the first three items of the FSI were used to measure fatigue intensity/severity (Donovan, Jacobsen, Small, Munster, & Andrykowski, 2008). Questions 5–11, which are referred to as the FSI-Interference Scale, were used to measure the degree to which fatigue has interfered with patients' daily activities in the past week. Each question on the FSI is answered using an 11-point Likert-type scale (0 = *not at all fatigued/no interference* to 10 = *as fatigued as I could be/extreme interference*). Interference in physical, cognitive, and emotional aspects of daily living are measured using the interference scale. Questions 1–3 and 5–11 were summed and then divided by the total number of items (3 and 7, respectively) to generate the intensity fatigue score and FSI-Interference Scale score, yielding scores ranging from 0 to 10. Higher scores reflect higher intensity of fatigue and more interference because of fatigue. The FSI-Interference Scale has excellent reliability as estimated by coefficient alphas ranging from 0.93 to 0.95 (Hann, Denniston, & Baker, 2000; Hann et al., 1998). Using the SF-36 vitality subscale as a comparison, Donovan et al. determined that an intensity score of ≥3 was reflective of clinically meaningful fatigue. In the current sample, reliability was strong for the FSI-Interference Scale ($\alpha = 0.93$) and the FSI intensity score ($\alpha = 0.86$).

Depressive Symptoms Depressive symptoms were measured using the Patient Health Questionnaire-9 (PHQ-9), which has been used in prior studies with cardiovascular patients (Fink et al., 2012; Lee, Lennie, Heo, & Moser, 2012). The PHQ is a nine-item self-report instrument with a 4-point Likert-type scale (0 = *not at all*; 1 = *several days*; 2 = *more than half the days*; 3 = *nearly every day*) for each question and was developed using the Diagnostic and Statistical Manual for Mental Disorders' criteria for major depression (American Psychiatric Association, 2013; Kroenke, Spitzer, & Williams, 2001). Scores of ≥10 indicate moderate/severe depressive symptoms; scores between 5 and 9 indicate minor depression. Using a structured mental health professional interview as the criterion standard, the sensitivity and specificity of the PHQ-9 (score ≥ 10) was 88% for detecting major depression (Kroenke et al., 2001). In this study, a score of ≥5 was used as the cutoff for the presence of depressive symptoms.

HRQoL HRQoL includes physical and mental health perceptions of positive and negative aspects of life (Centers for Disease Control and Prevention, 2012). The SF-36 has been extensively used to measure HRQoL and has established reliability and validity in numerous populations (McHorney et al.,

1993), including CHD populations (Fink et al., 2009; Hägglund et al., 2008). The SF-36 is a 36-item questionnaire that consists of eight subscales designed to measure quality of life in the domains of physical and mental functioning. The eight subscales are physical functioning, physical role limitation, emotional role limitation, vitality, mental health, social functioning, pain, and general health. The SF-36 generates eight subscale scores and two summary scores (physical component score and mental component score). Raw scores are standardized to range from 0 to 100, with lower scores indicating a lower level of functioning. Within the current study, reliability was good (α = .79-.88) for seven of the eight subscales, with a lower reliability for the general health subscale (α = .69).

Quantitative Analysis

Data were analyzed using the Statistical Package for the Social Sciences (Statistics for Windows, Version 19.0, IBM, Armonk, NY). A nominal alpha level of <.05 was designated for statistical significance. Chi-squared tests for independence and independent samples t tests were used to analyze demographic data and fatigue stratified by gender. Pearson's correlation and Spearman's rho were used to identify factors associated with fatigue. Multiple regression was used to identify predictors of fatigue.

Qualitative Measurement

Using scores from the FSI-Interference Scale, participants were identified as experiencing high ($\geq$2.5), moderate (1.15-2.4), or low (1.14) levels of interference from fatigue (Fink et al., 2010). Participants from each fatigue level were selected for the qualitative interview. Participants for the qualitative arm were interviewed within 3-5 weeks of enrollment. This time frame was selected to prevent potential recall bias and reduce the likelihood of participants experiencing cardiovascular events. Purposive sampling was used to achieve heterogeneity of the sample and to increase transferability of findings.

The principal investigator or research assistant completed all interviews, which lasted approximately 30 minutes. The principal investigator reviewed interviews completed by the research assistant to ensure consistency between interviewers. A semistructured interview guide was used to collect data. Questions included, "Describe a typical day," "What time of day do you feel most fatigued?" and "Describe your fatigue." Additional questions and probes were used to enhance the quality of the data. Field notes and an audit trail were maintained throughout data collection to ensure confirmability. Data saturation was reached after completing 13 interviews.

Qualitative Analysis

Interviews were digitally recorded and transcribed verbatim. Transcripts were imported into NVivo 9 (QSR International,

Burlington, MA) for coding and analysis. Transcripts were reviewed for accuracy by checking transcripts against the digitally recorded interview. Narrative analysis, which considers the potential for stories to give meaning to the data (Onwuegbuzie & Combs, 2010), was used as the primary analytic technique. Using the theory of unpleasant symptoms; themes of situational, psychological, and physiological factors; symptom description (timing, intensity, distress, quality); and performance (HRQoL) were analyzed. As data were coded, emerging themes were added, including an overall definition of fatigue, the worst part of being fatigued and aggravating/alleviating factors. To avoid biasing results, interviews were initially analyzed without regard to fatigue group. After all interview analyses were complete, within- and between-group analyses were done by comparing interviews from each group to determine similarities and differences between groups.

Mixed-Methods Analysis

After qualitative and quantitative analyses were complete, data were compared to determine patterns, enhance description, and address any discrepancies. Qualitative data were used to expand the overall depth of quantitative findings and provide a more thorough description of fatigue. If discrepancies were found, the authors reviewed discrepant data to determine if narrative data were revealing a concept not included on the standard instruments. Discrepancies in mixed-methods findings are generative, as they lead to further analysis and future research directions (Greene, 2007).

RESULTS

Demographic Characteristics

The mean age of participants (N = 102) was 65 years (SD = 11 years, range: 34-86 years). Most were men, non-Hispanic White, married, and had a high school education or greater (Table 1). The qualitative sample included nine men and four women (mean age = 67 years, SD = 12 years, range: 50-85 years); five participants reported low interference from fatigue, four reported moderate interference, and four reported high interference (Table 1).

Fatigue Intensity/Severity

Quantitative Analysis Women reported significantly higher levels of fatigue intensity (M = 4.38, SD = 2.16) than men (M = 3.43, SD = 2.16; t = 2.27, p = .003). Fifty-seven percent of men and 78.4% of women had clinically meaningful fatigue as indicated by an intensity score of $\geq$3. Fatigue intensity was significantly correlated with PHQ-9 score, smoking history, and income (Table 2). In a regression model, PHQ-9 (depressive symptoms) was the only predictor of fatigue intensity (Table 3).

TABLE 1. Demographic and Clinical Characteristics of the Sample

Variable	Total sample (N = 102)		Qualitative sample (n = 13)	
	N	%	n	%
Gender				
Men	65	63.7	9	69.2
Women	37	36.3	4	30.8
Race/ethnicity				
Non-Hispanic White	57	55.9	9	69.2
Black	36	35.3	4	30.8
Hispanic	4	3.9	0	0
Asian	2	2.0	0	0
Other	3	2.9	0	0
Marital status				
Married/long-term committed	60	58.8	10	76.9
Divorced/separated	23	22.5	1	7.7
Widowed	10	9.8	2	15.4
Single	9	8.8	0	0
Education				
Less than 12 years	17	16.8	2	15.4
High school diploma	38	37.3	4	30.8
Some college/associate degree	20	19.6	3	23.1
Baccalaureate degree	13	12.7	3	23.1
Graduate degree	13	12.7	1	7.7
Employment				
Full/part-time work	27	26.5	5	38.5
Retired	53	52.0	6	46.2
Disabled/unemployed/medical leave	18	17.6	1	7.7
Homemaker	2	2.0	0	0
Comorbid conditions				
Type 2 diabetes	40	39.2	5	38.5
Depression	12	11.8	2	15.4
Hypertension	91	89.2	11	84.6
Hyperlipidemia	95	93.1	12	92.3
Prior myocardial infarction	34	33.3	4	30.8
Prior percutaneous coronary intervention	79	77.5	11	84.6
Prior coronary artery bypass graft	24	23.5	3	23.1

Continues

TABLE 1. Continued

Variable	Total sample (N = 102)		Qualitative sample (n = 13)	
	N	%	n	%
Medications				
Aspirin	88	86.3	13	100
Ace inhibitor	60	58.8	9	69.2
Beta blocker	75	73.5	11	84.6
Lipid-lowering agent	88	86.3	13	100

Qualitative Analysis Participants in the qualitative arm of the study reported varying degrees of fatigue intensity. Some participants reported not recognizing fatigue until they "hit a wall" and did not want to do anything else. Others reported noticing a change from the past, stating, "I'd be able to doze off sitting up. I didn't used to be able to do that" (58-year-old woman, low fatigue interference) and "I'm more tireder (*sic*) this year than I was a year ago" (50-year-old man, high fatigue interference). One participant mentioned that she noticed an overall slowing down, "since I was sick." Most participants indicated a general slowing down but could not relate the change to any specific event. Of note, one participant stated, "I just get tired. Some

TABLE 2. Correlations: Fatigue Intensity and Interference With Demographic and Clinical Variables

Variable	Fatigue intensity		Fatigue interference	
	r	p	r	p
Age	−.08	.43	−.24	.02
Gender	.24	.02	.22	.02
PHQ-9 (depressive symptoms)	.56	<.0001	.66	<.0001
Income	−.20	.05	−.16	.12
Race	.09	.39	.09	.37
Education	−.16	.12	−.16	.12
Smoking history	.20	.05	.19	.06
Diabetes	.00	.99	−.03	.76
Hypertension	−.02	.82	−.13	.21
Myocardial infarction	−.13	.19	−.04	.67
PCI	.04	.71	.02	.81
Coronary artery bypass graft	.06	.540	.01	.93

Note. PHQ = Patient Health Questionnaire; PCI = percutaneous coronary intervention.

TABLE 3. Regression of Fatigue Intensity on Gender, Age, Income, History of Smoking, and Depressive Symptoms

Model	Predictors	b	t	p
1	Gender	.05	0.62	.54
	Income	.01	0.07	.99
	History of smoking	.04	0.41	.68
	PHQ-9	.54	5.80	<.0001
2	Gender	.05	0.60	.55
	Age	.03	0.38	.70
	PHQ-9	.55	6.15	<.0001

Note. PHQ = Patient Health Questionnaire. Model 1 variables were those correlated with fatigue intensity; $R^2 = .32$, adjusted $R^2 = .30$, SE = 1.73, $F_{2, 99} = 22.92$, and $p < .0001$. Model 2 variables were those hypothesized to be related to fatigue intensity; $R^2 = .32$, adjusted $R^2 = .30$, SE = 1.74, $F_{5, 96} = 15.20$, and $p < .0001$.

days I almost start crawling" (81-year-old man, low fatigue interference). This participant reported no interference from fatigue (score of 0 on FSI-Interference Scale), rated his worst fatigue severity as a 4 on an 11-point Likert scale, and consistently scored ≥50 (range: 0-100) on all HRQoL subscales. This incongruent finding may represent an accommodation to decreased physical capacity because of CHD.

Fatigue Interference

Quantitative Analysis Women reported significantly more interference from fatigue ($M = 3.28$, $SD = 2.71$; $t = 2.74$, $p = .007$) than men ($M = 1.99$, $SD = 2.03$). The FSI-Interference Scale score was significantly correlated with age and PHQ-9 score (Table 2). Depressive symptoms were the only predictor of interference from fatigue in a regression model (Table 4).

Qualitative Analysis A common theme was a general slowing down. "I have like a certain amount of energy in my bank account in the morning, and it just kind of gradually depletes during the day, and when it's gone, it's gone" (62-year-old man, moderate fatigue interference). Other participants reported rearranging their activities around the time of worst fatigue. "Then I arrange my day so that I can take my walk, come back and take a nap, and be fresh for the appointment. And that's the way I handle it" (81-year-old woman, high fatigue interference). Other descriptors of symptom distress included: "I remember I taught Grapes of Wrath. And ma would say, 'I'm sick tired,' you know.... You're almost sick, you're so tired" (74-year-old woman, moderate fatigue interference). Some participants described their distress in terms of activity, "like you want to lie down and take a nap" (50-year-old man, moderate fatigue interference). Participants who reported the lowest FSI-Interference Scale scores reported fewer instances of

daily fatigue but still reported having days when they were exhausted.

Timing of Fatigue

Quantitative Results Fatigue intensity was significantly correlated with the number of days per week participants experienced fatigue ($r = .63, p < .0001$) and the portion of the day participants felt fatigue ($r = .66, p < .0001$). Participants reported being fatigued a mean of 3.43 ($SD = 2.38$) days per week.

Qualitative Results Reports of the timing of fatigue varied. Some people reported fatigue every day at the same time: "Here lately it's been pretty much every day.... I get up and get [spouse] out to work...it feels like I'm drained" (85-year-old man, high fatigue interference). Other participants reported that fatigue only affected them after being busy and finally sitting down for the day, whereas some stated that there was no pattern. Two participants reported no fatigue on their quantitative measures, but they reported slowing down and needing more frequent breaks. One participant reported, "I take a nap...but as far as fatigue; I've got a lot of energy" (53-year-old man, low fatigue interference). Participants often did not relate slowing down, taking more frequent breaks, or needing naps to fatigue.

Quality of Fatigue

Qualitative Analysis The quality dimension of the theory of unpleasant symptoms refers to the symptom description, how the symptom manifests, or alleviating factors. Descriptors of fatigue included "I get winded a lot quicker," "going at a slower pace," and "a little aggravated and drained." Participants often reported that sitting down and resting was an alleviating factor. Many participants reported that simply going slower was helpful,

TABLE 4. Regression of Fatigue Interference on Gender, Age, and Depressive Symptoms

Model	Predictors	b	t	p
1	Gender	.07	0.90	.37
	Age	−.12	−1.54	.13
	PHQ-9	.61	7.56	<.0001
2	Gender	.07	0.90	.37
	Age	−.12	−1.54	.13
	PHQ-9	.61	7.56	<.0001

Note. PHQ = Patient Health Questionnaire. Model 1 variables were those correlated with fatigue interference; $R^2 = .46$, adjusted $R^2 = .43$, SE = 12.49, $F_{5, 96} = 16.07$, and $p < .0001$. Model 2 variables were those hypothesized to be related to fatigue interference; $R^2 = .45$, adjusted $R^2 = .42$, SE = 12.59, $F_{3, 98} = 19.60$, and $p < .0001$.

"so instead of working three hours, I should work two and then leave it" (79-year-old woman, low fatigue interference).

All participants in the qualitative arm were asked to define fatigue. Definitions included "being completely wore (*sic*) out," "different kind of fatigue," "bone weary," and "low energy, low mental processing." Participants often described it as being different than the feeling after a long day at work, "I've done a hard day's work before and not quite feel, wouldn't be the same.... I really don't know how to explain it...just more or less completely exhausted" (85-year-old man, high fatigue interference). Although the descriptions and definitions varied, it was obvious that fatigue was a physically and mentally taxing symptom that was affecting the individuals' daily lives. Definitions of fatigue did not vary whether participants experienced high, moderate, or low interference from fatigue.

HRQoL and Fatigue

Quantitative Analysis Fatigue intensity and interference from fatigue were negatively correlated with each of the SF-36 subscales that measure HRQoL (Table 5). Participants who reported more fatigue intensity and more interference from fatigue reported significantly worse scores on all eight subscales.

Qualitative Analysis Overall, participants reported that fatigue did not affect their enjoyment of life. Some participants reported feelings of jealousy when they saw people who were older doing things more easily than they could themselves: "I get jealous. Sometimes I'll see people in their 70s and 80s, and they're walking fast, like there's nothing wrong with them. They're full of piss and vinegar. It's like, 'wow I'm only 52'" (52-year old-man, high fatigue interference). Others reported finding ways to adapt to the fatigue by "unconsciously" planning their outings around times of worst fatigue.

TABLE 5. Correlations: Fatigue Intensity and Interference With Health-Related Quality of Life

HR-QoL[a]	Fatigue intensity	Fatigue interference
Physical functioning	−.54*	−.60*
Role limitation physical	−.50*	−.54*
Role limitation emotional	−.44*	−.53*
Vitality	−.65*	−.75*
Mental health	−.47*	−.60*
Social functioning	−.55*	−.65*
Pain	−.51*	−.52*
General health	−.53*	−.66*

Note. HR-QoL = health-related quality of life.
[a]HR-QoL variables are subscales from the SF-36.
*$p < .01$.

INTEGRATED ANALYSIS

There was concordance of findings between quantitative and qualitative measures on timing and distress dimensions of the theory of unpleasant symptoms. Table 6 summarizes the integrated analysis.

Participants with the highest FSI-Interference Scale scores tended to report the most difficulty with fatigue during qualitative interviews, with one exception: An 81-year-old man categorized as having low fatigue interference reported high fatigue during the interview. On the day of his interview, he reported he was "feeling pretty good" but described how bad he felt on his high fatigue days. It is possible that, when he completed the FSI, he was having a good day and did not answer the questions based on how he felt at any time other than the present.

Although participants during the qualitative interviews did not always acknowledge fatigue, they reported a general slowing, an increased frequency of breaks, and an overall tailoring of their lifestyle to avoid fatigue. All interviewed participants who reported low fatigue interference ($n = 5$) reported needing additional breaks. Neither the FSI fatigue severity score or interference score captured this phenomenon; therefore, without the addition of the qualitative component, important information might have been lost. The use of a partially mixed sequential dominant status design in which qualitative data enhance and expand data acquired through validated quantitative tools provided a deeper and contextualized picture of fatigue in patients with CHD.

DISCUSSION

A key finding of the study was that more than 50% of stable male and female participants with CHD reported clinically meaningful fatigue that occurred on an average of 3.43 days of the week. This indicates that patients with stable CHD experience a high degree of fatigue. Women ($M = 3.28$, $SD = 2.71$), but not men ($M = 1.99$, $SD = 2.03$), reported higher interference with activities because of fatigue than those reported by cancer patients undergoing active treatment ($M = 2.3$, $SD = 2.2$; Hann et al., 1998) and patients with reduced ejection fraction heart failure ($M = 2.9$, $SD = 2.7$; Fink et al., 2009).

The presence of depressive symptoms was the only predictor of fatigue intensity and interference among the potential contributors to fatigue. Interestingly, in the univariate analysis, women reported significantly greater fatigue intensity and interference compared with men; however, after controlling for depressive symptoms, there were no gender differences, indicating that depressed mood was a dominant factor. Finally, fatigue intensity and interference were correlated with poor HRQoL. Patients with higher PHQ-9 scores (depressive symptoms) reported more interference from fatigue and fatigue intensity. On the basis of the regression analysis, 45%

TABLE 6. Integrated Data Analysis

Fatigue dimension	Quantitative data (select)	Qualitative data (select)	Integrated analysis
Frequency and pattern	• 9.8% reported no fatigue in the past week • 47% reported fatigue 1–3 days in the past week • 43% reported fatigue ≥4 days in the past week • 20% reported fatigue worse in the morning • 21% reported fatigue worse in the afternoon • 28% reported fatigue worse in the evening • 23% reported no consistent pattern	• "Here lately it's been pretty much every day…" (high fatigue) • "…as far as fatigue, I've got a lot of energy." (low fatigue) • "…don't happen every day." (low fatigue) • "…sometimes in the afternoon, I'll get a little tired, and I'll lay down for a little bit. But most of the time it's more evenings…" (moderate fatigue) • "In the morning. And I usually have to end up stopping what I'm doing, getting up, and moving around." (moderate fatigue) • "It's no certain time. It varies." (high fatigue)	• Quantitative reports of frequency of fatigue correlated with qualitative comments such as "lots or energy" or "every day" • No consistent pattern of fatigue identified in qualitative or quantitative results
Distress	• 72% reported fatigue interfered with general activity • Nearly 65% reported that fatigue interfered with normal work activity, enjoyment of life, and mood. • Over 50% reported interference with relationships and ability to concentrate.	• "I felt that my medical condition had finally turned a corner, and so now I'm going to try to become more active…and then you find out you can't…" (low fatigue) • "I find myself nodding off…. Nobody saw me, did they? And it's embarrassing." (moderate fatigue)	• Even those participants who reported low fatigue on standardized instruments noted fatigue affecting daily life. • Standard instruments failed to capture the lifestyle tailoring that patients with stable CHD reported. • Providers need to ask more detailed questions about fatigue to determine if patients are compensating for the symptom.
Intensity	• Mean score of 5.44 (SD = 2.64) on the rating of most fatigue (range: 0–10) • Mean score of 3.71 (SD = 2.23) on the rating of average fatigue (range: 0–10) • Mean score of 2.17 (SD = 2.14) on the rating of least fatigue (range: 0–10)	• "I've been awful tired, and that usually is not me." (high fatigue) • "…you don't realize you were fatigued until…trying to go out and hanging on the cart keeping you up." (low fatigue)	• Rating of average fatigue intensity indicative of clinically meaningful fatigue • Qualitative reports of fatigue intensity did not differ significantly between high, moderate, and low fatigue groups.

Continues

TABLE 6. Continued

Fatigue dimension	Quantitative data (select)	Qualitative data (select)	Integrated analysis
Performance	• Participants classified as high fatigue using the FSI composite reported lower quality of life.	• "I'm going in there and get something done and get it done. Now you just kind of stretch it out." (moderate fatigue) • "…you just learn to accept it." (moderate fatigue)	• Consistent qualitative reports of adapting to fatigue and changing lifestyle to accommodate restrictions • Overall, patients reported that they adapted and did not allow fatigue to dictate the quality of life they lived.
(health-related quality of life)	• FSI scores were correlated with all of the SF-36 subscales.	• "I've got a lot to do, but just don't get it done…when you're feeling tired, you ain't got no business on a ladder." (high fatigue) • "I think that's what's the hardest on a guy that's like me…being shut down from what you used to be doing." (high fatigue) • "I can get out of the notion of going somewhere a lot easier." (low fatigue)	• It appears that patients with stable CHD adapt to a decreased functional capacity over time and do not allow quality of life to be dictated by the symptoms they experience.

of fatigue interference scores were explained by the presence of depressive symptoms. Even participants categorized as having mild depressive symptoms reported higher levels of fatigue. The link between fatigue and depression has been documented in patients with cardiovascular disease (Evangelista et al., 2008; Fennessy et al., 2010; Fink et al., 2012). Others have also indicated a strong relationship between fatigue and depression among patients attending primary care clinics. Skapinakis, Lewis, and Mavreas (2004) conducted a secondary analysis of data from the World Health Organization longitudinal collaborative study of psychological problems in general healthcare. Individuals with depression at baseline were 4 times more likely to develop new unexplained fatigue at the 12-month follow-up. In patients with cardiovascular disease, depressed mood or depression often coexist, and it remains to be determined if depression is the cause or consequence of fatigue.

Younger age was associated with higher fatigue interference but not fatigue intensity. It is possible that younger individuals find that fatigue interferes with daily activities, whereas older individuals are not as active or adapt more readily to fatigue by altering their activities. Kop, Appels, Mendes de Leon, and Bar (1996) found that younger age and female gender were significant predictors of vital exhaustion in patients with CHD.

Similar to others, fatigue intensity and fatigue interference were negatively correlated with all eight SF-36 subscales (HRQoL). Pragodpol and Ryan (2013) examined 17 studies and found that fatigue was a predictor of diminished HRQoL in patients with newly diagnosed CHD. In another study of patients with confirmed CHD and chronic angina, a symptom cluster containing fatigue, dyspnea, and chest pain frequency was found to be predictive of lower HRQoL (Kimble et al., 2011). Staniute, Bunevicius, Brozaitiene, and Bunevicius (2013) determined that poor HRQoL was associated with greater fatigue and reduced exercise capacity independent of mental health and severity of CHD. The findings validate the critical impact that the symptom of fatigue has on HRQoL.

All qualitative participants who reported low interference from fatigue on their standardized instruments ($n = 5$) reported fatigue during the interview. These individuals reported low levels of fatigue interference and severity but described not doing as much, tailoring their lifestyle to prevent fatigue, and moving at a slower pace. Lifestyle alterations in response to fatigue have been described in the heart failure literature (Jones, McDermott, Nowels, Matlock, & Bekelman, 2012). In an interpretive study of 26 patients with heart failure, emergent themes included descriptions of patients adapting to being tired and identifying ways to proactively prevent fatigue by rescheduling their days (Jones et al., 2012). This adaptation may also have occurred with patients in this study. It remains unknown if measurement error or other factors explain differences between quantitative and qualitative reports of fatigue in this study.

Strengths and Limitations

Although previous research has focused on determining if fatigue predicts CHD in healthy individuals and the prevalence of fatigue before and after AMI, this is the first study that specifically describes fatigue in a stable CHD population. This study is innovative in that the design included the use of mixed methods, which combined validated quantitative measures with in-depth qualitative interviews. The qualitative interviews complemented findings from the quantitative instruments and added rich descriptive details to the findings. Sampling an urban and rural population resulted in ethnic and geographic diversity, thus increasing the generalizability of findings. There were limitations to this study including the use of a convenience sample and the potential inclusion of patients with undiagnosed heart failure. Differences in reports of fatigue intensity between standardized instruments and interviews in the low fatigue group may indicate that the FSI-interference Scale is not as sensitive in individuals with lower interference from fatigue.

Conclusion

Fatigue was common in patients with stable CHD. Women experienced a greater burden from fatigue compared with men, and this was primarily because of the contribution of depressive symptoms. The use of mixed methods was beneficial to the study of fatigue in stable CHD and provided additional insight, especially in participants who reported low interference from fatigue. This study provides an important contribution to understanding fatigue as a possible symptom of stable CHD; however, these descriptive findings preclude determining if fatigue is an indicator of new onset or progressive CHD. Future research is needed to establish the mechanisms of fatigue in this population. In addition, longitudinal studies are essential to understand causal relationships between depression and fatigue. Further study is also needed to examine the effectiveness of interventions on reducing fatigue to improve HRQoL in patients with stable CHD.

Accepted for publication November 12, 2013.

The authors acknowledge that this research was supported in part by grants from the Midwest Nursing Research Society and Sigma Theta Tau International.

The authors have no conflicts of interest to disclose.

Corresponding author: Ann L. Eckhardt, PhD, RN, School of Nursing, Illinois Wesleyan University, P.O. Box 2900, Bloomington, IL 61702 (e-mail: aeckhard@iwu.edu).

REFERENCES

Aaronson, L. S., Teel, C. S., Cassmeyer, V., Neuberger, G. B., Pallikkathayil, L., Pierce, J., & Wingate, A. (1999). Defining and measuring fatigue. *Image: The Journal of Nursing Scholarship*, *31*, 45-50.

American Heart Association. (2013). Coronary artery disease. Retrieved from http://www.heart.org/HEARTORG/Conditions/More/MyHeartandStrokeNews/Coronary-Artery-Disease—The-ABCs-of-CAD_UCM_436416_Article.jsp

American Psychiatric Association. (2013). *Diagnostic and statistical manual of mental disorders* (5th ed.). Arlington, VA: American Psychiatric Publishing.

Centers for Disease Control and Prevention. (2012). Health-related quality of life (HRQOL). Retrieved from http://www.cdc.gov/hrqol/

DeVon, H. A., Ryan, C. J., Ochs, A. L., & Shapiro, M. (2008). Symptoms across the continuum of acute coronary syndromes: Differences between women and men. *American Journal of Critical Care*, *17*, 14-24.

Dittner, A. J., Wessely, S. C., & Brown, R. G. (2004). The assessment of fatigue: A practical guide for clinicians and researchers. *Journal of Psychosomatic Research*, *56*, 157-170. doi:10.1016/S0022-3999(03)00371-4

Donovan, K. A., Jacobsen, P. B., Small, B. J., Munster, P. N., & Andrykowski, M. A. (2008). Identifying clinically meaningful fatigue with the fatigue symptom inventory. *Journal of Pain and Symptom Management*, *36*, 480-487. doi:10.1016/j.jpainsymman.2007.11.013

Ekmann, A., Osler, M., & Avlund, K. (2012). The predictive value of fatigue for nonfatal ischemic heart disease and all-cause mortality. *Psychosomatic Medicine*, *74*, 464-470. doi:10.1097/PSY.0b013e318258d294

Evangelista, L. S., Moser, D. K., Westlake, C., Pike, N., Ter-Galstanyan, A., & Dracup, K. (2008). Correlates of fatigue in patients with heart failure. *Progress in Cardiovascular Nursing*, *23*, 12-17. doi:10.1111/j.1751-7117.2008.07275.x

Fennessy, M. M., Fink, A. M., Eckhardt, A. L., Jones, J., Kruse, D. K., VanderZwan, K. J., . . . Zerwic, J. J. (2010). Gender differences in fatigue associated with acute myocardial infarction. *Journal of Cardiopulmonary Rehabilitation and Prevention*, *30*, 224-230. doi:10.1097/HCR.0b013e3181d0c493

Fink, A. M., Eckhardt, A. L., Fennessy, M. M., Jones, J., Kruse, D., VanderZwan, K. J., . . . Zerwic, J. J. (2010). Psychometric properties of three instruments to measure fatigue with myocardial infarction. *Western Journal of Nursing Research*, *32*, 967-983. doi:10.1177/0193945910371320

Fink, A. M., Gonzalez, R. C., Lisowski, T., Pini, M., Fantuzzi, G., Levy, W. C., & Piano, M. R. (2012). Fatigue, inflammation, and projected mortality in heart failure. *Journal of Cardiac Failure*, *18*, 711-716. http://dx.doi.org/10.1016/j.cardfail.2012.07.003

Fink, A. M., Sullivan, S. L., Zerwic, J. J., & Piano, M. R. (2009). Fatigue with systolic heart failure. *Journal of Cardiovascular Nursing*, *24*, 410-417. doi:10.1097/JCN.0b013e3181ae1e84

Goblirsch, G., Bershow, S., Cummings, K., Hayes, R., Kokoszka, M., Lu, Y., Sanders, D., & Zarling, K. (2013). Stable coronary artery disease. Institute for Clinical Systems Improvement. Retrieved from https://www.icsi.org/_asset/t6bh6a/SCAD.pdf

Greene, J. C. (2007). *Mixed methods in social inquiry*. San Francisco, CA: Jossey-Bass.

Högglund, L., Boman, K., Stenlund, H., Lundman, B., & Brulin, C. (2008). Factors related to fatigue among older patients with heart failure in primary health care. *International Journal of Older People Nursing*, *3*, 96-103.

Hann, D. M. vDenniston, M. M., & Baker, F. (2000). Measurement of fatigue in cancer patients: Further validation of the fatigue symptom inventory. *Quality of Life Research*, *9*, 847-854. doi:10.1023/A:1008900413113

Hann, D. M., Jacobsen, P. B., Azzarello, L. M., Martin, S. C., Curran, S. L., Fields, K. K., . . . Lyman, G. (1998). Measurement of fatigue in cancer patients: Development and validation of the Fatigue Symptom Inventory. *Quality of Life Research*, *7*, 301-310. doi:10.1023/A:1024929829627

Jones, J., McDermott, C. M., Nowels, C. T., Matlock, D. D., & Bekelman, D. B. (2012). The experience of fatigue as a distressing symptom of heart failure. *Heart & Lung: The Journal of Acute and Critical Care, 41*, 484–491. doi:10.1016/j.hrtlng.2012.04.004

Kimble, L. P., Dunbar, S. B.vWeintraub, W. S., McGuire, D. B., Manzo, S. F., & Strickland, O. L. (2011). Symptom clusters and health-related quality of life in people with chronic stable angina. *Journal of Advanced Nursing, 67*, 1000–1011. doi:10.1111/j.1365-2648.2010 .05564.x

Kop, W. J., Appels, A. P. W. M., Mendes de Leon, C. F., & Bar, F. W. (1996). The relationship between severity of coronary artery disease and vital exhaustion. *Journal of Psychosomatic Research, 40*, 397–405.

Kroenke, K., Spitzer, R. L., & Williams, J. B. W. (2001). The PHQ-9: Validity of a brief depression severity measure. *Journal of General Internal Medicine, 16*, 606–613. doi:10.1046/j.1525-1497.2001.016009606.x

Lee, K. S., Lennie, T. A., Heo, S., & Moser, D. K. (2012). Association of physical versus affective depressive symptoms with cardiac event-free survival in patients with heart failure. *Psychosomatic Medicine, 74*, 452–458. doi:10.1097/psy.0b013e31824a0641

Leech, N. L., & Onwuegbuzie, A. J. (2009). A typology of mixed methods research designs. *Quality & Quantity, 43*, 265–275. doi:10.1007/s11135-007-9105-3

Lenz, E. R., Pugh, L. C., Milligan, R. A., Gift, A., & Suppe, F. (1997). The middle-range theory of unpleasant symptoms: An update. *Advances in Nursing Science, 19*, 14–27.

Lindeberg, S. I., Rosvall, M., & østergren, P.-O. (2012). Exhaustion predicts coronary heart disease independently of symptoms of depression and anxiety in men but not in women. *Journal of Psychosomatic Research, 72*, 17–21. doi:10.1016/j.jpsychores.2011.09.001

McHorney, C. A., Ware, J. E., & Raczek, A. E. (1993). The MOS 36-item short-form health survey (SF-36): II. Psychometric and clinical tests of validity in measuring physical and mental health constructs. *Medical Care, 31*, 247–263.

McSweeney, J. C., & Crane, P. B. (2000). Challenging the rules: Womens prodromal and acute symptoms of myocardial infarction. *Research in Nursing & Health, 23*, 135–146. doi:10.1002/ (SICI)1098-240X(200004)23:2<135::AID-NUR6>3.0.CO;2-1

Onwuegbuzie, A. J., & Combs, J. P. (2010). Emergent data analysis techniques in mixed methods research: A synthesis. In TashakkoriA.TeddlieC. (Eds.), *Handbook of mixed methods in social and behavioral research* (2nd ed., pp. 397–430). Los Angeles, CA: Sage.

Pragodpol, P., & Ryan, C. (2013). Critical review of factors predicting health-related quality of life in newly diagnosed coronary artery disease patients. *Journal of Cardiovascular Nursing, 28*, 277–284. doi:10.1097/JCN.0b013e31824af56e

Ream, E., & Richardson, A. (1996). Fatigue: A concept analysis. *International Journal of Nursing Studies, 33*, 519–529. doi:10.1016/0020-7489(96)00004-1

Shaffer, J. A., Davidson, K. W., Schwartz, J. E., Shimbo, D., Newman, J. D., Gurland, B. J., & Maurer, M. S. (2012). Prevalence and characteristics of anergia (lack of energy) in patients with acute coronary syndrome. *American Journal of Cardiology, 110*, 1213–1218. doi:10.1016/j.amjcard.2012.06.022

Skapinakis, P., Lewis, G., Mavreas, V. (2004). Temporal relations between unexplained fatigue and depression: Longitudinal data from an international study in primary care. *Psychosomatic Medicine, 66*, 330–335. doi:10.1097/01.psy.0000124757.10167.b1

Staniute, M., Bunevicius, A., Brozaitiene, J., & Bunevicius, R. (2013). Relationship of health-related quality of life with fatigue and exercise capacity in patients with coronary artery disease. *European Journal of Cardiovascular Nursing*. doi:10.1177/1474515113496942

Zimmermann-Viehoff, F., Wang, H. X., Kirkeeide, R., Schneiderman, N., Erdur, L., Deter, H. C., & Orth-Gomer, K. (2013). Womens exhaustion and coronary artery atherosclerosis progression: The Stockholm female coronary angiography study. *Psychosomatic Medicine, 75*, 478–485. doi:10.1097/PSY.0b013e3182928c28

Read Updated Reviewer Guidelines

Nursing Research the Reviewer Guidelines on the publisher's website here: http://journals.lww.com/nursingresearchonline/Pages/reviewerguidelines.aspx

Care Transition Experiences of Spousal Caregivers: From a Geriatric Rehabilitation Unit to Home

Qualitative Health Research
XX(X) 1–17
© The Author(s) 2011
Reprints and permission:
sagepub.com/journalsPermissions.nav
DOI: 10.1177/1049732311407078
http://qhr.sagepub.com
⑤SAGE

Kerry Byrne,[1] Joseph B. Orange,[2] and Catherine Ward-Griffin[2]

Abstract

The purpose of this study was to develop a theoretical framework about caregivers' experiences and the processes in which they engaged during their spouses' transition from a geriatric rehabilitation unit to home. We used a constructivist grounded theory methodology approach. Forty-five interviews were conducted across three points in time with 18 older adult spousal caregivers. A theoretical framework was developed within which reconciling in response to fluctuating needs emerged as the basic social process. Reconciling included three subprocesses (i.e., navigating, safekeeping, and repositioning), and highlighted how caregivers responded to the fluctuating needs of their spouse, to their own needs, and to those of the marital dyad. Reconciling was situated within a context shaped by a trajectory of prior care transitions and intertwined life events experienced by caregivers. Findings serve as a resource for scientists, rehabilitation clinicians, educators, and decision makers toward improving transitional care for spousal caregivers.

Keywords

aging, caregivers / caregiving; grounded theory; health care; rehabilitation; relationships; relationships, primary partner; theory development

Recent initiatives in care for older persons with disabilities include geriatric rehabilitation units (GRUs). Care transitions into and out of GRUs involve both the older person/patient and his or her family members (Fredman & Daly, 1998). Several researchers have called for the inclusion of family caregivers and their goals (e.g., knowledge of and access to services) in GRU assessment and rehabilitation programs (Aminzadeh et al., 2005; Bradley et al., 2000; Demers, Ska, Desrosiers, Alix, & Wolfson, 2004; Hills, 1998). When family caregivers agree with recommendations made for their relatives during geriatric assessments, adherence to the recommendations is more likely to occur (Bogardus et al., 2004). Despite a primary focus on the older adults in the GRU, their family caregivers often require their own health-related support in addition to information about how best to care for their relatives (Demers et al.; Hills); however, little is known about how family caregivers experience their relative's transition from the GRU to home, and about the processes engaged in during care transitions.

Current models and theories of family caregiving (Lazarus & Folkman, 1984; Pearlin, Mullan, Semple, & Skaff, 1990; Schumacher, 1995; Skaff, Pearlin, & Mullan, 1996) and

transitions (Chick & Meleis, 1986; Meleis, Sawyer, Im, Hilfinger Messias, & Schumacher, 2000; Schumacher, Jones, & Meleis, 1999) include, in part, concepts and processes related to caregiving during transitions from hospital to home settings. However, none focus on the processes enacted by caregivers during the experiences of their relative's transition from a GRU to home. As a result, rehabilitation researchers, clinicians, and policy makers have few conceptual resources to help them understand how caregivers experience the transition of their husband or wife from a GRU hospital based setting to home or, moreover, what caregivers actually "do" during these transitions. The purpose of our study was to develop a theoretical framework illustrating how spousal caregivers experience the transition

[1]University of British Columbia, Vancouver, British Columbia, Canada
[2]University of Western Ontario, London, Ontario, Canada

Corresponding Author:
Kerry Byrne, University of British Columbia Department of Sociology,
1314-6303 N.W. Marine Drive, Vancouver, British Columbia,
V6T 1Z1, Canada
Email: Kerry.Byrne@ubc.ca

151

of their husband or wife from a GRU hospital-based setting to the home.

Literature Review
Spousal Caregiving

Spouses, more than any other caregiver, are likely to provide care during periods of disability and illness, and are likely to continue doing so even as their own health declines (Chappell, 1992; Hess & Soldo, 1985). A study commissioned by Health Canada (2002) found that family caregivers are most likely to provide care to a spouse or partner (38%). Spousal caregivers experience adverse emotional and physical health, caregiving burden, and challenges with the role of caregiving (Braun, Mikulincer, Rydall, Walsh, & Rodin, 2007; Connell, Janevic, & Gallant, 2001; Jacobi et al., 2003). Fredman and Daly (1998) reported that 46% of caregivers are the spouses of individuals who are discharged from GRUs. Given the extent to which spouses engage in caregiving and the difficulties they encounter during transitional care, the present study focused specifically on spousal caregivers.

Transitional Care

Transitional care is defined as "a set of actions designed to ensure the coordination and continuity of health care as patients transfer between different locations or different levels of care within the same location" (Coleman, Boult, & American Geriatrics Society Health Care Systems Committee, 2003, p. 556). The study of transitional care is crucial to optimize quality care for older adults with complex care needs (Coleman et al.). Coleman and Williams (2007) proposed several key elements of a research agenda designed to improve the quality of transitions out of hospitals for older adults. They called for greater recognition of the integral role of family caregivers during care transitions. Older adults and their family caregivers encounter numerous difficulties during care transitions (from acute care to home and into long-term care), such as not feeling prepared for the transition, a lack of communication with health care providers, difficulty obtaining needed information (e.g., medical aspects of care), and access to resources (Bull, 1992; Bull, Maryuyama, & Luo, 1995; Davies & Nolan, 2003, 2004; Grimmer & Moss, 2001). These difficulties contribute to family caregivers' negative experiences of care transitions.

Current definitions of and approaches to transitional care (Coleman et al., 2003; Holland & Harris, 2007) focus on patients' experiences of moving between and among a range of health care settings. Unfortunately, caregivers' experiences often are not highlighted in definitions and current approaches. In several recent interventions aimed at improving care transitions, caregivers' experiences, their characteristics, and outcomes during transition were not reported and/or distinguished from patients' perspectives and experiences (Naylor, 2002; Naylor et al., 2007, Parry, Kramer, & Coleman, 2006). Although patients' perspectives of care transitions obviously are critically important, grouping patient and caregiver perspectives makes it very difficult to discern concerns specific to each group. The blending clouds our understandings of caregivers' experiences of their relatives' transitions to and from health care settings. A recent exception is the study by Shyu, Chen, Chen, Wang, and Shao (2008), in which the investigators examined the outcomes of a caregiver-oriented care transition intervention for family caregivers of individuals who had suffered a stroke. They found that their intervention resulted in higher self-evaluations of preparation and better satisfaction of discharge needs in comparison to a control group who received only routine care.

Caregiving During Care Transitions From Hospital-Based Settings to Home

Several investigators have demonstrated that caregiver needs, concerns, relationships, and burdens are salient and change throughout the transition from hospital to home for caregivers of older adult care recipients (e.g., Bull, 1990; Grimmer, Falco, & Moss, 2004; Kane, Reinardy, Penrod, & Huck, 1999; Naylor, Stephens, Bowles, & Bixby, 2005; Shyu, 2000a). Many of these authors identified "issues" that occur during transitions from hospital to home, but few identified how caregivers respond to the difficulties, changes, and unmet needs that arise during the transition. Notable exceptions include five studies that explored processes engaged in during care transitions from hospital to home (Bull, 1992; Bull & Jervis, 1997; Li & Shyu, 2007; Shyu, 2000a, 2000b, 2000c), and whose authors put forth theoretical frameworks (Bull, 1990; Li & Shyu; Shyu, 2000b) to understand what caregivers are "doing" during periods of transitional care.

The published articles reporting on these studies offer useful findings; however, they provide limited information about how spousal caregivers experience their husband's or wife's transition. First, none of the authors considered the transition from a GRU unit to home. GRUs are an increasingly common type of health care setting for older adults, and differ from acute care settings, where the majority of care transition work has been completed. Second, the majority of studies group experiences of spousal caregivers with other types of caregivers (e.g., adult children, daughters-in-law, siblings), even though research findings suggest that spouses experience caregiving differently (Barnes, Given, & Given, 1992; Frederick & Fast, 1999; George & Gwyther, 1986; Hayes, Zimmerman, & Boylstein, 2010; Navon & Weinblatt, 1996). The grouping reduces our ability to understand fully the issues specific to spousal caregivers' experiences of care transitions. Third, the experiences of spousal caregivers aged 65 years and older are underrepresented. For instance, the average age of caregivers in studies that identified "how" they manage transitions are always below 60 years (Bull, 1992; Bull & Jervis, 1997; Li & Shyu, 2007; Shyu, 2000b, 2000c). Finally, the experiences of caregivers prior to the discharge of their relative from a hospital-based setting were addressed only by Shyu (2000b, 2000c). Despite the important collective efforts of these investigators, we are left with little knowledge about how spousal caregivers prepare for the transition home from a GRU.

Recent attempts to describe transitions to care for family caregivers of older adults have yielded no theoretical or conceptual framework that specifically addresses older adult spousal caregivers' experiences of their relative's transition from a GRU to home. Such a framework would help guide education, research, and practice in rehabilitation settings. The aim of our study was to develop a theoretical understanding of the processes engaged in by spousal caregivers during the transfer of their husband/wife from a GRU to home. We gathered the perspectives of spousal caregivers who cared for older adult husbands or wives with and without cognitive impairment or dementia.

Methodology

A constructivist grounded theory methodology was used because it emphasizes the examination of processes and the creation of interpretive understandings (Charmaz, 2006). Ontologically, a constructivist approach highlights how the processes enacted during transition for caregivers are viewed as both individually experienced and socially constructed via interactions with other people. Grounded theory is an ideal methodology to understand actions and processes through transitions (Morse, 2009), and has been used by qualitative researchers to study processes engaged in by patients (Grant, St John, & Patterson, 2009) and family caregivers (Bull & McShane, 2008; Holtslander & Duggleby, 2009).

Sampling and Recruitment

A 36-bed inpatient GRU housed within a larger long-term care hospital in Ontario, Canada served as the recruitment site. The first author (Byrne) contacted spousal caregivers only after they indicated to a GRU team member who was not affiliated with the study that they were willing to participate. Spousal caregivers participated in three interviews (i.e., 48 hours prior to discharge, 2 weeks post-discharge, and 1 month postdischarge). In keeping with grounded theory methodology, both initial and theoretical sampling techniques were used to guide data collection

(Charmaz, 2006; Cutcliffe, 2000). Initial sampling criteria included spousal caregivers returning home with their husband or wife, and spouses (both men and women) caring for their partner who did or did not have cognitive impairment or dementia.

Participants

Eighteen caregivers participated in the study (9 men, 9 women). Caregivers' mean age was 77.4 years (range 65 to 89). They were married, on average, 47 years (range 8 to 60). Four caregivers were in a second marriage (M =19.5 years, range 8 to 36), and 14 were in their first marriage (M = 54.9 years, range 44 to 60). Eleven caregivers reported receiving home care services, and 5 did not receive any home care services. Two caregivers were not available for followup postdischarge (see below). Care recipients' mean age was 78.7 years (range 65 to 90). Five care recipients had a diagnosis of dementia, 4 had other cognitive impairments (e.g., delirium, mild cognitive impairment), and 9 had no identified cognitive issues. The mean length of stay on the GRU for care recipients was 41 days (range 22 to 77). Reasons for admission to the GRU included deconditioning (some from acute care), hip fracture, hip replacement, stroke, and knee joint replacement.

Data Collection

The first author conducted 45 face-to-face interviews with 18 spousal caregivers on the GRU and in their homes. Interviews lasted between 35 and 120 minutes. Fifteen of 18 caregivers were interviewed more than once (i.e., across time); of these 15, total interview time per participant ranged from 1.5 to 5 hours.

Sensitizing concepts, based on previous research on caregiving and transitions (e.g., Grimmer et al., 2004; Kneeshaw, Considine, & Jennings, 1999; Showalter, Burger, & Salyer, 2000) such as changes in relationship and social supports, were used as points of departure for the interview guide and also guided the initial analysis. As recommended by Charmaz (2006), these concepts were incorporated into specific questions in the initial interview guide and were used as tentative tools to develop ideas about the processes in our data. For instance, participants were asked how they would describe their relationship with their spouse currently (at the time of interview) in comparison to before they were admitted to the GRU, and about who had been especially helpful to them in caring for their spouse. We were particularly attuned and sensitive to these concepts during initial coding and debriefing, as well.

Three time points for data collection were planned: 48 hours prior to discharge from the GRU, 2 weeks postdischarge, and 4 to 6 weeks postdischarge. These time periods were based on previous research on care transitions (Bull, 1992; Bull & Jervis, 1997; Lin, Hung, Liao, Sheen, & Jong, 2006; Naylor, 2000). Minor changes to the initial intended time points were made for several participants because of loss to follow up and scheduling conflicts. Twelve caregivers were interviewed at all three time points. Three caregivers were interviewed at two points in time ($n = 1$ at 2 weeks and 1 month postdischarge; $n = 2$ prior to discharge and 2 weeks postdischarge); of these, 1 caregiver was not available prior to discharge, 1 did not want to be followed up for a third interview, and 1 could not be reached for a third interview. Three caregivers were interviewed only once ($n = 2$ prior to discharge; $n = 1$ at 2 weeks post discharge); of these, 2 were not discharged as planned and so could not be followed up, and 1 was not available at the other points in time (i.e., prior to discharge or 1 month postdischarge). First interviews were conducted between 72 and 48 hours prior to discharge ($n = 12$) and 1 to 6 days postdischarge ($n = 6$). Second interviews occurred between 14 and 21 days postdischarge (one of the second interviews was conducted 29 days postdischarge because of scheduling conflicts). Third interviews were conducted between 28 and 64 days postdischarge. Data collection began September 2006 and continued until November 2007.

In accordance with theoretical sampling, the categories noted to be relevant to the development of the emerging theoretical framework guided the sampling process rather than particular sample characteristics such as demographics. For example, as we tried to understand how and when caregivers "shifted the boundaries" (an element in the theoretical framework), it emerged that this experience might be different for men caregivers. Therefore, the last few caregivers who were interviewed were deliberately men so that elements of how and when they shifted the boundaries and how this differed from the experiences that emerged for women caregivers could be explored.

Interviews were digitally audio-recorded by the first author, transcribed verbatim by an experienced transcriptionist, and verified by the first author. In keeping with grounded theory methodology, data generation and data analysis occurred simultaneously, which supported follow-ups with participants about emergent codes and categories.

Observations

Observations of interactions between spouses and care recipients were made prior to, during, and after interviews, and were recorded in a field notebook (guided by Charmaz, 2006; Morse & Field, 1995). Specific observation times were not established a priori. The interviewer (first author) was "finely tuned in" to look for interactions that would help elucidate processes and categories emerging from the data (Charmaz). Throughout the duration of the study, an electronic field notebook was used to record observations, reflexive journal entries, audit trail details, and field notes about each interview.

Care recipient spouses were included in observations but were not interviewed. We wanted spousal caregivers to be able to speak candidly about their relationships, and thus provided the option for them to be interviewed either without partners present or outside of their homes. If care recipients were present, we did not want to miss the opportunity to observe interactions; thus, we included an observational component and included the care recipient in this method of data collection. This approach proved to be fruitful, as the interviewer was able to "see" the actions engaged in by caregivers during the interviews in which partners were present.

Analysis

The first author engaged in line-by-line coding. As data collection and analysis progressed, all authors contributed to focused coding, followed by theoretical coding (Charmaz, 2006) using the constant comparative method with all units of data. For example, in the early stages of data collection and analysis, we noticed that caregivers continually used the phrase "I don't know," and thus an open code by this name was created to capture this aspect of the data. As data collection and analysis proceeded, we engaged in focused coding using the term *knowing/not knowing* to reflect these instances in the data. The following comment by Marie,[1] was coded as knowing/not knowing, but through theoretical coding was understood to be part of the process of navigating:

> I don't know how long it [medication for dementia] will last, I can't find out. I've asked different doctors and nurses and they don't know, don't say how long it'll, but I hope it's years. You know, asked those questions. Why and how long do they think, maybe they can't tell, I don't know, how long do they think that they can give it to him?

To develop this category further, caregivers were asked how they became informed and what helped or did not help them to do so. We began to understand how navigating was critical to safekeeping (theoretical coding). Constant comparison entailed comparing incident to incident and comparing incidents over time between and within participants. Charmaz (2006) encouraged looking for implicit actions and meanings, comparing statements at one point, and comparing incidents at different points in time. Tables were created to compare instances across time. Once the theoretical code of navigating was identified, quotations from participants that reflected the various elements of this process (such as negotiating paths) were put into a table so we could examine the change in processes across time.

Moving from line-by-line coding to focused coding was not a linear process. As we engaged with the data, we returned to the data collected to explore new ideas and conceptualizations of codes. The simultaneous actions of collecting and analyzing data supported the discovery of gaps in the data, which were then filled by going back to existing participants and conducting interviews with new participants.

When a code was raised to the level of a category, the first author created a memo describing the category, the elements contained in the category, illustrative quotes that reflected the category, and further ideas on which to follow up to ensure theoretical saturation of the category. These memos were shared and discussed among authors. This process continued until we had no new elements to add to a category. To foster theoretical sensitivity, memos focused on actions and processes, and gradually incorporated relevant literature (e.g., theoretical perspectives on transition; Charmaz, 2006). We used diagramming (Lofland, Snow, Anderson, & Lofland, 2006) throughout data generation and analysis to help us understand the relationships between and within the emerging processes.

Criteria for Rigor

The criteria and techniques we used to evaluate the rigor of this study were a combination of those deemed to be important for (a) qualitative research in general, (b) constructivist approaches, and (c) grounded theory methodology. Techniques to establish reflexivity, transparency, authenticity, and credibility (Ballinger, 2004; Beck, 1993; Charmaz, 2006; Chiovitti & Piran, 2003; Guba & Lincoln, 1989) included peer debriefing, reflexive journal entries, postinterview notes, an audit trail, theoretical sampling, memoing, constant comparison methods, triangulation, and member checking.

The paradigm of our research was constructivist, and assumed multiple realities; consequently, the repeatability of the research itself was not relevant (Sandelowksi, 1993). However, techniques traditionally associated with repeatability and confirmability, such as triangulation and member checks, were used and conceptualized according to a constructivist perspective. Our use of member checking facilitated a fuller understanding of the experiences of participants. The preliminary theoretical framework was shared with five caregivers (who had participated in earlier interviews) to explore whether or not their experiences of transition were reflected in the emergent framework. Caregivers reported being able to "see" their own experience of transition in the processes presented. In addition, the framework was further refined to reflect the

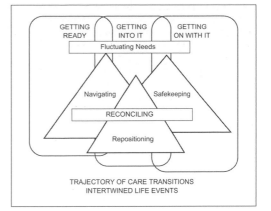

Figure 1. Theoretical framework of reconciling

feedback from these participants. For example, the phase of getting ready was focused on largely relative to the physical and environmental preparations that must be made throughout transition; however, during reflections about the findings presented, caregivers discussed the need to be mentally and emotionally prepared during the phase of getting ready. On returning to the data generated for the study and considering participant experiences, emotional aspects of this phase and the framework in general were explored more fully and included in the final theoretical framework. Similarly, we used triangulation not to confirm existing data, but rather to enhance completeness (Redfern & Norman, 1994). This was achieved through our use of in-depth interviews, observations, and detailed field notes.

The University of Western Ontario Ethics Board for Health Sciences Research Involving Human Subjects (HSREB) and the hospital ethics board at the GRU approved the procedures for interviewing and consent. Participants received a detailed letter of information (LOI) and were informed that they had the right to withdraw from the study at any time. Direct and clear wording in the LOI indicated that participant information would be treated confidentially and used only for the purposes of the study. Participants were informed that there would be no identifiable individual data in published findings, and participants' names and other identifying demographic information would be altered to ensure participants' anonymity.

Findings
Overall Framework: Reconciling

The findings from this study describe the basic social process of reconciling (see Figure 1) enacted by caregivers to integrate and merge the dissonance between their past and present knowledge, skills, roles, relationships (e.g., marital relationships), beliefs, routines, and life circumstances. Reconciling occurred

- Within a context shaped by a trajectory of prior care transitions and intertwined life events
- Across three overlapping phases: getting ready, getting into it, and getting on with it
- Through three subprocesses: navigating, safekeeping, and repositioning

Reconciling captures spousal caregivers' interactions with their husband's or wife's health care providers, families, and friends, and advances a theoretical understanding of the strategies caregivers used during their relative's transition from the GRU to home. The following excerpt from Eileen, who cared for her husband with dementia, illustrates the basic social process of reconciling:

> But you adjust somehow. It's amazing what you can adjust to, it's amazing how you can say, "Well, this is the way it is." I'm not a person that goes around feeling bitter or down or depressed or anything like that, you just deal with what you got dealt, as they say. So it's just getting, my getting used to somebody who moves differently. I mean it takes him a long time to get up out of his chair, and to get to the bathroom or to the bedroom. And I have to allow for that. I can't operate mentally in the same way that I used to because it ain't going to happen. It's different now.

Why did caregivers engage in reconciling? They did so in response to fluctuating needs, including the physical, medical, emotional, and social needs of the caregivers themselves, their spouse, and the marital dyad. Caregivers' needs included information, skills, and directives about medications and medical aspects of care (e.g., how to use a condom catheter); exercise regimes; cognitive impairment; dementia; transportation options; services in the community (e.g., how to "get out" in public with their spouse and the walker; caregiver respite; how to connect with other caregivers); food preparation (e.g., how to prepare low-sodium food); how to work through their own emotions of anxiety, guilt, and feeling unappreciated; and finally, their own social needs and those of their partner. Needs fluctuated for a variety of reasons. Prior to leaving the GRU, during the phase of getting into it, several caregivers did not discuss a lot of needs; however, once caregivers were home with their husband or wife and were getting into it, needs surfaced and caregivers realized they were missing essential knowledge required to care for their spouse or themselves. In some cases, changing circumstances, such as declining function or increased depression, necessitated the need for information about the decline or how to cope with the psychological changes caregivers were observing.

Understanding the Context
That Shapes the Process of Reconciling

As depicted in Figure 1, reconciling from the GRU to home was embedded within (a) a trajectory of prior care and resultant health care setting transitions, and (b) the context of ongoing intertwined life events that were often the result of the caregivers' own aging-related experiences.

Reconciling within the context of a trajectory of care transitions. During the first interview (generally 48 hours prior to the discharge of their spouse) it became apparent that even though caregivers were in the midst of preparing to take their spouse home from the GRU, they were still coping with issues that occurred in other health care settings. For instance, Tony spent much time reflecting on his experiences during the time his wife was in acute care. During this period he was told that his wife would likely not survive, but that if she did she would require long-term care. Although neither of these scenarios materialized, during the first interview with Tony, he was still reconciling these experiences:

> The rough time, the really, really rough time was when she was at [acute care unit], when she was really sick. That was the rough time. I mean, many a time I'd come home crying, and I would just lay in bed and just let it go.

Similarly, to understand how Marie experienced the GRU-to-home transition, it was critical to understand the context of the multiple care settings from which she and her husband had emerged. A year before Marie's first interview, her husband was admitted to acute care and then discharged to a long-term care facility under the following circumstances, as explained by Marie:

> Yeah because they wouldn't do nothing [at acute care]. And then they, the bed come up at [nursing home], which I didn't want but you can't say no. They said you have no say, if a bed comes and you refuse it you pay for the hospital bed. And I couldn't refuse it, I had nothing to say, he had to go. Wherever they said, what they come up with. So I had to sign and let him go there.

Marie worked steadily from that point forward to get her husband home, and part of that work was getting him into the GRU. She explained her struggle:

> Well there's a lot in the family that didn't want me to bring him, but I said, "No, he's coming home.

He's not staying. Why would he have to stay in there," I said? It's not for him. All the while he's okay, he's got his mind now, why would I put him in there to stay? I wanted him home with me, I really missed him. So I would never ask her [sister], or anyone else. I'd have to figure it out myself, that's the only way you can do things. You can't rely on anyone. I can't. I can't depend on anyone. I have people tell me I'm selfish. Do you think I'm selfish for wanting to bring him home?

Marie's decision to work toward having her husband at home influenced her experience of reconciling during the transition from the GRU to home, namely the lack of support she received from her family, who did not think she should be caring for her husband at home. Consequently, her experience of reconciling from the GRU to home was shaped by a lack of support, a feeling of isolation, and her decision not to rely on anyone. Understanding the process of reconciling for caregivers is a matter of placing the GRU-to-home transition within the context of where they have come "from."

Reconciling within the context of intertwined life events. It was not only the multiple care transitions that were most salient in shaping the process of reconciling; rather, caregivers were reconciling within a context of ongoing, intertwined life events (i.e., intertwined with GRU-to-home transitions). These interwoven life events often involved larger life transitions such as relocating their home to new living circumstances (e.g., downsizing to an apartment or condominium); coping with their own health issues, illnesses, and transitions within their own marriage; and other family and friend relationships. Individual caregiving circumstances meant that some caregivers were relocating to new living circumstances, coping with an alcoholic partner or the death of a child, and handling adverse relationships with other family members. These intertwined life events served to facilitate or undermine reconciling. For several years prior to the interview Jessica had been dealing with her husband, who was an alcoholic. This "dealing with" influenced tremendously her experience of reconciling. Jessica revealed what it was like to be home with her husband after the admission to the GRU:

Well it's probably a lot calmer. See, I haven't told you [that] the initiating problem here was acute alcoholism, and so life hasn't been very peaceful. And now he's been off it for four months, and he's also been on antidepressants, so he's not as he was, so he's not as difficult and cranky to deal with. He's much calmer. Certainly so that makes it easier, yeah. So however, it's nice to see him sober for a change.

Relocating to smaller living arrangements was paramount for several caregivers. Some caregivers were in the process of relocating while their spouses were on the GRU, whereas others had moved just prior to the GRU admission. In addition, caregivers were reconciling within a context shaped by their own ongoing health and illness experiences. Declines in the their own health and function were a very real worry, because many knew that if something happened to them, their spouse would end up in long-term care. Sean expressed his worry: "The only concerns that I got right now, dear, is if I stay healthy. That's my biggest concern." A detailed examination of contextual forces shaping the process of reconciling enabled us to increase our understanding of the meanings of past forces on transitions. In the next sections we describe the three phases of reconciling.

Three Phases of Reconciling

Each of the three phases of reconciling (getting ready, getting into it, getting on with it) was differentiated by (a) the saliency of each subprocess (i.e., navigating, safekeeping, and repositioning) within a phase, and (b) the patterns among the subprocesses engaged in within each phase across time. The three phases, though not mutually exclusive on a time scale, corresponded approximately to spousal caregivers' experiences prior to discharge home (i.e., getting ready), the first 2 to 3 weeks home postdischarge (i.e., getting into it), and several weeks postdischarge (i.e., getting on with it). The phases were not necessarily linear, but rather overlapped one another. Movement from one phase to another was subtle, particularly the shift between getting into it and getting on with it.

The first phase of reconciling, getting ready, was characterized by spousal caregivers' multifaceted preparations, including physical, emotional, and environmental, which were aimed at optimizing the care provided for their spouses. Tony explained:

There's getting ready emotionally, getting ready physically, and then getting the house ready. 'Cause a lot of people coming out of [the GRU], you have to make a lot of changes to the house. So to me, getting ready can be multifaceted.

For the most part, caregivers were pleased to be taking their spouse home. However, they also were aware of how difficult it would be and aware of the need to prepare themselves emotionally. Jack revealed how, in some ways, it was easier for him to have his wife on the GRU: "I didn't have to worry about caring for her [at home] . . . so actually going to the hospital was easier for me, because I didn't have to look after her." In the getting-ready phase, spousal caregivers were juggling numerous pieces of information and were meeting with a range of health care providers. This occurred while they prepared themselves emotionally for their spouse to return home and made needed physical changes to their home to ensure safety (e.g., installed wheelchair ramps, grab bars, and so forth).

The second phase of reconciling, getting into it, began when husbands or wives were discharged home and spousal caregivers assumed the majority of care. The preparations and knowledge gleaned (or not) influenced caregivers on a day-to-day basis. The getting-into-it phase was the busiest of the three phases for caregivers, during which time they coped with multiple demands surrounding care for their spouse.

Movement from the second phase of getting into it to the third phase of getting on with it was relatively insidious. The third phase of reconciling, getting on with it, represented a subtle shift from a focus that included GRU-related issues, such as illness and impairments, to a focus on striving for predictability, enabling the social health of their spouse and shifting the care boundaries that caregivers set previously for themselves. The phase of getting on with it was demarcated by the focus of caregivers on not just the medical aspects of care, but rather on a distinct attention to facilitate and enable opportunities for social participation both within and outside of the home for themselves, their spouse, and them as a couple. The three phases, and the second and third in particular, are best explained and understood through an exploration of the various subprocesses enacted by spouses during this care transition.

Subprocesses Enacted Across Phases of Reconciling

Caregivers were reconciling through the three phases by enacting three interdependent subprocesses including navigating, safekeeping, and repositioning. These three subprocesses encompassed a range of strategies that changed over time, in response to the fluctuating needs of caregivers, the needs of their spouse, and their marriage. A brief overview of each subprocess and associated strategies is provided in the following section; however, a more detailed discussion of these subprocesses can be found in Byrne (2008), and will be the topic of forthcoming articles.

Navigating. Navigating emerged as a subprocess whereby caregivers were locating, evaluating, creating, and integrating past and current sources of knowledge. Through navigating, caregivers were reconciling previous knowledge with new knowledge needed to care for their spouse, themselves individually, and as a couple. Navigating was accomplished through three strategies, including negotiating paths to knowledge formulation, maneuvering obstacles, and making decisions. Caregivers negotiated paths that were merging, connecting, and diverging toward the formulation of the knowledge base they needed. A merging path resulted when caregivers used knowledge and skills gleaned from previous experiences with health care providers and/or providing care for their spouse.

Connecting paths resulted when caregivers received much-needed new knowledge to meet the needs of their spouse, themselves, and the marital dyad. Kathleen explained:

> Yeah, that you got all, because usually when you leave the hospital they give you your list of prescriptions to get filled and everything. But I think if your husband isn't walking great, well, you have to have a walker and things; for the bathroom to sit on, he's got a higher seat to sit on, and he's got a seat in the bathtub for when he's getting a bath. He doesn't have to stand all the time, and he has safety bars all around the shower to hold on to. But they did ask me at the GRU what I had and what I didn't have, to make sure I had everything.

Divergent paths, conversely, resulted when caregivers did not receive needed knowledge. Paths were divergent when knowledge for caregivers was absent, incorrect, difficult to understand, conflicting, or when it is was provided at the wrong time:

> But just somebody to say, "How are you doing? How are things going? Is there anything you need that you're not getting?" and just like I could use somebody, I mean, somebody to come in and help with the housework, to clean, and but, just some support for caregivers, that's what you need, and I don't think it's available, to get it in terms of your, of your needs for your client. But there's no support for the caregiver. Does that make sense? Yeah, like this is what I did when I had this, or has anybody got any suggestions for that, or just a time to have a cup of coffee with somebody that's going through the same thing.

In response to these diverging paths, caregivers maneuvered obstacles by taking actions such as sorting multiple sources of knowledge, looking for directions, and learning through experiences. Jessica explained:

> And here's CCAC [community care access center], and everybody was coming in to his room at once. And um, so I came home and I had to sit down immediately and make out huge charts of, especially his medication chart, and uh, who was coming when, and try to sort out all this information that I got, that last day, which might have been perhaps a good idea to have had that a couple days before he went home, so I'd have time to work it out. But anyway I got it straightened away.

Caregivers made decisions based on the information and services that were available, and based on what was perceived as best for their husband or wife or themselves. Several caregivers turned down services they were offered because the services did not meet their specific needs, or they felt that the services were not needed. Deborah commented on her decision to not accept help from Meals on Wheels (an organization that provides home-delivered meals):

And the social worker said what about Meals on Wheels, and I said oh no, I'm not going to sit and wait for somebody, if it's snowing. Well last week there was no Meals on Wheels, nobody got meals, it stopped. So I said, Meals on Wheels, I says no, I said I'm quite capable. So we eat when we want to, not because we have to. No, no, no they did send somebody down and were insisting on home, Meals on Wheels, and somebody to do your laundry. And I thought God's sake, no—I'd be sitting here waiting for somebody, I'd have it done.

Elements of navigating changed over time across phases. For example, during the phase of getting ready, caregivers most often faced an absence of sources of knowledge related to how their spouse would progress once discharged from the GRU, and which types of services would be received in the home. However, during the phase of getting into it, caregivers often did not have information about medications, dietary restrictions, and home care services, among other service related information. It was only once their spouse was discharged home, and care was placed squarely on the shoulders of the caregivers, that the caregivers then realized the extent of what they did not know.

Safekeeping. Safekeeping, the second subprocess of reconciling, highlights how caregivers protected, promoted, and enhanced the emotional, physical, and social health of their spouse. Caregivers engaged in safekeeping when there was a risk or perceived threat to their spouse's safety, or to the maintenance of or improvement in physical, emotional, or social health and well-being. Three strategies were used by caregivers during safekeeping, including advocating, shielding, and enabling physical and social health. Caregivers advocated on behalf of their spouse by challenging health care providers or other family members to ensure that their spouse received proper care and requisite services. Sean discussed how he felt the home care services were not meeting his wife's needs, and how he was handling the situation:

Yeah, they do, some of them are pretty good, but there's more of them that are just, I don't know. They, they come in and they just, sometimes I wonder if they, see they're supposed to brush her teeth, they're supposed to comb her hair, they're supposed to give her a, a sponge bath if she doesn't get in the

tub, and they're supposed to give her a bath twice a week, and I got after them last week. She had two baths last week, but I got after them because I wanted her, her bathed twice a week at least, a sponge bath. A sponge bath is not the same as a shower or baths, is it, eh? They're not doing, there's a couple of them there is not doing their job, I'll tell you that right now, and one of these days I'm going to get mad. I don't get mad, but when I do . . . .

In addition, caregivers, particularly for individuals with cognitive impairment or dementia, shielded the emotional health of their spouse. During interviews, caregivers did not want to discuss aspects of dementia while their spouse was present, stating that they did not talk about the "memory problems" or use the word *dementia* in front of him or her. For instance, while interviewing Marie, she stated,

Yeah, well I'm hoping the Aricept [medication] will keep on working. And they're always coming out with new drugs [lowers her voice and looks at husband who is sitting across the room]. I don't talk to him too much about it, so . . . .

Observations revealed that caregivers shielded their partners from the interview process itself. This manifested, for example, as whispering or speaking in lowered, hushed tones during the interview. Enabling emerged as a strategy by which caregivers promoted, demanded, facilitated, or encouraged courses of action to benefit the physical and/or social health of their spouse and themselves. Jack explained:

And it's quite easy to say, well, the caregiver to say, well the heck with the exercises, why bother? Or well, I'm going out, I'll bring someone in to look after you, and don't push, or let's go ourselves. You got to do a lot of pushing to get the person going. That's another thing I think a lot of people find difficult.

Enabling was intended to keep partners safe, to serve as a limit on caregivers' own worry and anxiety, and to meet the social needs of both their spouse and themselves. Several instances of enabling were observed while the first author was present in caregivers' homes. For instance, Patrick instructed his wife to uncross her legs, whereas Nicholas demonstrated to his wife how and when she should keep the brakes on her walker. Enabling health was affected by the knowledge barriers faced by caregivers. Kevin explained how not knowing influenced his ability to enable the physical health of his wife:

I don't know when to push her. She gets out here and takes her walker and walks to the end of the driveway and back, and then she says, "I'm tired." I don't know whether to say, "Do it again." Who am I to say that when she says she's tired? Unless I knew what I was doing, and I don't, I can't say that to her. I said, "Honey, leave it up to the day hospital. Whatever they tell you, that's what you should be doing."

Safekeeping manifested differently across phases depending on the strategy employed by caregivers. For instance, one of the major differences between the phases of getting into it and getting on with it was that spousal caregivers shifted from a focus of enabling physical health to a focus on enabling social health. Once caregivers mastered enabling physical health they began enabling social health for their spouse and themselves by engaging in social outings.

Repositioning. Repositioning, the third subprocess, was used by caregivers to alter, shift, and modify either temporarily or permanently their geographical space and place, relationships, and social positions. Positions for caregivers included locations, roles, beliefs, and attitudes, and encompassed geographical, emotional, and social aspects. Caregivers engaged in repositioning to reconcile the dissonance between past and present beliefs, and roles regarding, for example, what their marriages "used to be like" in relation to what their relationship was currently like. Repositioning strategies included vowing to care, anticipating, shifting the boundaries, and striving for predictability. The strategy of vowing to care was permeated with beliefs that providing care was part of the duty to the couple's relationship. Sean talked about caring for his wife with dementia:

Well, I, I, geez, that's, why do I do it? Why do I do it? Well, the way I look at it is, I've been married to her now for 52 years. I love the woman, and that's probably why I do it. I got, I don't find no other reason to do it, that's just, that's the reason, that's the reason why I do it, because I don't want to see nothing happen to her, or anything like that, as far as that, at least I hope not. And if I could do anything for her I'd gladly do it, if I could help her in any way, even if I can help her, you know, get rid of this dementia or Alzheimer's [disease], but I can't do that. The only one that can do that is the one up above. I can't do that. I just got to do the best I can and live with it.

In some cases, caregivers discussed how they repositioned their relationship from that as husband and wife to that of parent and child or brother and sister. Caregivers described power differentials that developed within their relationship, role reversals, absent sexual relationships, and the need to learn how to operate as a single person. Changes to the spousal relationship, despite vowing to care, were not always viewed positively, but as an occurrence that had to happen out of necessity. It was difficult for caregivers to accept and cope with changing marital relationships from emotional perspectives. Irene explained: "I think because now he's become sort of like the child and I'm the parent. And I don't like that situation. I'd like to be an equal partner."

Anticipating emerged as a second strategy whereby caregivers envisioned immediate and long-term situations. Anticipating was critical to the entire process of reconciling, because it "paved the way" for merging and integrating past, present, and potential future circumstances. Anticipating was related to several other processes. As examples, caregivers anticipated what types of safekeeping they would engage in once home. They anticipated what kinds of activities they would enable once home. They anticipated the need for routines, and used anticipation as a strategy for maneuvering barriers (e.g., planning or waiting to look for directions). Without the proper sources of knowledge, or without understanding of information received, caregivers had a difficult time anticipating. For example, caregivers were unsure as to how their spouse would progress once home, and without information about potential progress once home from GRU team members it was difficult to anticipate what the coming situations (i.e., at home with their spouse) would entail.

Shifting the boundaries emerged as a third strategy of setting and shifting limits for "self" based on beliefs, feelings, and comfort levels. Caregivers adjusted their own activities outside of the home for fear that something bad would happen while they were gone, and/or for fear that their spouse would feel neglected if left on his or her own. During the phase of getting on with it, men and women differed in their responses relative to the strategy of shifting the boundaries, particularly for their own activities and participation. Men expressed the desire and the need for their own social life outside the marriage. Kevin illustrated how, although he wanted to participate in activities with his wife, he still needed to have his own life within the marriage:

We are definitely going to go to join something. I think it would be beneficial for my wife and could be beneficial for me to meet some people. What I gather is that the men go off and play darts and the women play euchre [game] or whatever they do. I think it's kind of necessary for caregivers and their spouses to get a little separate time from each other. My wife has always been insecure. If I go anywhere, she wants to come with me. If I am going to Canadian Tire she'll say, can I come? Sometimes I would like to go to be by myself. Part of my wife's being hospitalized, I would take walks by myself around the grounds of the hospital. I miss a lot of the male comradeship now, just don't have time for it really.

For women, however, guilt persisted about leaving their husband alone, even as time since discharge progressed. One month postdischarge, Phyllis explained:

Because it sort of hurts and it's an effort he doesn't want to particularly do it, so. Like for instance, he said, well my daughter asked us out for New Year's. [He said], "I couldn't go out again, I just, I'm not gonna go. You go." But uh, whether I'll go or not, I don't know, cause I'll feel badly leaving him. So I might go for a couple of hours or something.

Striving for predictability emerged as the fourth strategy, which included integrating predictable courses of action into day-to-day life. Caregivers were striving for predictability in response to the need for order and routine.

While spouses were on the GRU, most caregivers took daily trips to the hospital as a means of maintaining normalcy and providing emotional comfort for their spouse and for themselves. Once home, caregivers strove for predictability to integrate previous daily patterns, with the need to establish new patterns such as incorporating exercise regimes and new diets or, for some caregivers, making their spouse incorporate their assistive devices (e.g., walkers) into their life. Deborah commented, "But I have a routine that keeps me going," and Irene said, "But it's just to try and get some predictability in my routine, to know what, what's happening."

Discussion

Consistent with the aims of constructivist theorizing (Charmaz, 2006), the framework developed in this study provides a plausible account of the processes experienced by spousal caregivers during transition; highlights patterns and connections not previously considered; and provides new ways of thinking about the processes engaged in by spousal caregivers' to inform rehabilitation clinicians, researchers, and policy makers. This investigation is the first to explore the processes enacted by spousal caregivers during the transition of their relative from a GRU to home. Prior research describing the processes engaged in by family members during their relatives' hospital-to-home transition included processes directed mainly at medical aspects (Bull, 1992; Bull & Jervis, 1997) and, in a select few studies, the emotional and relational processes

involved in providing care (Bull, 1992; Shyu, 2000b, 2000c). However, none of the authors of the resulting articles mentioned the social aspects of providing care, such as enabling social health of the care recipients, or setting and shifting boundaries for their own social participation, as was identified in our findings. Reconciling was not simply about integrating past and present medical care routines or engaging in the more medical and physical aspects of caregiving, but rather reflected a strong emotional and social component, as well. This has not been addressed adequately in prior research. The needs, processes, and strategies engaged in by spousal caregivers highlight the medical, physical, emotional, and social elements of reconciling, and the biopsychosocial nature of care transitions as experienced by spousal caregivers.

Furthermore, in a theory of transition developed by Meleis and colleagues (2000), several patterns of transition, including single, multiple, sequential, simultaneous, related, or unrelated, are discussed. These patterns characterize the potential multiplicity and complexity of transitions as identified in their theory. Our framework supports the multidimensional and complex nature of transitions put forth by Meleis et al., and our findings show the influence of multiple sequential (health care setting transitions) and simultaneous (relocating, declining health of caregiver, changing spousal relationship) transitions on the experience of the transition from hospital to home (i.e., process of reconciling). It is the patterns among all of these different transitions that support a comprehensive understanding of the hospital-to-home transition itself, and elucidate the complexity of the process of reconciling. For example, Phyllis' experience of reconciling from hospital to home was influenced by her own declining health as she was feeling depressed about her health while simultaneously caring for her spouse and meeting his physical needs. Trying to come to terms with the present situation was complicated by her concerns about her own physical and emotional health.

Although the present study incorporated only a single care transition (i.e., from GRU to home), it highlights how experiences during prior health care setting trajectories influenced caregivers' engagement in the process of reconciling. This was particularly salient for caregivers who almost lost their spouse in acute care health settings, or who had particularly stressful experiences in acute care. In a study exploring caregivers' experiences of transition to long-term care, Reuss, Dupuis, and Whitfield (2005) reported that many of the families in their study (including spousal caregivers) experienced multiple transfers between different settings prior to their relatives' placement in a long-term care facility. They called for longitudinal research to explore the experiences of multiple transitions for families and their relatives. Our study supports this contention, and provides insight into one of the many potential care transitions (hospital to home) that can precede caregivers' experiences of the transfer of their relative to long-term care.

The process of reconciling identified in the present study was influenced not only by a range of caregiving contexts, but also by caregivers' experiences of intertwined life events. For example, in our findings, the death of a family member, marital discord, and conflicts with other family members influenced caregivers' experiences of reconciling. Intertwined life events share similarities with the concept of "linked lives" in Elder's life course theory, which addresses the interdependent nature of social life and relationships (Elder, 1998; Elder & Johnson, 2003). The emergence of the influence of intertwined life events during the transition from the GRU has important implications for the need to explore the experiences of older adults (65 and older) providing care during their older adult relatives' transition from hospital to home. Older adult caregivers are an underrepresented group of caregivers in other studies of hospital-to-home transitions. Spousal caregivers were experiencing transitions in other aspects of life that are common to aging individuals, such as relocation (Firbank & Johnson-Lafleur, 2007). Intertwined life events influenced the transition. For example, if caregivers had relocated recently, then they had greater difficulty reconciling, particularly with regard to striving for predictability. In addition, anticipating the need for relocation was perceived as stressful for some caregivers, especially if it involved the placement of their spouse in long-term care. Declining self-health was another key consideration regarding the process of reconciling for older adult caregivers, because they worried about whether or not their health status would allow them to provide care for their husband or wife. Moreover, the older adult caregivers worried about who would care for their husband or wife if they could not do so in the future because of their own declining health. Our study, unlike other research about care transitions, emphasized these unique aspects of care transitions experienced by older adult spousal caregivers.

Our findings contribute to the growing body of literature aimed at demonstrating the importance of needs assessments for family caregivers (Guberman, Keefe, Fancey, & Barylak, 2007; Nolan, Lundh, Grant, & Keady, 2003) by illustrating the fluctuating medical, physical, emotional, and social needs of spousal caregivers during the transition of their relative from the GRU to home. However, in addition to assessing caregiver needs, the strategies engaged in during hospital-to-home transitions might be an important part of a comprehensive caregiver assessment, and could be amenable to intervention (e.g., when caregivers were informed, they were able to enable physical health). Whereas the assessment of "needs" is

critical, recognizing that caregivers are engaging in multiple strategies to meet these needs during the transition from hospital to home also is essential. In addition to the changing types of needs of caregivers over time (Bull, 1990; Grimmer et al., 2004; Shyu, 2000b), our findings highlight how needs fluctuate in intensity over time. Several caregivers reported low levels of need prior to leaving the GRU, but once they returned home with their spouse their needs intensified. Thus, whereas the GRU is an ideal place in the continuum of care to ascertain caregiver needs, the process of needs assessment itself needs to be ongoing, not a one-time endeavor.

Aside from shielding, which caregivers to spouses with CI or dementia engaged in more frequently than other caregivers, the types of processes enacted by spousal caregivers to individuals with CI or dementia were relatively similar to those engaged in by caregivers to individuals without CI or dementia. However, the intensity of the need to engage in the processes differentiated these two groups. Caregivers of individuals with dementia often discussed more unknowns, particularly around the disease progression and disease-related medications. These caregivers required increased efforts to navigate, and needed to create a knowledge base that was much more diverse than that required of the other caregivers. These two findings are consistent with the broader caregiving–dementia literature which highlights that caregiving for those with dementia often is more demanding than caring for individuals without dementia (Ory, Hoffman, Yee, Tennstedt, & Schulz, 1999). The care recipients in this study who had dementia were in the mild-to-moderate clinical stages, as is the case for the majority of those on geriatric rehabilitation units (Wells, Seabrook, Stolee, Borrie, & Knoefel, 2003). Therefore, different experiences for those caring for individuals with and without CI or dementia might not be as salient within the context of this study.

Although gender differences are not identified in transitional care literature, research in the broader caregiving literature suggests that for caregiving wives, the exchange of emotional support with their care recipient husbands is related to decreased caregiver burden and higher levels of marital satisfaction, and that wife caregivers are more depressed and report higher levels of burden (Pruchno & Resch, 1989; Wright & Aquilino, 1998). In our study, both men and women discussed changes to their relationships; however, women were more apt to comment on the loss of conversation, missing how "life used to be," were more apt to discuss power differentials that developed within their relationship, and were more likely to identify shifts from partnership in marriage to dependency (e.g., Eileen, who described her relationship as akin to a parent–child relationship). This finding is similar to those of Jansson, Nordberg, and Grafstrom (2001), who reported that spousal caregivers undergo a transition from being an equal partner in marriage to "caregiver," requiring caregivers to sacrifice their own time to take care of their husband or wife. These findings point to a need for health care professionals to work with both husband and wife caregivers, paying careful attention to the emotional and relationship needs of caregiving wives, and ensuring that both men and, particularly women spousal caregivers, are assisted in shifting the boundaries they set for themselves around their own activities and participation.

Two prominent care-transition interventions for patients (Coleman et al., 2004; Naylor et al., 2004; Parry, Coleman, Smith, Frank, & Kramer, 2003) have demonstrated promising results for patient (e.g., positive perception of quality of care) and health care system outcomes (decreased rehospitalization). Whereas family caregivers were identified as integral to the success of both interventions, and were involved in the implementation of these interventions, their experiences with the transition intervention and their outcomes were not included. The effectiveness of these interventions for influencing caregiver experiences or outcomes during the transition of relatives from hospital to home is not known. Coleman and Williams (2007) proposed an approach to involve caregivers in transitional care that defined the type and intensity of roles that caregivers play; namely, the types of contributions caregivers make, including financial, advocacy, care coordination, emotional support, and direct care provision (creating the acronym FACED). Acknowledging the role of caregivers, and providing information to health care providers about the contributions of caregivers, is important to transitional care. What has not been emphasized adequately in this approach is how the care transition and potential transition interventions influence outcomes specific to caregivers, such as their own feelings of preparation and physical, psychological, and social health. Caregivers have their own unmet needs that occur during transition. A focus for future studies might include how to fulfill caregivers' needs, and to help them engage in the strategies they are using to care for their spouse, themselves, and the marital dyad. Such a focus would be critical to the design of interventions aimed at improving caregiver-specific outcomes.

Shyu and colleagues (2008) designed a caregiver-oriented transition intervention that included individualized health education, follow-up phone calls, and home visits for family caregivers following the discharge of their relative from a hospital setting. They demonstrated how focusing on caregiver-specific needs resulted in better self-evaluations of preparation, and better satisfaction of discharge needs after the intervention. Our theoretical framework might be useful to inform the development of future caregiver-oriented interventions during transition from a GRU to home, aimed at helping caregivers with what they are "doing" during transitions. For instance, interventions aimed at helping caregivers to navigate, safekeep, and reposition, with a focus on ways to enhance and improve the strategies engaged in by caregivers, would provide meaningful and useful skills and approaches.

Although the purpose of the present study was to highlight the experiences of spousal caregivers through transition from a GRU to home, a potential limitation is that the care recipient spouse was not interviewed. Changes in the nature of the relationship between caregivers and care recipients during the transition from hospital to home have been identified in previous studies (Shyu, 2000b, 2000c). In addition, our limited consideration of the complexity of social networks—in particular how the social interactions between spousal caregivers; care recipients and other family members (e.g., adult children); friends; and formal care providers might shape the phases and processes of reconciliation—is a limitation. Future research should expand the focus to include other individuals in the social networks of spousal caregivers to understand better the complexity of interactions and processes involved during care transitions. Our research provides insight into the importance of considering the trajectory of multiple care transitions experienced by caregivers. However, further research is needed that incorporates a longitudinal perspective whereby caregivers are recruited in acute care settings and followed through multiple care transitions across the care continuum. Another limitation, and an implication for future research, is that our study did not include caregivers from a range of cultural backgrounds, thereby limiting a consideration of how the experiences and processes might be different for caregivers in non-Western cultures (Li & Shyu, 2007).

The theoretical framework developed in this study provides a means of understanding the relationships and patterns among the processes engaged in by caregivers during the period of their relative's transition from a GRU to home. Helping caregivers to reconcile and meet their transitional-based needs will require a commitment on the part of both GRU team members and community health care professionals. The theoretical framework provides a resource to health care scientists, health care clinicians, educators, and decision makers regarding how they must work together to improve transitional care for spousal caregivers.

Acknowledgments

We thank the caregivers, GRU clinicians, and research team for their invaluable contributions to the study. The guidance and support of Ingrid Connidis and Margaret Cheesman is also acknowledged. We thank Catherine Craven for her help with the preparation of this article.

Authors' Note

Portions of this article were presented at the Canadian Association on Gerontology conference, October, 2008, London, Canada, and the British Society of Gerontology conference, September 2009, Bristol, United Kingdom.

Declaration of Conflicting Interests

The authors declared no conflicts of interest with respect to the authorship and/or publication of this article.

Funding

The authors disclosed receipt of the following financial support for the research and/or authorship of this article: Dr. Byrne was funded by a doctoral award from the Social Sciences and Humanities Research Council of Canada, and a Graduate Research Award from the Alzheimer Society of London Middlesex.

Note

1.   All participant names are pseudonyms.

References

Aminzadeh, F., Byszewski, A., Dalziel, W. B., Wilson, M., Deane, N., & Papahariss-Wright, S. (2005). Effectiveness of outpatient geriatric assessment programs: Exploring caregiver needs, goals, and outcomes. *Journal of Gerontological Nursing, 31*(12), 19-25. Retrieved from http://www.jognonline.com/view.asp?rid=4673

Ballinger, C. (2004). Writing up rigour: Representing and evaluating good scholarship in qualitative research. *British Journal of Occupational Therapy, 67,* 540-546. Retrieved from http://www.ingentaconnect.com/content/cot/bjot/2004/00000067/00000012/art00004

Barnes, B., Given, C., & Given, B. (1992). Caregivers of elderly relatives: Spouses and adult children. *Health and Social Work, 17,* 282-289. Retrieved from http://www.ncbi.nlm.nih.gov/pubmed/1478554

Beck, C. T. (1993). Qualitative research: The evaluation of its credibility, fittingness and auditability. *Western Journal of Nursing Research, 15,* 263-266. doi:10.1177/019394599301500212

Bogardus, S. T., Jr., Bradley, E. H., Williams, C. S., Maciejewski, P. K., Gallo, W. T., & Inouye, S. K. (2004). Achieving goals in geriatric assessment: Role of caregiver agreement and adherence to recommendations. *Journal of the American Geriatrics Society, 52,* 99-105. doi:10.1111/j.1532-5415.2004.52017

Bradley, E. H., Bogardus, S. T., Jr., van Doorn, C., Williams, C. S., Cherlin, E., & Inouye, S. K. (2000). Goals in geriatric assessment: Are we measuring the right outcomes? *Gerontologist, 40,* 191-196. doi:10.1093/geront/40.2.191

Braun, M., Mikulincer, M., Rydall, A., Walsh, A., & Rodin, G. (2007). Hidden morbidity in cancer: Spouse caregivers. *Clinical Oncology, 25,* 4829-4834. doi:10.1200/JCO.2006.10.0909

Bull, M. J. (1990). Factors influencing family caregiver burden and health. *Western Journal of Nursing Research, 12,* 758-770. doi:10.1177/019394599001200605

Bull, M. J. (1992). Managing the transition from hospital to home. *Qualitative Health Research, 2,* 27-41. doi:10.1177/104973239200200103

Bull, M. J., & Jervis, L. L. (1997). Strategies used by chronically ill older women and their caregiving daughters in managing posthospital care. *Journal of Advanced Nursing, 25,* 541-547. doi:10.1046/j.1365-2648.1997.1997025541

Bull, M. J., Maruyama, G., & Luo, D. (1995). Testing a model for posthospital transition of family caregivers for elderly persons. *Nursing Research, 44,* 132-138. Retrieved from http://journals.lww.com/nursingresearchonline/Abstract/1995/05000/Testing_a_Model_for_Posthospital_Transition_of.2.aspx

Bull, M. J., & McShane, R. E. (2008). Seeking what's best during the transition to adult day health services. *Qualitative Health Research, 18,* 597-605. doi:10.1177/1049732308315174

Byrne, K. (2008). *Spousal caregivers' during their husbands'/wives' transition from a GRU to home.* (Unpublished doctoral dissertation). University of Western Ontario, London, ON, Canada.

Chappell, N. L. (1992). *Social support and aging.* Toronto, ON, Canada: Butterworths.

Charmaz, K. (2006). *Constructing grounded theory: A practical guide through qualitative analysis.* Thousand Oaks, CA: Sage.

Chick, N., & Meleis, A. I. (1986). Transitions: A nursing concern. In P.L. Chinn (Ed.), *Nursing research methodology: Issues and implementation* (pp. 237-257). Rockville, MD: Aspen.

Chiovitti, R. F., & Piran, N. (2003). Rigour and grounded theory research. *Journal of Advanced Nursing, 44,* 427-435. doi:10.1046/j.0309-2402.2003.02822

Coleman, E. A., Boult, C., & American Geriatrics Society Health Care Systems Committee. (2003). Improving the quality of transitional care for persons with complex care needs. *Journal of the American Geriatrics Society, 51,* 556-557. doi:10.1046/j.1532-5415.2003.51186

Coleman, E. A., Smith, J. D., Frank, J. C., Min, S. J., Parry, C., & Kramer, A. M. (2004). Preparing patients and caregivers to participate in care delivered across settings: The care transitions intervention. *Journal of the American Geriatrics Society, 52,* 1817-1825. doi:10.1111/j.1532-5415.2004.52504

Coleman, E. A., & Williams, M. V. (2007). Executing high-quality care transitions: A call to do it right. *Journal of Hospital Medicine, 2,* 287-290. doi:10.1002/jhm.276

Connell, C. M., Janevic, M. R., & Gallant, M. P. (2001). The costs of caring: Impact of dementia on family caregivers. *Journal of Geriatric Psychiatry, 14,* 179-187. doi:10.1177/089198870101400403

Cutcliffe, J. R. (2000). Methodological issues in grounded theory. *Journal of Advanced Nursing, 31,* 1476-1484. doi:10.1046/j.1365-2648.2000.01430

Davies, S., & Nolan, M. (2003). 'Making the best of things': Relatives' experiences of decisions about care-home entry. *Ageing & Society, 23*, 429-450. doi:10.1017/S0144686X03001259

Davies, S., & Nolan, M. (2004). Making the move: Relatives' experiences of transition to a care home. *Health and Social Care in the Community, 12*, 517-526. doi:10.1111/j.1365-2524.2004.00535

Demers, L., Ska, B., Desrosiers, J., Alix, C., & Wolfson, C. (2004). Development of a conceptual framework for the assessment of geriatric rehabilitation outcomes. *Archives of Gerontology and Geriatrics, 38*, 221-237. doi:10.1016/j.archger.2003.10.003

Elder, G. H., Jr. (1998). The life course and human development. In R. M. Lerner (Ed.), *Handbook of child psychology: Volume 1. Theoretical models of human development* (pp. 939-991). New York: Wiley.

Elder, G. H., Jr., & Johnson, M. K. (2003). The life course and aging: Challenges, lessons, and new directions. In R. A. Setterson, Jr. (Ed.), *Invitation to the life course: Toward new understandings of later life* (pp. 48-81). Amityville, NY: Baywood.

Firbank, O. E., & Johnson-Lafleur, J. (2007). Older persons relocating with a family caregiver: Processes, stages, and motives. *Journal of Applied Gerontology, 26*, 182-207. doi:10.1177/0733464807300224

Frederick, J., & Fast, J. (1999). Eldercare in Canada. Who does how much? *Canadian Social Trends, 53*, 26-32. Retrieved from http://www.statcan.gc.ca/pub/11-008-x/1999002/article/4661-eng.pdf

Fredman, L., & Daly, M. P. (1998). Enhancing practitioner ability to recognize and treat caregiver physical and mental consequences. *Topics in Geriatric Rehabilitation, 14*, 36-44.

George, L., & Gwyther, L. (1986). Caregiver well-being: A multidimensional examination of family caregivers of demented adults. *Gerontologist, 26*, 253-259. doi:10.1093/geront/26.3.253

Grant, S., St John, W., & Patterson, E. (2009). Recovery from total hip replacement surgery: "It's not just physical." *Qualitative Health Research, 19*, 1612-1620. doi:10.1177/1049732309350683

Grimmer, K., Falco, J., & Moss, J. (2004). Becoming a carer for an elderly person after discharge from an acute hospital admission. *Internet Journal of Allied Health Sciences & Practice, 2*(4). Retrieved from http://ijahsp.nova.edu/articles/vol2num4/grimmer-carer%20issues.pdf

Grimmer, K., & Moss, J. (2001). The development, validity and application of a new instrument to assess the quality of discharge planning activities from the community perspective. *International Journal for Quality in Health Care, 13*, 109-116. Retrieved from http://intqhc.oxfordjournals.org/cgi/reprint/13/2/109

Guba, E., & Lincoln, Y. (1989). *Fourth generation evaluation.* Beverly Hills, CA: Sage.

Guberman, N., Keefe, J., Fancey, P., & Barylak, L. (2007). 'Not another form!': Lessons for implementing carer assessment in health and social service agencies. *Health and Social Care in the Community, 15*, 577-587. doi:10.1111/j.1365-2524.2007.00718.x

Hayes, J., Zimmerman, M., & Boylstein, C. (2010). Responding to the symptoms of Alzheimer's disease: Husbands, wives, and the gendered dynamics of recognition and disclosure. *Qualitative Health Research, 20*, 1101-1115. doi:10.1177/1049732310369559

Health Canada. (2002). *National profile of family caregivers in Canada—Final report.* Retrieved from http://www.hc-sc.gc.ca/hcs-sss/pubs/home-domicile/2002-caregiv-interven/index-eng.php

Hess, B. B., & Soldo, B. J. (1985). Husband and wife networks. In W. J. Sauer & R. T. Coward (Eds.), *Social support networks and the care of the elderly: Theory, research and practice* (pp. 67-92). New York: Springer.

Hills, G. A. (1998). Caregivers of the elderly: Hidden patients and health team members. *Topics in Geriatric Rehabilitation, 14*, 1-11.

Holland, D. E., & Harris, M. R. (2007). Discharge planning, transitional care, coordination of care, and continuity of care: Clarifying the concepts and terms from the hospital perspective. *Home Health Care Services Quarterly, 26*(4), 3-19. doi:10.1300/J027v26n04_02

Holtslander, L. F., & Duggleby, W. D. (2009). The hope experience of older bereaved women who cared for a spouse with terminal cancer. *Qualitative Health Research, 19*, 388-400. doi:10.1177/1049732308329682

Jacobi, C. E., van den Berg, B., Boshuizen, H. C., Rupp, I., Dinant, H. J., & van den Bos, A. M. (2003). Dimension-specific burden of caregiving among partners of rheumatoid arthritis patients. *Rheumatology, 42*, 1226-1233. doi:10.1093/rheumatology/keg366

Jansson, W., Nordberg, G., & Grafstrom, M. (2001). Patterns of elderly spousal caregiving in dementia care: An observational study. *Journal of Advanced Nursing, 34*, 804-812. Retrieved from http://www3.interscience.wiley.com/cgi-bin/fulltext/118983178/PDFSTART

Kane, R. A., Reinardy, J., Penrod, J. D., & Huck, S. (1999). After the hospitalization is over: A different perspective on family care of older people. *Journal of Gerontological Social Work, 31*, 119-141. doi:10.1300/J083v31n01_08

Kneeshaw M. F., Considine R. M., & Jennings, J. (1999). Mutuality and preparedness of family caregivers for elderly women after bypass surgery. *Applied Nursing Research, 12*, 128-135. doi:10.1016/S0897-1897(99)80034-2

Lazarus, R. S., & Folkman, S. (1984). *Stress, appraisal, and coping.* New York: Springer.

Li, H. J., & Shyu, Y. I. (2007). Coping processes of Taiwanese families during the postdischarge period for an elderly family member with hip fracture. *Nursing Science Quarterly, 20*, 273-279. doi:10.1177/0894318407303128

Lin, P. C., Hung, S. H., Liao, M. H., Sheen, S. Y., & Jong, S. Y. (2006). Care needs and level of care difficulty related to hip fractures in geriatric populations during the post-discharge transition period. *Journal of Nursing Research, 14*, 251-259. doi:10.1097/01.JNR.0000387584.89468.30

Lofland, J., Snow, D., Anderson, L., & Lofland, L. H. (2006). *Analyzing social settings: A guide to qualitative observation and analysis.* Florence, KY: Wadsworth.

Meleis, A. I., Sawyer, L. M., Im, E. O., Hilfinger Messias, D. K., & Schumacher, K. (2000). Experiencing transitions: An emerging middle-range theory. *Advances in Nursing Science, 23*, 12-28. Retrieved from http://journals.lww.com/advancesin nursingscience/Abstract/2000/09000/Experiencing_Transi tions__An_Emerging_Middle_Range.6.aspx

Morse, J. M. (2009). Exploring transitions. *Qualitative Health Research, 19*, 431.doi:10.1177/1049732308328547

Morse, J. M., & Field, P. A. (1995). *Qualitative research methods for health professionals.* Thousand Oaks, CA: Sage.

Navon, L., & Weinblatt, N. (1996). The show must go on—Behind the scenes of elderly spousal caregiving. *Journal of Aging Studies, 10*, 329-342. doi:10.1016/S0890-4065(96)90005-5

Naylor, M. D. (2000). A decade of transitional care research with vulnerable elders. *Journal of Cardiovascular Nursing, 14*(3), 1-14. Retrieved from http://ovidsp.tx.ovid.com/sp-3.2/ovid-web.cgi?&S=HLANFPLFEGDDDKLCNCDLDCGCECH NAA00&Link+Set=S.sh.15.17.22.27%7c4%7csl_10

Naylor, M. D. (2002). Transitional care of older adults. *Annual Review of Nursing Research, 20*, 127-147. Retrieved from http://www.ingentaconnect.com/content/springer/ arnr/2002/00000020/00000001/art00007

Naylor, M. D., Brooten, D. A., Campbell, R. L., Maislin, G., McCauley, K. M., & Schwartz, J. S. (2004). Transitional care of older adults hospitalized with heart failure: A randomized, controlled trial. *Journal of the American Geriatrics Society, 52*, 675-684. doi:10.1111/j.1532-5415.2004.52202.x

Naylor, M. D., Hirschman, K. B., Bowles, K. H., Bixby, M. B., Konick-McMahan, J., & Stephens, C. (2007). Care coordination for cognitively impaired older adults and their caregivers. *Home Health Care Services Quarterly, 26*(4), 57-78. doi:10.1300/J027v26n04_05

Naylor, M. D., Stephens, C., Bowles, K. H., & Bixby, M. B. (2005). Cognitively impaired older adults: From hospital to home. *American Journal of Nursing, 105*, 52-61. Retrieved from http://journals.lww.com/ajnonline/Citation/2005/ 02000/Cognitively_Impaired_Older_Adults__From_Hos pital.28.aspx

Nolan, M. R., Lundh, U., Grant, G., & Keady, J. (Eds.). (2003). *Partnerships in family care: Understanding the caregiving career.* Maidenhead, UK: Open University Press.

Ory, M. G., Hoffman, R. R., Yee, J. L., Tennstedt, S., & Schulz, R. (1999). Prevalence and impact of caregiving: A detailed comparison between dementia and nondementia caregivers. *Gerontologist, 39*, 177-185. doi:10.1093/geront/39.2.177

Parry, C., Coleman, E. A., Smith, J. D., Frank, J., & Kramer, A. M. (2003). The care transitions intervention: A patient-centered approach to ensuring effective transfers between sites of geriatric care. *Home Health Care Services Quarterly, 22*(3), 1-17. doi:10.1300/J027v22n03_01

Parry, C., Kramer, H. M., & Coleman, E. A. (2006). A qualitative exploration of a patient-centered coaching intervention to improve care transitions in chronically ill older adults. *Home Health Care Services Quarterly, 25*(3-4), 39-53. doi:10.1300/J027v25n03_03

Pearlin, L. I., Mullan, J. T., Semple, S. J., & Skaff, M. M. (1990). Caregiving and the stress process: An overview of concepts and their measures. *Gerontologist, 30*, 583-594. doi:10.1093/geront/30.5.583

Pruchno, R. A., & Resch, N. (1989). Husbands and wives as caregivers: Antecedents of depression and burden. *Gerontologist, 29*, 159-165. doi:10.1093/geront/29.2.159

Redfern, S. J., & Norman, I. J. (1994). Validity through triangulation. *Nurse Researcher, 2*, 41-56.

Reuss, G. F., Dupuis, S. L., & Whitfield, K. (2005). Understanding the experience of moving a loved one to a long-term care facility: Family members' perspectives. *Journal of Gerontological Social Work, 46*, 17-46. doi:10.1300/J083v46n01_03

Sandelowksi, M. (1993). Rigor or rigor mortis—The problem of rigor in qualitative research revisited. *Advances in Nursing Science, 16*(2), 1-8.

Schumacher, K. L. (1995). Family caregiver role acquisition: Role-making through situated interaction. *Scholarly Inquiry for Nursing Practice, 9*, 211-226.

Schumacher, K. L., Jones, P. S., & Meleis, A. (1999). Helping elderly persons in transition: A framework for research and practice. In E. Swanson & T. Tripp-Reimer (Eds.), *Life transitions in the older adult: Issues for nurses and other health professionals* (pp. 1-26). New York: Springer.

Showalter, A., Burger, S., & Salyer, J. (2000). Patients' and their spouses' needs after total joint arthroplasty: A pilot study. *Orthopaedic Nursing, 19*, 49-62.

Shyu, Y. I. (2000a). The needs of family caregivers of frail elders during the transition from hospital to home: A Taiwanese sample. *Journal of Advanced Nursing, 32*, 619-625. Retrieved from http://www3.interscience.wiley.com/cgi-bin/ fulltext/119010648/PDFSTART

Shyu, Y. I. (2000b). Role tuning between caregiver and care receiver during discharge transition: An illustration of role function mode in Roy's adaptation theory. *Nursing Science Quarterly, 13*, 323-331.doi:10.1177/08943180022107870

Shyu, Y. I. (2000c). Patterns of caregiving when family caregivers face competing needs. *Journal of Advanced Nursing, 31*, 35-43. Retrieved from http://www3.interscience.wiley.com/ journal/121440743/abstract

Shyu, Y. L., Chen, M., Chen, S., Wang, H., & Shao, J. (2008). A family caregiver-oriented discharge planning program for older stroke patients and their family caregivers. *Journal of Clinical Nursing, 17,* 2497-2508. Retrieved from http://www3.inter science.wiley.com/cgi-bin/fulltext/121377510/PDFSTART

Skaff, M. M., Pearlin, L. I., & Mullan, J. T. (1996). Transitions in the caregiving career: Effects on sense of mastery. *Psychology and Aging, 11,* 247-257.

Wells, J. L., Seabrook, J. A., Stolee, P., Borrie, M. J., & Knoefel, F. (2003). State of the art in geriatric rehabilitation. Part II: Clinical challenges. *Archives in Physical Medicine and Rehabilitation, 84,* 898-903. doi:10.1016/S0003-9993(02) 04930-4

Wright, D. L., & Aquilino, W. S. (1998). Influence of emotional support exchange in marriage on caregiving wives' burden and marital satisfaction. *Family Relations, 47,* 195-204. Retrieved from http://www.jstor.org/stable/585624?cookieSet=1

Bios

Kerry Byrne, PhD, is a postdoctoral fellow in the Department of Sociology at the University of British Columbia, Vancouver, British Columbia, Canada.

Joseph B. Orange, PhD, is an associate professor in and the director of the School of Communication Sciences and Disorders in the Faculty of Health Sciences at the University of Western Ontario at London, Ontario, Canada.

Catherine Ward-Griffin, RN, PhD, is a professor and acting chair of graduate programs in the Arthur Labatt Family School of Nursing, the University of Western Ontario, London, Ontario, Canada.

Nursing Research • November/December 2011 • Vol 60, No 6, 386–392

Sharing a Traumatic Event

The Experience of the Listener and the Storyteller Within the Dyad

Jeanne Cummings

▶ **Background:** Individuals who have experienced traumatic events often share their experiences in story form. This sharing has consequences for both storytellers and listeners. Understanding the experience of both members of the listener–storyteller dyad is of value to nurses who are often the listener within the nurse–patient dyad.

▶ **Objective:** The aim of this study was to illuminate the experiences of the listener and the storyteller when a traumatic event is shared within the dyad.

▶ **Methods:** The phenomenon was explored using an interpretive phenomenological approach. Participants consisted of 12 dyads, each with a storyteller and a listener. The storytellers were individuals who had been involved in U.S. Airways Flight 1549 when it crash-landed in the Hudson River in January 2009. Each storyteller identified a listener who had listened to them share their story of this event, dubbed *The Miracle on the Hudson.* In-depth interviews were conducted with each storyteller and each listener.

▶ **Results:** Five essential themes emerged from the data: Theme 1, The Story Has a Purpose; Theme 2, The Story as a Whole May Continue to Change as Different Parts Are Revealed; Theme 3, The Story Is Experienced Physically, Mentally, Emotionally, and Spiritually; Theme 4, Imagining the "What" as well as the "What If"; and Theme 5, The Nature of the Relationship Colors the Experience of the Listener and the Storyteller. Roy's Adaptation Model of Nursing was found to be applicable to the findings of this study.

▶ **Discussion:** For the participants in this study, the experience of sharing a traumatic event involved facts, feelings, and images. The story evolved as it was remembered, told, and listened to in a nonlinear, multifaceted way. The listener and the storyteller collaborated, adapted, and responded physically, mentally, emotionally, and spiritually.

▶ **Key Words:** dyad · Flight 1549 · listening · Miracle on the Hudson · nursing · storytelling · trauma

T rauma is any distressing event or psychological shock from experiencing a disastrous event (Webster's Dictionary, 2001, p. 760). The surgeon general has recognized trauma as a major public health risk (Courtois & Gold, 2009). Individuals can directly experience a trauma or can be indirectly traumatized through witnessing or other forms of secondhand exposure (Courtois, 2002). In a national survey of the general population, 60% of men and 51% of women reported having experienced at least one traumatic event in their lifetime (Kessler, Sonnega, Bromet, Hughes, & Nelson, 1995).

People who have experienced traumatic events may tell trauma stories that are fragmented and disjointed, and understanding these stories can be complicated and challenging (Leydesdorff, Dawson, Burchardt, & Ashplant, 2009). Trauma is experienced subjectively; its meaning is very personal (BenEzer, 2009): "for a trauma survivor, putting the story and its imagery into words is the goal of recovery" (Herman, 1992, p. 177). Being asked to share traumatic experiences lets storytellers know that listeners recognize them and their suffering (Rosenthal, 2003). The absence of an invitation to share may convey the message that these experiences are unspeakable or unbearable to listen to; in addition, delayed disclosure and negative reactions to disclosure have been associated with poor adjustment (Ullman, 2007). When people avoid talking about a traumatic event with a victim, the victim may interpret it as a lack of concern and support (Guay, Billette, & Marchand, 2006). Esposito (2005) found that women who had been raped failed to disclose the rape during many subsequent encounters with healthcare providers because no one ever asked them about it. In a study of veterans, it was reported that when healthcare providers asked them about previous trauma, 71% disclosed a history of trauma; nearly 45% remembered receiving a negative response to their disclosure and 30% felt they had not been believed (Leibowitz, Jeffreys, Copeland, & Noel, 2008). Symonds (1980), who worked with crime victims, described *the second wound*, which he defined as "the victim's perceived rejection by and lack of expected support from the community, agencies, family, friends, and society in general" (p. 37). Nurses and other healthcare professionals risk creating a second wound if they do not acknowledge trauma, fail to invite the patient to share, or respond in a way that does not feel meaningful to the patient.

For nurses, listening is one way of responding and adapting to patients within the nurse-patient relationship. The essence of nursing through the ages has been rooted in the relationship between nurse and patient (Roy, 1988).

Jeanne Cummings, DNS, RN, NP, CS, BC, is Visiting Professor, The Graduate Center, City University of New York.

DOI: 10.1097/NNR.0b013e3182348823

169

In Roy's Adaptation Model of Nursing, the person is conceptualized as an adaptive system functioning toward a purpose (Roy, 1988). In Roy's theory, it is proposed that, as adaptive systems, humans respond to stimuli to initiate a coping process, which has an effect on behavior that leads to responses that are either adaptive or ineffective (Perrett, 2007).

Nurses who bear witness to trauma survivors should keep in mind that "just talking without being listened to is not enough; the one that talks must find someone who will listen" (Vajda, 2007, p. 90). In addition, as Bunkers (2010) observed, there is more to listening than hearing the words of another person. When nurses are listeners for storytelling patients, a dyad is formed. In a dyad, each person must relate directly to the other; thoughts and feelings are engaged (Moreland, 2010). The act of listening enables humans to be present and to bear witness to one another (Kagan, 2008). By remaining present, listeners can create a space for storytellers to reveal themselves, the experience, and the story. "Stories are told with, not only to, listeners" (Frank, 2000, p. 354). Pasupathi and Rich (2005) found that storytellers told shorter stories and experienced negative emotions when listeners were distracted. They also found that, when listeners did not respond to the meaning in the story, storytellers had problems completing the story.

Listening to the patient's story is part of the emotional labor of healthcare (Barrett et al., 2005). Repeatedly listening to trauma stories is not without effect on listeners. Exposure to accumulated stress and secondary trauma can result in compassion fatigue; individuals can become fatigued, depressed, and withdrawn and can lose interest. They can experience recurrent thoughts and images, somatic symptoms, and anger (Showalter, 2010). Shortt and Pennebaker (1992) found that, as dyads of listeners and storytellers shared a story of the Holocaust, the listeners' heart rate increased and the storytellers' heart rate decreased. Nurses and social workers were reported to have strong physical sensations when doing traumatic clinical work (Raingruber & Kent, 2003). Baird and Kracen (2006) documented secondary stress reactions and posttraumatic stress disorder symptoms in trauma therapists. These reactions may affect the treatment process as well as the therapist's own experience (Canfield, 2005). Listening to trauma stories may affect the listener; the storyteller may sense this and adapt by changing the way they share.

Nurse practitioners have described listening as the most valuable skill they have (Parrish, Peden, & Staten, 2008). Hearing the patient's story helps in understanding the patient as a person (Barrett et al., 2005). In spite of the emphasis in nursing education on the importance of listening to the patient, "there is a paucity of nursing literature on listening" (Kagan, 2008, p. 109). Little information is available on what listening to stories of traumatic events is like for nurses, how they may be affected by such stories, and how the patient experiences the nurse as listener. This study sought to illuminate the experience of the listener and the storyteller when a traumatic event is shared within the dyad by interviewing individuals who told their story of being involved in the crash-landing of a plane and the people who listened to them. The knowledge gained from this study has implications for individuals who share stories of traumatic events and the nurses and other healthcare professionals who listen to them.

> *Sharing a traumatic event has consequences for both listener and storyteller.*

Methods

Design

An interpretive phenomenological research approach, as outlined by van Manen (1997), guided this study. Van Manen believed that lived experience was the starting and ending point of phenomenological research (van Manen, 1997). This approach was chosen as a way to gain a deeper understanding of the lived experience of individual participants. The personal experiences that were part of the public traumatic event may not have been known by others. This study was done to illuminate the experience of the listener and the storyteller when a traumatic event was shared within the dyad.

Setting and Sample

The context was the crash-landing of a plane, which was the traumatic event. On January 15, 2009, U.S. Airlines Flight 1549, bound for Charlotte, North Carolina, took off from a New York airport carrying 150 passengers and 5 crew members. The plane lost engine thrust shortly after takeoff when a flock of Canadian geese flew into the engines. It crash-landed in the Hudson River in New York City, and all those on board survived. The good news of this event, which the media dubbed *Miracle on the Hudson*, spread throughout the country. Despite its outwardly happy ending, the event would be considered traumatic for the individuals involved.

Data Collection

A purposive sample was obtained in that individuals were sampled in order to purposefully inform an understanding of the phenomenon under study (Creswell, 2007). As primary investigator (PI), I obtained institutional review board approval from my academic setting. I then sent an invitation to participate to potential participants. It was sent via e-mail to 20 potential storyteller participants by an individual who had contact with those involved in Flight 1549. The invitation contained an overall description of the study, including the purpose, and the PI's name, background, and contact information. The 12 storyteller participants who responded and agreed to be in the study then asked someone who had listened to them tell their story previously if he or she would be interested in participating in the study as the listener member of the storyteller–listener dyad. If the listener agreed, he or she responded via e-mail. Listeners were then sent the original e-mail invitation.

The purposive sample consisted of 24 participants forming 12 dyads, each with a storyteller and a listener. These spouse, friend, sibling, and parent dyads included 9 men and 15 women, with ages ranging from 29 to 74 years. Signed consent, including permission to be audiotaped, was obtained from all participants who were made aware that their participation was voluntary and that they had the right to stop participation or withdraw from the study at any time without penalty. Information regarding the availability of mental health counseling was also provided to participants.

In-depth interviews were done face to face with 21 participants; the remaining three interviews were conducted on the telephone because of participant availability. Each storyteller and each listener were asked to speak about what their experience was like when the traumatic event was shared within the dyad. Each storyteller was asked, "Tell me what it was like to tell your story to [name of listener]." Each listener was asked, "Tell me what it was like listening to [name of storyteller] tell you [his or her] story." The interviewer encouraged participants to share their experiences by asking nonleading questions such as "Tell me more about your experience" until participants felt they had no more to say on the topic. The interviews were audiotaped, assigned pseudonym titles, and downloaded individually to a secure server. Each audiotape was transcribed verbatim by a transcriptionist who had completed the Human Subjects Research in Social and Behavioral Sciences module as well as the Research Integrity module. Names were removed during transcription. After the transcription was completed, each transcript was reviewed for completeness and to ensure that all identifying information was removed.

Data Analysis

Data analysis was carried out according to the process described by van Manen (1997). The following steps were taken to achieve rigor; preconceived notions and beliefs were put aside about the phenomenon under study. A holistic reading was done of each transcript to get a sense of it as a whole and then read again to see what statements or phrases seemed to best represent the experience of the participants. During these readings, notes were made in the margins, using different color highlighters for what appeared to be different categories of statements. Each of the statements or phrases was listed in categories that seemed to be related. After repeatedly reviewing and dwelling with the data, five essential themes were identified, after determining that the phenomenon would lose its meaning without the inclusion of these themes.

As a way to further maintain rigor, the PI collaborated with two professional colleagues and expert qualitative researchers who reviewed transcripts and findings; each had more than 20 years of experience in qualitative research. A journal was kept to record additional observations and personal reflections. Findings were presented and clarified with participants to assess whether the transcripts were accurate and whether the identified themes resonated with them. According to Lincoln and Guba (1985), "The criterion for objectivity is intersubjective agreement; if multiple observers agree on a phenomenon, then their collective judgment can be said to be objective" (p. 292). Saturation, as described by Lincoln and Guba (1985), was achieved upon interviewing nine dyads, as there was no new or different information emerging; however, a total of 12 dyads were interviewed to confirm redundancy and maintain rigor. There was intersubjective agreement on themes between the PI, participants, and expert qualitative researchers. Five essential themes were supported in the form of narrative excerpts from participants.

Results

The five essential themes and the data to support them are discussed in the sections that follow.

Essential Theme 1: The Story Has a Purpose for the Listener and the Storyteller

Purposes identified included sharing the facts and the special story, giving inspiration, and providing a benefit to the storyteller and the listener. Personal experience often differed from public media presentation. One storyteller noted, "I guess there's almost this compulsion to set the record straight and say, 'It's still a wonderful story, and we are so fortunate, and it could have been so much worse, but let me tell you, it wasn't as easy as you think.'"

Storytellers wanted to inspire: "I've seen the really, really strong inspirational impact it had on certain people. That's the kind of impact I want to have when I tell it because that's the most rewarding for me." In turn, many listeners described experiencing a feeling of awe while listening. Storytellers and listeners spoke of feeling that the story was special. A listener smiled and whispered, "I love the story." A storyteller described the story, "It's a little bit, maybe, too big of a word—sacred—but just special, very special." Many felt that an incomplete version was disrespectful. One storyteller felt that "the worst thing that can happen when you are telling somebody about something like this, it's either dismissiveness or indifference."

It was revealed repeatedly that the storytellers did not mind telling their story and felt that telling was helpful to them. One storyteller said, "I could probably go on a ramble about it as long as anybody would listen." She went on to say, "It was very therapeutic, saying it over and over; it helped me remember things." Another storyteller explained, "Talking about it was actually a way for me to release, not to keep it in, because I think I know myself enough: I keep it in, and it will just burn a hole." In some dyads, the listeners had the impression that the storyteller preferred to avoid telling the story. A listener shared her belief, "I know she did not want to tell it all the time." Another commented, "I did not have a sense that he needed to share or get support." These statements revealed that listeners sometimes had a different perception of the storyteller's desire to tell the story and were unaware of the benefit of doing so.

Another benefit of telling the story was reflected in the fact that, as time went on, listeners and storytellers noticed that the more they shared, the easier it got. They felt less emotionally and physically reactive. A storyteller explained, "Over time, I feel less bad about it. The trauma of the actual event has subsided some." A listener found that her responses had changed as well: "You know, I still get the chills on occasion, but it's not as emotional as it was for the first few months." A storyteller explained, "Going through it over and over and over again, it got easier and easier. I don't think I could have healed without—and I really feel that I healed from it." All participants spoke about learning and gaining a sense of understanding as they shared. A listener recalled, "Each time we'd share, we'd learn a little something." A storyteller recalled that, "Telling it, it helped me process it to a certain extent."

Essential Theme 2: The Story That Is Known as a Whole May Continue to Change as Different Parts of It Are Revealed

Participants talked about how the story was remembered, told, and listened to in bits and pieces—that there was a "worst part" to the story and that the story evolved as information was gathered. All participants were drawn to fill in the holes of the story or elaborate on specific parts. A storyteller explained, "So in the beginning, it was probably a lot of—I was probably—definitely more scattered. So I maybe couldn't have told it in a linear fashion." She remembered things as she shared: "So it was a progression to where my story is today, and I—it may change; I don't know that it's complete. I suspect there will be continued learnings, there will be the evolution." Listeners also were aware of the evolution of the story: "Listening in those respects over the next 4 or 5 months when bits and pieces would come in, it would be more of an unveiling of something." The listener and the storyteller often collaborated to piece the story together, accepting what they knew in the present moment to be the story while being open to the possibility of change in the future.

Even though parts of the story changed as information was gathered, the part of the story that was identified as the worst part never changed. A listener revealed the worst part for her: "He thought he was going to die. But the most painful was the next day, when I got to process it more." There is no way to know what the worst part was for each individual without asking them. A storyteller recounted what was the worst part for him: "We're going down, and he's already told us to brace for impact, and I start thinking about what I was thinking then.... That would get me choked up every time."

Essential Theme 3: The Story Is Often Experienced Physically, Mentally, Emotionally, and Spiritually

Both members of the dyad were aware of physical manifestations of emotion reflected in the body, the face, and the eyes of the other as the story was shared. Simultaneous listener–storyteller nonverbal communication added to the collaborative nature of the experience within the dyad. The observation, perception, and interpretation of these nonverbal cues affected the creation, cessation, and modification of dialogue as well as the images, emotions, and physical sensations experienced. For example, the responses of the listener often validated the storyteller: "Just to see the reaction on other people's faces makes you realize exactly how traumatic the experience was." This storyteller described her awareness of the listener as she spoke: "I do notice if I feel like they're actually interested in listening to what I'm saying or not. I notice it in people's faces." She found herself responding to these nonverbal cues: "I'm very big on mannerisms and stuff like that. If I felt like they were losing interest, then I probably would just quit talking about it."

Participants also had physical reactions to the experience. One listener remembered "that nonstop crying and the throwing up." A storyteller noted, "I can get varying degrees of physical response, tightening, tensing up, or I found myself fidgeting and stuff like that; the heart rate starts to go up a little bit." The listener in this dyad remembered she would "get goose bumps at a certain point when he would talk about it."

Listeners and storytellers experienced the story mentally through images. This occurred spontaneously at times, and at other times, the participant actively tried to picture things. In one dyad, the storyteller recalled, "So when I started telling about it was—it was the pictures playing over and over in my head." In the same dyad, the listener revealed, "I could almost tell you what she looked like; I could picture her there." Another listener talked about "seeing" the storyteller's experience as she escaped the cabin of the plane. "You know, getting out on that wing, I almost—it's almost like, you know, I can almost—I can see the light." He imagined being there: "I'll be thinking about it, and maybe listening to her, and at the same time maybe trying to imagine what it's like being right alongside of her." Participants often described a sense of derealization as they shared the story of the traumatic event. A storyteller felt as though he was "dreaming." A listener recalled thinking, "This is surreal."

While telling or listening, participants experienced the story emotionally. A storyteller elaborated: "When I talk about it and remind her how much she means, it definitely gets her emotional, I know it does. And I, in turn, get emotional." The listener in this dyad was clear about the emotional impact that listening had on her: "I was, like, traumatized by this, you know, by listening to it." She called her experience an "emotional roller coaster." Both listeners and storytellers reported feeling as though they were reliving the experience as it was shared. A storyteller recalled, "When I'm going through the narrative, it's like in a lesser degree as time has gone on—but it's kind of happening again, and instead of just talking about the emotional part, it's more like you're feeling the emotional part." A listener felt that things came alive as she listened: "And so as he speaks, and I'm listening, then I am, if you will, reprocessing. I'm reliving, I'm recounting. I'm—it's real."

Participants also had spiritual experiences. As one listener put it, "God was providing me a moment by moment peace" as the storyteller shared bits of what had happened early on. Another listener felt a presence. She had a "feeling wash over her" and felt as if "someone was trying to comfort me—like maybe it was the Holy Ghost."

Essential Theme 4: Imagining the "What" as Well as the "What If" Is Done by Both Listener and Storyteller

Many participants found themselves imagining what happened as well as what could have happened. When a storyteller imagined the what if, he thought about "the things I was going to miss out on, I wouldn't—all those missed-out-on things that haven't happened yet. And every time I'd think about that, and how lucky I am to do some of those things, I just get choked up." One storyteller imagined what it would be like to lose his wife, the listener, and, at the same time, what it would have been like for her to lose him: "I always try to reflect in other people's shoes, and if I lost my wife, it would be devastating. It would have been very painful for her [to lose me]. Still painful for her [to contemplate], I'm sure, but it didn't work out that way."

Many listeners imagined what had happened and what it was like for the storytellers by putting themselves in their shoes. A listener revealed, "Every time she was telling it, I would think—I would picture myself in her situation. I see me doing it. I wasn't listening as much as I was picturing myself in it." One listener imagined two aspects of walking in the other's shoes. First, she imagined how the storyteller had experienced the event: "It was amazing to listen and then try to put myself in his shoes to really try and comprehend the thought processes that he was describing." Second, she imagined experiencing the event herself: "Once I get a feel for things I step into a role, but I'm going to—so as he tells the story, then I try and put myself in his shoes, and how would I have reacted?"

Some participants, in contrast, felt that they could never imagine putting themselves in the shoes of the other: "There is no way you can understand; there's no way, even if you'd had a similar experience, that you can put yourself in their shoes." They may have understood the facts but have been unable to achieve a deeper understanding of the lived experience.

Essential Theme 5: The Nature of the Relationship Colors the Experience of the Listener and the Storyteller When a Traumatic Event Is Shared Within the Dyad

The listener, the context, the type of relationship, and the amount of time the dyad spent together affected the experience of sharing. A storyteller observed, "A lot of that storytelling has to do with the listener, too." He said that he "tells the story differently depending on who he is talking to." Sometimes storytellers altered the story to protect the listener. One storyteller told me, "I didn't want to burden her. I didn't want to—I just didn't want to upset *her*." The listener in this dyad explained, "She doesn't want me to really know how it really was…and she was worried about me." Other listeners felt that they had listened so often they knew the story by heart: "It's become very familiar, and I could almost, you know, recite at least parts of it."

Storytellers always made decisions about whom to share their story with: "It's almost like because it's such a personal and deep experience, you sort of don't want to waste it on people…. It's precious, like a piece of gold." They considered the reactions of listeners: "When somebody acknowledges your feelings—and not just acknowledges; somebody says, 'Oh, this must have been this and that'—it makes you more willing to discuss your feelings that maybe you were a little more reserved about before."

That some listeners felt they had had enough of listening and wanted to move on was evident in the study findings. A listener explained, "It's not so therapeutic for me to keep reliving that, I guess." Another listener described being "sick of hearing the story" and expressed a desire to "move on, some normalcy." As a way to cope, another listener revealed an attempt to actively try not to listen: "I just think I knew I'd heard it, and I didn't want to have to get it in my mind again." Another listener became "exhausted, definitely exhausted" after fully listening for a very long time. However, she was one of several listeners who said they would continue to listen if the storyteller needed them to: "I mean, I was there to support, as I still am, and that's just what you do." Adding, "I wouldn't have done anything differently."

Sharing stories of traumatic events is one way of responding and adapting to the stimulus of trauma.

Continuing to listen for the sake of the other despite feeling as though they had had enough of listening may affect listeners as well as storytellers. Storytellers had some awareness of listener saturation and desire to move on. One storyteller believed that, after initially hearing the entire story, the listener had met her capacity for listening and had become saturated; he said, "She doesn't really want to hear it." Another storyteller worried about the effect on the listener: "I would not want to bore people…I don't want to wear somebody out with it."

All storytellers noted that when they were with other people who had shared the traumatic experience, they felt understood: "That's the best-case scenario because they really understand what's going on…because they understand what I went through." One storyteller added, "Unless you've lived it, there's no comparison."

Integrated Essential Essence

The meaning of phenomenological description lies in its interpretation, its aim to transform lived experience by breathing meaning into a textual expression of its essence (van Manen, 1997). A textual interpretative statement was formulated from essential themes as a summary of the experience. An integrated essential essence was created to capture the essence of the experience of the listener and the storyteller when a traumatic event is shared within the dyad. The Integrated Essential Essence is as follows. The traumatic event is lived by an individual who, in an attempt to understand his or her own experience and to eventually have it understood by another, forms a story about the event and his or her experience and shares it with a listener, forming a unique dyad. Seeking physical, psychic, and spiritual integrity, the listener and the storyteller collaborate, sharing the story of the traumatic event and the experience in a complex, nonlinear multifaceted way, continuously adapting while attempting to create a sense of meaning through the experience.

Discussion

Implications for Nursing

For nurses, inviting an individual to share his or her experience of a traumatic event is a way to say, "I see *you*; come, share your story with me, and I will listen." Initial assessments are not complete without this invitation. This study revealed a collaborative, adaptive process between listener and storyteller, consistent with Roy's Adaptation Model. It was revealed that the listener and the storyteller acted as interdependent parts, collaborating as they shared the story of the traumatic event within the dyad. Participant's individual patterns of adaptation and individual attempts at coping were illuminated, providing a deeper understanding of the lived experiences of these individuals.

Sharing stories of traumatic events is one way of responding and adapting to the stimulus of trauma. In this study, the results showed that despite feeling as though they had had enough of listening and wanted to move on, some listeners adapted by continuing to try to listen. Nurses may do the same. Just as some athletes develop stress injuries, some nurses who listen repeatedly to stories of traumatic events may develop stress injuries. This pattern may carry a risk for both nurse and patient. Nurses may continue to listen for the sake of their patients; however, they may experience compassion fatigue and, as a result, may tire, withdraw, and lose interest. Patients may sense this and adapt by altering their trauma story or by not sharing it at all. Focusing more intensively on listening within nursing curricula may be of value. Preventing stress injury, exploring ways to promoting resilience, and illuminating ways for nurses to be with patients so they are able to share their stories of traumatic events are of value to nursing.

Implications for Future Research

Nursing education includes the topic of therapeutic communication. However, few studies have explored how the patient experiences the nurse during this communication and what it is like for nurses to be fully present while listening. Further dyadic studies exploring the experience of sharing a traumatic event within the nurse–patient dyad may reveal patterns related to listening, being heard, presencing, resilience, and burnout or compassion fatigue.

Future studies exploring the experience of sharing a traumatic event in specific relationship dyads may reveal different patterns. For example, veterans are returning from war having experienced traumatic events. Exploring what it is like for these individuals and their significant others to share these events may add to the understanding of their experience.

Also highlighted in the results of this study was the sense of understanding that often exists among individuals who have shared similar experiences. Nurses who have experienced traumatic events and work-related stress injuries may benefit from sharing these with other nurses who have had similar experiences. This sense of mutual understanding may be a protective factor in recovery from work-related stress, burnout, and compassion fatigue.

Strengths and Limitations

A strength of this dyadic study was that it enabled the perspective of both listener and the storyteller to be illuminated. The findings may be of value to the nurse–patient dyad, because the nurse is often the listener to the patient storyteller when a traumatic event is shared. The fact that three participants were interviewed on the telephone may have changed what was shared; however, there did not seem to be any differences in the findings among these participants. A potential bias is that the PI's brother was a passenger on the plane. He was not a participant in the study.

Conclusions

This study illuminates the experience of the listener and the storyteller when a traumatic event is shared within the dyad. In this study, it was revealed that, when the traumatic event is shared, the story includes more than factual events; it is accompanied by feelings and images. The story evolved as it was remembered, told, and listened to in a nonlinear, multifaceted way. When the traumatic event is shared within the dyad, the listener and the storyteller collaborate, adapt, and respond physically, mentally, emotionally, and spiritually. ▼

Accepted for publication August 15, 2011.

The author thanks her brother (a passenger on Flight 1549) for his assistance in providing access to potential participants. The author also thanks the participants for generously sharing their experiences. The author has no funding or conflicts of interest to disclose.

Corresponding author: Jeanne Cummings, DNS, RN, NP, CS, BC, The Graduate Center, City University of New York, Doctor of Nursing Science Program, 365 Fifth Avenue, New York, NY 10016-4309 (e-mail: JCummings225@gmail.com).

References

Baird, K., & Kracen, C. (2006). Vicarious traumatization and secondary traumatic stress: A research synthesis. *Counselling Psychology Quarterly, 19*, 181–188. doi: 10.1080/09515070600811899.

Barrett, C., Brothwick, A., Bugeja, S., Parker, A., Vis, R., & Hurworth, R. (2005). Emotional labour: Listening to the patient's story. *Practice Development in Health Care, 4*, 213–223. doi: 10.1002/pdh.17.

BenEzer, G. (2009). Trauma signals in life stories. In K. L. Rogers, S. Leydesdorff, & G. Dawson (Eds.). *Life stories of survivors of trauma* (pp. 29–44). New Brunswick, NJ: Transaction Publishers.

Bunkers, S. S. (2010). The power and possibility in listening. *Nursing Science Quarterly, 23*, 22–27. doi: 10.1117/0894318409353805.

Canfield, J. (2005). Secondary traumatization, burnout, and vicarious traumatization: A review of the literature as it relates to therapists who treat trauma. *Smith College Studies in Social Work, 75*, 81–101. doi: 10.1300/j497v75n02_06.

Courtois, C. A. (2002). Traumatic stress studies: The need for curricula inclusion. *Journal of Trauma Practice, 1*, 33–57. doi: 10.1300/J189v01n01_03.

Courtois, C. A., & Gold, S. (2009). The need for inclusion of psychological trauma in the professional curriculum: A call to action. *Psychological Trauma: Theory, Research, Practice, and Policy, 1*, 3–23. doi: 10.1037a0015224.

Cresswell, J. (2007). *Qualitative inquiry & research design, choosing among five approaches*. Lincoln, NE: Sage.

Esposito, N. (2005). Manifestations of enduring during interviews with sexual assault victims. *Qualitative Health Research, 15*, 912–927. doi: 10.117/1049732305279056.

Frank, A. W. (2000). The standpoint of the storyteller. *Qualitative Health Research, 10*, 354–365. doi: 10.1177/104973200129118499.

Guay, S., Billette, V., & Marchand, A. (2006). Exploring the links between posttraumatic stress disorder and social support: Processes and potential research avenues. *Journal of Traumatic Stress, 19*, 327–338. doi: 10.1002/jts.20124.

Herman, J. (1992). *Trauma and recovery*. New York, NY: Basic Books.

Kagan, P. N. (2008). Listening: Selected perspectives in theory and research. *Nursing Science Quarterly, 21*, 105–110. doi: 10.1177/0894318408315027.

Kessler, R. C., Sonnega, A., Bromet, E., Hughes, M., & Nelson, C. (1995). Posttraumatic stress disorder in the national comorbidity study. *Archives of General Psychiatry, 52*, 1048–1060.

Leibowitz, R. Q., Jeffreys, M. D., Copeland, L. A., & Noel, P. H. (2008). Veterans' disclosure of trauma to healthcare providers. *General Hospital Psychiatry, 30*, 100–103. doi: 10.1016/j.genhosppsych.2007.11.004.

Leydesdorff, S., Dawson, G., Burchardt, N., & Ashplant, T. G. (2009). Trauma and life stories. In K. L. Rogers, S. Leydesdorff, &

G. Dawson (Eds.), *Life stories of survivors of trauma* (pp. 1–26). New Brunswick, NJ: Transaction Publishers.

Lincoln, Y., & Guba, E. (1985). *Naturalistic inquiry*. Newbury Park, CA: Sage.

Moreland, R. (2010). Are dyads really groups? *Small Group Research, 41*, 251–267. doi: 10.1177/1046496409358618.

Parrish, E., Peden, A., & Staten, R. (2008). Strategies used by advanced practice psychiatric nurses in treating adults with depression. *Perspectives in Psychiatric Care, 44*, 232–240. doi: 10.1111/j.1744-6163.2008.00182.x.

Pasupathi, M., & Rich, B. (2005). Inattentive listening undermines self verification in personal storytelling. *Journal of Personality, 73*, 1051–1086. doi: 10.1111/j.1467-6494.2005.00338.x.

Perrett, S. E. (2007). Review of Roy Adaption Model-based qualitative research. *Nursing Science Quarterly, 20*, 349–356. doi: 10.1177/0894318407306538.

Raingruber, B., & Kent, M. (2003). Attending to embodied responses: A way to identify practice-based and human meanings associated with secondary trauma. *Qualitative Health Research, 13*, 449–468. doi: 10.1177/1049732302250722.

Rosenthal, G. (2003). The healing effects of storytelling on the conditions of curative storytelling in the context of research and counseling. *Qualitative Inquiry, 9*, 915–933. doi: 10.1177/1077800403254888.

Roy, C. Sr. (1988). An explication of the philosophical assumptions of the Roy Adaptation Model. *Nursing Science Quarterly, 1*, 26–34. doi: 10.1177/089431848800100108.

Shortt, J., & Pennebaker, J. (1992). Talking versus hearing about Holocaust experiences. *Basic and Applied Psychology, 13*, 165–179. doi: 10.1207/s15324834basp1302_2.

Showalter, S. (2010). Compassion fatigue: What is it? Why does it matter? Recognizing the symptoms, acknowledging the impact, developing the tools to prevent compassion fatigue and strengthen the professional already suffering from the effects. *American Journal of Hospice and Palliative Medicine, 27*(4), 239–242. doi: 10.1177/1049909109354096.

Symonds, M. (1980). The second injury to victims. *Evaluation and Change, 4*, 36–38.

Ullman, S. E. (2007). Relationship to perpetrator, disclosure, social reactions, and PTSD symptoms in child sexual abuse survivors. *Journal of Child Sexual Abuse, 16*, 19–36. doi: 10.1300/j070v16n01-02.

Vajda, J. (2007). Two survivor cases: Therapeutic effect as side product of the biographical narrative interview. *Journal of Social Work Practice, 21*, 89–102. doi: 10.1080026505306011173664.

van Manen, M. (1997). *Researching lived experience* (2nd ed.). Winnipeg, Manitoba, Canada: Althouse Press.

Webster's dictionary. (4th ed.). (2001). New York, NY: Ballentine Books.

Journal of Cardiovasvcular Nursing. 2016 Jul–Aug; 31(4): 357–66

The Effectiveness of Medication Adherence Interventions Among Patients With Coronary Artery Disease
A Meta-analysis

Jo-Ana D. Chase, PhD, APRN-BC; Jennifer L. Bogener, BSN; Todd M. Ruppar, PhD, RN; Vicki S. Conn, PhD, RN, FAAN

Background: Despite the known benefits of medication therapy for secondary prevention of coronary artery disease (CAD), many patients do not adhere to prescribed medication regimens. Medication nonadherence is associated with poor health outcomes and higher healthcare cost. **Objective:** The purpose of this meta-analysis was to determine the overall effectiveness of interventions designed to improve medication adherence (MA) among adults with CAD. In addition, sample, study design, and intervention characteristics were explored as potential moderators to intervention effectiveness. **Methods:** Comprehensive search strategies helped in facilitating the identification of 2-group, treatment-versus-control–design studies testing MA interventions among patients with CAD. Data were independently extracted by 2 trained research specialists. Standardized mean difference effect sizes were calculated for eligible primary studies, adjusted for bias, and then synthesized under a random-effects model. Homogeneity of variance was explored using a conventional heterogeneity statistic. Exploratory moderator analyses were conducted using meta-analytic analogs for analysis of variance and regression for dichotomous and continuous moderators, respectively. **Results:** Twenty-four primary studies were included in this meta-analysis. The overall effect size of MA interventions, calculated from 18,839 participants, was 0.229 ($P < .001$). The most effective interventions used nurses as interventionists, initiated interventions in the inpatient setting, and informed providers of patients' MA behaviors. Medication adherence interventions tested among older patients were more effective than those among younger patients. The interventions were equally effective regardless of number of intervention sessions, targeting MA behavior alone or with other behaviors, and the use of written instructions only. **Conclusions:** Interventions to increase MA among patients with CAD were modestly effective. Nurses can be instrumental in improving MA among these patients. Future research is needed to investigate nurse-delivered MA interventions across varied clinical settings. In addition, more research testing MA interventions among younger populations and more racially diverse groups is needed.

KEY WORDS: coronary artery disease, medication adherence, meta-analysis, patient compliance

Jo-Ana D. Chase, PhD, APRN-BC
Assistant Professor, S343 School of Nursing, University of Missouri, Columbia.
Jennifer L. Bogener, BSN
Nursing Student, School of Nursing School of Health Professions, University of Missouri, Columbia.
Todd M. Ruppar, PhD, RN
Assistant Professor, S423 School of Nursing, University of Missouri, Columbia.
Vicki S. Conn, PhD, RN, FAAN
Potter-Brinton Professor and Associate Dean for Research, S317 School of Nursing University of Missouri Columbia.

Supported by Award Number R01NR011990 (Conn-PI) from the National Institute of Nursing Research. The content is solely the responsibility of the authors and does not necessarily represent the official views of the National Institute of Nursing Research or the National Institutes of Health.
The authors have no conflicts of interest to disclose.

Correspondence
Jo-Ana D. Chase, PhD, APRN-BC, S343 School of Nursing, University of Missouri, Columbia, MO 65211 (chasej@missouri.edu).

DOI: 10.1097/JCN.0000000000000259

Introduction

Heart disease is the leading cause of death among adults in the United States.[1,2] Coronary artery disease (CAD), the most common form of heart disease, is responsible for 385,000 deaths and $108.9 billion in healthcare expenditures annually.[1,2] Secondary prevention for CAD is a multi-intervention approach involving therapeutic lifestyle changes and evidence-based medical therapies, such as prescribed medications. Between 1980 and 2000, these therapies have contributed to a 50% reduction in CAD-related deaths.[3] Research suggests that the greatest contributor to this reduction is medications for secondary prevention of CAD.[3]

Unfortunately, medication nonadherence is highly prevalent.[4] Approximately one-third of patients who have had a myocardial infarction do not adhere to prescribed

177

medication regimens.[5] Nonadherence is associated with increased risk for all-cause and cardiovascular mortality, revascularization procedures, hospitalization, and higher healthcare cost.[6–8] Effective interventions to improve medication adherence (MA) in this population are critically needed.

Efficacy of MA interventions varies.[9–14] Few systematic reviews have focused on MA interventions among patients with CAD.[15–18] Prior reviews have been limited by narrow search strategies, unclear inclusion criteria, lack of a quantitative synthesis, or absent exploration of potential moderating variables.[16] To date, no current meta-analyses addressing MA intervention effectiveness among patients with CAD exist. Thus, the overall effectiveness of MA interventions in this population is unclear; furthermore, the most effective types of interventions are yet unknown.

A meta-analysis and moderator analysis of MA interventions among patients with CAD could promote efficiency in developing future interventions and provide clinicians with guidance to promote MA in clinical practice. The purposes of this systematic review and meta-analysis were to describe and quantify the overall effectiveness of the body of MA intervention research among patients with CAD and to explore potential moderators of intervention effectiveness. In addition, we identified limitations in the extant research and suggested areas for future study.

The following research questions guided this study:

1) What is the overall effectiveness of MA interventions on MA outcomes among patients with CAD?
2) Does intervention effectiveness vary based on intervention, sample, or design characteristics?

Methods

The systematic review and meta-analysis were performed using standard meta-analysis techniques and PRISMA guidelines.[19,20] This project was part of a larger parent study examining MA outcomes of MA interventions across multiple chronic and acute illnesses.

Search Strategies

We consulted an expert health sciences reference librarian to ensure comprehensive search strategies.[21] Databases that were searched included the following: MEDLINE, PubMED, PsychINFO, CINAHL, EBSCO, PQDT, Cochrane Central Trials Register, Cochrane Database of Systematic Reviews, IndMed, ERIC, International Pharmaceutical Abstracts, EBM Reviews-Database of Abstracts of Reviews of Effects, as well as Communication and Mass Media. Broad MeSH terms were used, which included the following: *patient compliance*, *medication adherence*, *drugs*, *prescription drugs*, *pharmaceutical preparations*, *generic*, *dosage*, *compliant*, *compliance*, *adherent*, *adherence*, *noncompliant*, *noncompliance*, *nonadherent*,

nonadherence, *medication(s)*, *regimen(s)*, *prescription(s)*, *prescribed*, *drug(s)*, *pill(s)*, *tablet(s)*, *agent(s)*, *improve*, *promote*, *enhance*, *encourage*, *foster*, *advocate*, *influence*, *incentive*, *ensure*, *remind*, *optimize*, *increase*, *impact*, *prevent*, *address*, *decrease*. Fifty-seven relevant journals were hand-searched, and author searches and ancestry searches of prior reviews' bibliographies were conducted to identify additional potentially eligible studies.

Inclusion Criteria

We included 2-group, treatment-versus-control comparison studies testing interventions to increase MA in patients 18 years or older with a diagnosis of CAD, defined by the primary studies. Medication adherence interventions are deliberate actions performed or directed by investigators to increase adherence to specified medication regimens. Examples include education, reminders, and special packaging. Studies with varied types of MA measurement (eg, electronic monitoring devices, pharmacy refills, self-report) were included, given the diversity of MA measures in this research area. Eligible studies needed to contain enough data to calculate an effect size (ES). The research team attempted to contact corresponding authors to obtain missing outcome data.

Data Extraction

To extract relevant data from primary studies, a coding strategy was developed from prior research and expert consultations. The codebook was developed through an iterative process and pilot tested. Data extracted included the primary study source, publication date, dissemination type (eg, journal article, dissertation), presence of funding, participant demographics (eg, age, gender, ethnicity, comorbidities), research methods, intervention details, and MA outcomes. Multiple descriptors of primary study research methods were coded, such as sample size, randomization, and intention-to-treat analyses. Method of MA measurement and follow-up interval were recorded. Varied intervention characteristics were coded, including content (eg, problem solving, self-monitoring, goal setting), delivery (eg, face-to-face, telephone), dose (eg, length/number of sessions), and setting (eg, clinic, home).

Included studies were independently coded by 2 extensively trained research specialists, then compared and discussed until consensus was reached. A doctorally prepared senior research specialist supervised the coding process to ensure coding integrity and reviewed all ES data. Questionable items were resolved in team meetings with the study principal investigator.

Data Analysis

All data were analyzed using Comprehensive Meta-Analysis Software.[22] Standardized mean difference effect sizes (d, ES) were calculated for each 2-group treatment-versus-control posttest comparison. The standardized mean difference ES between the groups was calculated by dividing the difference between treatment and control group postintervention means by the pooled standard deviation. Additional ES analyses were conducted within the groups by subtracting the outcome scores from the baseline scores and dividing by the baseline standard deviation. Effect sizes were weighted by the inverse of variance to account for sample size and adjust for bias, then synthesized using a random-effects model.[23] A random-effects model was chosen a priori, given the expected within- and between-study variance across primary studies. Data were examined for possible outliers on the basis of standardized residuals of each primary study's ES. Publication bias was examined by assessing the symmetry of a funnel plot constructed by plotting each primary study's standard error against its ES.[23]

Homogeneity of variance was tested using a conventional heterogeneity statistic (Q), to quantify observed heterogeneity across studies, and I^2 to determine the proportion of observed heterogeneity due to true differences in effects across studies.[23] Exploratory moderator analyses were used to examine possible associations between study characteristics and intervention effectiveness. Dichotomous variables were evaluated using subgroup analysis, and continuous variables were evaluated using meta-regression.[23]

Results

Twenty-four primary reports were eligible for analysis.[9–14,24–41] Additional coding information was found in 4 companion reports about the same primary studies.[42–45] Three primary study reports contained multiple comparison groups.[33,36,37] There were 28 treatment-versus-control-group posttest comparisons, 9 treatment group pretest-posttest comparisons, and 6 control group pretest-posttest comparisons. Few smaller studies with negative findings were included, indicating evidence of publication bias.

Primary Study Characteristics

The primary studies that were included in this meta-analysis included 24 journal articles, 3 dissertations, and 1 presentation. Six studies were disseminated before 2000. Seventeen studies were supported by funding.

Primary study characteristics are presented in Table 1. Majority of the samples were males. The median of the mean age for participants was 62.9 years. Only 7 studies reported data on ethnicity. Of those, most subjects were white. Some studies reported additional chronic diseases among their subjects including the following: hypertension ($k = 17$), undifferentiated diabetes ($k = 16$), hyperlipidemia ($k = 12$), heart failure ($k = 4$), stroke ($k = 3$), lung disease ($k = 3$), renal disease ($k = 2$), osteoarthritis ($k = 1$), asthma ($k = 1$), atrial fibrillation ($k = 1$), nephritic syndrome ($k = 1$), thyroid disorder ($k = 1$), and cerebral vascular disease ($k = 1$).

Primary studies reported diverse methods. The median number of intervention sessions was 2 ($k = 17$). The median number of days for MA intervention duration was 35 ($k = 23$). Only 1 study reported intervention session duration. Outcome data of MA were collected with a median of 124.5 days after intervention ($k = 14$). Studies reported diverse methods of collecting MA outcomes including pharmacy refill ($k = 7$), self-report ($k = 18$), biological measures ($k = 2$), and pill counts ($k = 1$).

Overall Effects of Medication Adherence Interventions of Medication Adherence Outcomes

Overall MA ESs are presented in Table 2. The ESs were calculated for 28 treatment-versus-control-group comparisons containing 18,839 subjects. The overall ES for these comparisons was 0.229 ($P < .001$), indicating significant improvements in MA outcomes in the treatment over the control group (Figure). When the 3 largest sample studies were excluded, the ES for these comparisons demonstrated minimal change ($d = 0.269$, $P < .001$). The ESs were significantly heterogeneous.

We also calculated overall ESs for the 9 treatment group pretest-posttest comparisons and for the 6 control group pretest-posttest comparisons. Although the former ES was positive (0.183) and the latter negative (-0.014), neither were statistically significant. Lack of

TABLE 1 Characteristics of Primary Studies Included in Medication Adherence Meta-analyses						
Characteristic	k	Min	Q_1	Median	Q_3	Max
Treatment group sample size	28	4	18.75	86.5	246.5	3635
Control group sample size	24	5	21	82	562	3010
Percentage attrition	23	0	0	4.545	14.646	65.282
Percentage of females	23	0	25	40	51.05	67.4
Percentage underrepresented group subjects	7	7	24.1	48	90.4	92.9
Mean age, y	21	53.7	58.4	62.9	64	72.22
Median number of intervention sessions	17	1	1	2	5	12
Median duration of interventions, d	23	1	1	35	126	365
Median duration postintervention for MA outcome data collection, d	14	12	40.25	124.5	175.5	700

k, number of comparisons in which characteristic was reported; Min, minimum; Max, maximum; Q_1, first quartile; Q_3, third quartile.

TABLE 2 **Overall Effects of Medication Adherence Interventions Among Patients With Coronary Artery Disease**

Comparison	k	d	P (d)	95% Confidence Interval	SE	Q	I²	P (Q)
Treatment vs control groups at posttest[a]	28	0.229	<.001	0.138–0.321	0.047	78.201	65.474	<.001
Treatment vs control groups at posttest[b]	25	0.269	<.001	0.135–0.403	0.068	65.384	63.294	<.001
Treatment group pretest vs posttest	9	0.183	.106	−0.039 to 0.405	0.113	69.462	88.483	<.001
Control group pretest vs posttest	6	−0.014	.887	−0.208 to 0.180	0.099	11.124	55.052	.049

d, standardized mean difference effect size; I², proportion of observed variance across effect size due to true differences in effects; k, number of comparisons; Q, conventional homogeneity statistic; SE, standard error.
[a]All studies included.
[b]Three larger sample studies excluded.

statistical significance may reflect low power from the small number of comparisons.

Moderator Analyses

Continuous and dichotomous moderator analyses are displayed in Tables 3 and 4, respectively. Although all studies from the main analysis were examined for moderating variables, only those moderators reported for a

sufficient number of comparisons were included in the analyses.

Intervention Moderators

Studies in which health care providers were given information about subjects' MA revealed a significantly greater ES (0.387) than when the providers were not given information on MA (0.151). An example of this type of intervention component could involve using a

Study name	Std diff in means	Standard error	Lower limit	Upper limit
2012	0.516	0.228	0.069	0.962
2012	0.140	0.164	-0.182	0.462
2012	0.075	0.164	-0.245	0.396
2012	-0.077	0.174	-0.418	0.265
2011	0.383	0.694	-0.977	1.742
2011	0.151	0.026	0.099	0.202
2011	-0.411	0.369	-1.134	0.312
2010	-0.021	0.139	-0.294	0.251
2010	0.455	0.425	-0.378	1.288
2009	0.598	0.142	0.319	0.876
2008	0.382	0.812	-1.208	1.973
2008	0.541	0.796	-1.019	2.100
2008	-0.020	0.213	-0.438	0.397
2008	0.114	0.195	-0.268	0.496
2007	0.194	0.078	0.040	0.348
2007	0.284	0.156	-0.021	0.589
2006	0.143	0.381	-0.602	0.889
2006	0.242	0.432	-0.605	1.089
2005	0.375	0.158	0.065	0.685
2004	0.979	0.193	0.600	1.358
2004	0.132	0.057	0.019	0.244
2001	0.059	0.042	-0.023	0.142
2000	0.000	0.503	-0.986	0.986
1998	0.424	0.077	0.274	0.574
1990	-0.153	0.283	-0.708	0.402
1988	0.739	0.387	-0.019	1.497
1986	0.132	0.330	-0.515	0.780
1985	2.521	0.585	1.374	3.668
Summary Effect	0.229	0.047	0.138	0.321

FIGURE. *Forest plot of main effects. Forest plot of meta-analysis of two-group posttest comparisons of medication adherence outcomes listed by year of publication. Effect sizes calculated using a random effects model. Study weight is proportional to the area of each square.*

TABLE 3	Continuous Moderator Results			
Moderator	k	B	SE	P
Report and methods moderators				
Year of publication	28	−0.005	0.004	.205
Sample size	28	−0.000	0.000	.004
Sample attribute moderators				
Age	21	0.014	0.004	.001
Percentage of women	23	−0.000	0.002	.968
Underrepresented groups	7	0.000	0.001	.810
Intervention feature moderator				
No. sessions	17	−0.013	0.013	.304
Duration of intervention	23	−0.000	0.000	.972
Time point for MA outcome data collection	14	−0.000	0.000	.213

B, meta-regression coefficient (unstandardized); k, number of comparisons; p, value for B; SE, standard error.

questionnaire on participants' baseline MA and barriers to MA.[24] Studies with nurse interventionists (0.428) reported significantly higher MA than studies without nurse interventionists (0.127). Studies with and without physician and pharmacist interventionists had similar ESs. Interventions started when participants were inpatients had significantly larger effects (0.590) than interventions that did not start with inpatients (0.141); however, there was little difference when the intervention was delivered at home versus in the clinic. With regards to the mode of intervention delivery, we saw no significant differences among telephone, written materials only, or face-to-face delivery. Interventions using mail delivery were less effective (0.060) than interventions without mail delivery interventions (0.292). There were several nonsignificant variables, including: utilization of theory, number of sessions, duration of intervention, time point for measuring outcome MA, goal setting, interventions delivered at home, interventions delivered in clinic, problem solving, succinct written instructions, any written instructions, behavior target (MA or multiple behaviors), physician or pharmacist interventionists, telephone and face-to-face delivery, and written instructions only.

Report and Sample Moderators
The age of subjects had a significant positive slope (0.014), revealing that MA interventions led to greater adherence improvement in samples of older patients. Interventions were equally effective regardless of publication status, funding, and location. Other nonsignificant moderators included year of publication, percentage of women and underrepresented groups, and socioeconomic status.

Design and Methods Moderators
Although sample size had a statistically significant negative slope, this finding is not clinically substantive. Other potential moderators related to design, such as blinding, allocation concealment, random assignment, and intention-to-treat analyses, were not associated with MA effectiveness.

Discussion
Findings from this meta-analysis, which is the first of its kind, that suggest interventions to increase MA among participants with CAD were significantly effective. These positive findings are similar to prior meta-analyses examining MA outcomes from MA interventions among underrepresented groups and from packaging intervention effects.[46,47] Although poor MA has been linked to negative health outcomes in patients with CAD,[4,6,7] consensus on how much MA is needed to improve varied CAD-related outcomes is not yet clear. Prior research exploring MA and blood pressure outcomes[48,49] as well as cardiovascular disease risk exists.[49] However, further research is needed to quantify the amount of MA needed to mitigate additional CAD-related outcomes. Moreover, the dose of MA intervention needed to change MA behavior among patients with CAD is yet to be determined. Due to the small number of comparisons using similar measures of MA, we were unable to convert the ES to a clinical metric of adherence. Future MA intervention research among patients with CAD should include explicit information regarding intervention dose.

Moderator Findings
We found several interesting moderators. Interventions in which healthcare providers were given information regarding participants' MA were more effective than interventions without this component. Awareness of patients' MA behavior can motivate and guide providers to address issues related to MA. Clinicians working with patients with CAD should assess issues with or barriers to MA to identify the possible need to intervene. Future research might directly compare an intervention that provides patient MA status to healthcare providers to a similar intervention without this provision.

Medication adherence interventions delivered by nurses were especially effective. Nurses have considerable access to patients with CAD in outpatient settings, such as cardiac rehabilitation and clinics. In addition, nurses working in the inpatient setting spend approximately 25% to 37% of their time providing direct patient care and 11% to 21% of their time in medication-related tasks.[50,51] In addition to substantial access to this patient population, nurses also have clinical skills to promote MA. For example, nurses have delivered efficacious MA interventions through counseling,[52] follow-up communication,[27,53,54] and case management.[55,56] Nurses should play an active role in developing and implementing MA interventions among patients with CAD. Research exploring nursing interventions to increase MA among patients with CAD could focus on testing or comparing specific intervention strategies such as education, counseling, and managing barriers. Specific nurse type and training were not clearly reported among the studies, hindering the comparison of

TABLE 4	Dichotomous Moderator Results				
Moderator	***k***	***d***	**SE**	***Q*₈**	***P***
Report moderators					
Publication status				1.267	.260
Unpublished (eg, dissertation, presentation)	4	0.724	0.474		
Published article	24	0.189	0.037		
Presence of funding for research				1.911	.167
Unfunded	11	0.452	0.192		
Funded (any funding reported or acknowledged)	17	0.182	0.040		
Socioeconomic status				0.194	.660
Not reported as low income	24	0.237	0.046		
Reported as low income	4	0.352	0.259		
Location				0.531	.466
Not North America	7	0.380	0.125		
North America	21	0.182	0.045		
Research methods moderators					
Allocation to treatment and control groups				0.200	.655
Not random assignment	8	0.199	0.068		
Random assignment	20	0.244	0.072		
Allocation concealment				1.222	.269
Allocation not concealed	15	0.188	0.050		
Allocation concealed	13	0.319	0.108		
Theory				0.167	.683
No theory	23	0.239	0.050		
Any theory	5	0.184	0.124		
Data collectors blinded				0.481	.488
Data collectors not blinded	18	0.207	0.052		
Data collectors blinded	10	0.293	0.112		
Intention-to-treat				0.000	.997
No intention-to-treat	23	0.236	0.063		
Intention-to-treat	5	0.237	0.097		
Intervention feature moderators					
Goal setting				0.095	.758
No goal setting	23	0.227	0.050		
Goal setting	5	0.183	0.135		
Healthcare provider given information about MA				3.899	.048
Healthcare provider NOT given information about MA	20	0.151	0.042		
Healthcare provider given information about MA	8	0.387	0.112		
Intervention delivered at home				0.676	.411
Not at home	23	0.254	0.053		
At home	5	0.129	0.143		
Intervention delivered at clinic				0.705	.401
Not at clinic	23	0.213	0.049		
At clinic	5	0.320	0.118		
Intervention started while subjects were inpatients				8.448	.004
Not inpatients	19	0.141	0.037		
Inpatients	9	0.590	0.150		
Problem solving				0.307	.580
No problem solving	22	0.245	0.054		
Problem solving	6	0.188	0.088		
Self-monitoring of medications				1.198	.274
No self-monitoring	25	0.195	0.045		
Self-monitoring	3	0.492	0.267		
Succinct written instructions				1.820	.177
No succinct written instructions	22	0.255	0.054		
Succinct written instructions	6	0.124	0.080		
Any written instructions				2.868	.090
No written instructions	19	0.287	0.065		
Any written instructions	9	0.149	0.049		
Behavior target				1.212	.271
Multiple behaviors	11	0.306	0.109		
MA only	17	0.179	0.038		

(continues)

TABLE 4 Dichotomous Moderator Results, Continued					
Moderator	**k**	**d**	**SE**	**Q_B**	**P**
Part of intervention delivered to providers				0.476	.490
Not delivered to providers	24	0.213	0.053		
Delivered to providers	4	0.311	0.131		
Nurse interventionist				6.502	.011
No nurse	18	0.127	0.020		
Any nurse	10	0.428	0.116		
Physician interventionist				0.397	.529
No physician	21	0.223	0.050		
Physician	7	0.322	0.148		
Pharmacist interventionist				0.310	.578
No pharmacist	21	0.240	0.056		
Pharmacist	7	0.193	0.062		
Mail delivery				10.845	.001
No mail delivery	23	0.292	0.059		
Mail delivery	5	0.060	0.038		
Telephone delivery				0.701	.403
No telephone delivery	14	0.192	0.065		
Telephone delivery	14	0.280	0.082		
Written materials ONLY				2.985	.084
No written intervention	26	0.248	0.049		
Written intervention	2	0.008	0.130		
Face-to-face delivery				2.604	.107
No face-to-face	7	0.143	0.048		
Face-to-face	21	0.288	0.076		

k, number of comparisons; d, standardized mean difference effect size; SE, standard error; Q_B, sum of weighted sum of squares of subgroup means about overall mean; p, value for Q_B

MA intervention effectiveness across different types of nurses. Investigators of future studies should explicitly identify types of nurses delivering MA interventions among patients with CAD.

Medication adherence interventions initiated in the inpatient setting were more effective. The inpatient setting may provide an opportunity for clinicians to inform patients and families about the importance of medications for secondary prevention of CAD as well as strategies for MA. Moreover, the dire nature of hospitalization may influence patient and family receptivity to MA interventions. Most MA interventions initiated in the inpatient setting included follow-up intervention content after discharge. Continued reinforcement of MA after discharge may positively affect MA outcomes. For those patients who may start medications outside the hospital, interventions delivered at home or in the clinic were equally effective. Future research might directly compare MA interventions initiated in the inpatient setting to MA interventions initiated after hospitalization.

Regarding sample characteristics, only age appeared to impact intervention effectiveness. As the age of the sample increased, so did the intervention effectiveness. These findings support prior research related to statin MA and low-density lipoprotein goal attainment.[57,58] Chi and colleagues[57] postulated that older individuals are more likely to have multiple comorbidities and may be more attentive to prescribed medication regimens. Additional primary research is needed to identify effective MA interventions among younger populations with CAD. Furthermore, more primary research involving more diverse samples is needed. Deaths related to CAD are higher among African Americans than whites and other groups.[2,59] Rates of MA for various chronic diseases also differ across race and ethnicity, with minority groups being less adherent to prescribed medications.[60,61] However, few primary studies included in this meta-analysis reported racially or ethnically diverse groups. Thus, future primary research testing MA interventions among patients with CAD must strive to include minority groups to reduce this disparity.

We found some interesting nonsignificant moderators. Interventions focusing solely on MA were as effective as interventions that had multiple behavioral foci. Thus, clinicians may take the opportunity to introduce strategies for MA while discussing other health behaviors with CAD patients. The use of only written material did not impact intervention effectiveness, suggesting that providers should consider using more than this type of delivery when promoting MA among patients with CAD. Future MA intervention research among patients with CAD should incorporate additional forms of intervention delivery beyond written materials. Number of intervention sessions did not appear to be a significant moderator. It is possible that even 1 or 2 intervention sessions may be effective in changing MA behavior among patients with CAD. However, additional research testing or comparing various aspects of intervention dose could help identify the most effective dose needed to change MA behavior. We did not identify any specific

---

What's New and Important

- Interventions designed to increase MA among patients with CAD are modestly effective.
- In this patient population, nurse-delivered MA interventions were more effective than interventions not delivered by nurses.
- Among patients with CAD, MA interventions initiated in the inpatient setting can be more effective than interventions initiated in the outpatient setting.

---

intervention strategy that increased MA intervention effectiveness; however, lack of statistical significance of these moderators may be related to the small number of comparisons.

Medication adherence interventions delivered by physicians or pharmacists were equally effective as interventions not delivered by these providers. Although these findings suggest that involving these providers may not increase MA intervention effectiveness, the number of studies incorporating these types of interventionists was small. Future research could directly compare similar MA interventions among patients with CAD delivered by different clinicians. Additional research may also explore variations in MA intervention delivery across diverse healthcare providers.

This meta-analysis was limited by some primary study characteristics. Although efforts were made to contact corresponding authors, some studies were excluded because critical data were missing from primary study reports. Primary study reporting limits the generalizability of this study's findings to more diverse populations. Primary study quality is an important issue in meta-analysis work. Multiple strategies are recommended to manage primary study quality.[62,63] We used specific inclusion criteria to capture reports with more rigorous study designs, employed analysis techniques accounting for study heterogeneity, and explored study quality empirically through moderator analyses. Some publication biases were present. Smaller, negative studies are less likely to be published; therefore, access to these studies is limited. Despite extensive search strategies, capturing these relevant studies was a challenge.

Primary study reporting affected the ability to identify effective combinations of MA components. Several studies used multiple intervention strategies; however, combinations of strategies were inconsistent. Thus, determining the most effective combination of MA intervention strategies was not possible.

Measurement error within the primary studies could have introduced bias toward overestimation of MA intervention effects. Objective measures are the most sensitive and specific means of measuring MA[64,65]; however, most included studies used self-reported MA, which is known to overestimate patients' MA.[66] Future MA intervention research conducted among patients with CAD

should consider using objective measures of MA to reduce bias.

Meta-analyses are observational studies. The moderator findings of this study are intended to promote additional exploration in this area of study. The scope of this meta-analysis is limited to MA among patients with CAD. Therefore, interpretation of these findings may not be possible among patients with other chronic illnesses or other forms of heart disease.

Conclusion

Medication management is an important aspect of secondary prevention for CAD. Nonadherence to prescribed medications for CAD has been linked with multiple poor outcomes. Findings from this meta-analysis suggest that MA interventions among patients with CAD are effective, especially among older patients. Clinicians working with patients with CAD evaluate patients' MA behavior before initiating interventions to improve MA. Nurses are on the front lines of health behavior promotion among these patients and can be effective MA interventionists. Future research is needed to explore MA interventions among younger populations and more racially diverse groups.

REFERENCES

1. Centers for Disease Control and Prevention. *Heart Disease Facts*. 2014. http://www.cdc.gov/heartdisease/facts.htm. Accessed July 16, 2014.
2. National Heart, Lung, and Blood Institute. *Morbidity and Mortality: 2012 Chart Book on Cardiovascular, Lung, and Blood Diseases*. Washington, DC: National Institutes of Health; 2012.
3. Ford ES, Ajani UA, Croft JB, et al. Explaining the decrease in U.S. deaths from coronary disease, 1980–2000. *N Engl J Med.* 2007;356(23):2388–2398.
4. Ho PM, Bryson CL, Rumsfeld JS. Medication adherence its importance in cardiovascular outcomes. *Circulation.* 2009; 119(23):3028–3035.
5. Naderi SH, Bestwick JP, Wald DS. Adherence to drugs that prevent cardiovascular disease: meta-analysis on 376,162 patients. *Am J Med.* 2012;125(9):882–887.
6. Chowdhury R, Khan H, Heydon E, et al. Adherence to cardiovascular therapy: a meta-analysis of prevalence and clinical consequences. *Eur Heart J.* 2013;34(38):2940–2948.
7. Sokol MC, McGuigan KA, Verbrugge RR, Epstein RS. Impact of medication adherence on hospitalization risk and healthcare cost. *Med Care.* 2005;43(6):521–530.
8. Ho PM, Magid DJ, Shetterly SM, et al. Medication nonadherence is associated with a broad range of adverse outcomes in patients with coronary artery disease. *Am Heart J.* 2008; 155(4):772–779.
9. Kelly JM. Sublingual nitroglycerin: improving patient compliance with a demonstration dose. *J Am Board Fam Pract.* 1988;1(4):251–254.
10. Nicoleau, CM. *Evaluation of a comprehensive cardiac rehabilitation program* [dissertation]. New York, NY: Yeshiva University; 1985.
11. Zhao Y. Effects of a discharge planning intervention for elderly patients with coronary heart disease in Tianjin, China:

a randomized controlled trial. 2004. http://search.proquest
.com.proxy.mul.missouri.edu/pqdt/docview/305041963/
abstract/CE2FD56D4F7B49F2PQ/1?accountid=14576.
Accessed June 11, 2014.

12. Costa e Silva R, Pellanda L, Portal V, Maciel P, Furquim A,
Schaan B. Transdisciplinary approach to the follow-up of
patients after myocardial infarction. *Clin Sao Paulo Braz.*
2008;63(4):489–496.

13. Lourenco L, Rodrigues RCM, Gallani CB, Spana TM. Effectiveness of the combination of planning strategies in adhering to
the drug therapy and health related quality of life among coronary heart disease outpatients. Paper presented at: International
Nursing Intervention Conference; 2011; Montreal, Canada.

14. Miller P, Wikoff R, Garrett MJ, McMahon M, Smith T.
Regimen compliance two years after myocardial infarction.
Nurs Res. 1990;39(6):333–336.

15. Ara S. A literature review of cardiovascular disease management programs in managed care populations. *J Manag Care
Pharm.* 2004;10(4):326–344.

16. Cutrona SL, Choudhry NK, Fischer MA, et al. Targeting
cardiovascular medication adherence interventions. *J Am
Pharm Assoc (2003).* 2012;52(3):381–397.

17. Maddox TM, Ho PM. Medication adherence and the patient with coronary artery disease: challenges for the practitioner. *Curr Opin Cardiol.* 2009;24(5):468–472.

18. Schadewaldt V, Schultz T. Nurse-led clinics as an effective
service for cardiac patients: results from a systematic review.
Int J Evid Based Healthc. 2011;9(3):199–214.

19. Cooper H, Hedges LV, Valentine JC, eds. *The Handbook of
Research Synthesis and Meta-Analysis.* 2nd ed. New York, NY:
Russell Sage Foundation; 2009.

20. Moher D, Liberati A, Tetzlaff J, Altman DG. Preferred reporting items for systematic reviews and meta-analyses: the PRISMA
statement. *BMJ.* 2009;339:b2535.

21. Reed JG, Baxter PM. Using reference databases. In: *The
Handbook of Research Synthesis and Meta-Analysis.* 2nd ed.
New York, NY: Russell Sage Foundation; 2009:73–101.

22. Borenstein M, Hedges LV, Higgins JPT, Rothstein HR. *Comprehensive Meta-Analysis.* Englewood, NJ: Biostat; 2005.

23. Borenstein M, Hedges LV, Higgins JPT, Rothstein HR. *Introduction to Meta-Analysis.* 1st ed. West Sussex, UK: Wiley; 2009.

24. Calvert SB, Kramer JM, Anstrom KJ, Kaltenbach LA,
Stafford JA, Allen LaPointe NM. Patient-focused intervention
to improve long-term adherence to evidence-based medications:
a randomized trial. *Am Heart J.* 2012;163(4):657–665.

25. Campbell N, Ritchie L, Thain J, Deans H, Rawles J, Squair J.
Secondary prevention in coronary heart disease: a randomised
trial of nurse led clinics in primary care. *Heart.* 1998;80(5):
447–452.

26. Choudhry NK, Avorn J, Glynn RJ, et al. Full coverage for
preventive medications after myocardial infarction. *N Engl
J Med.* 2011;365(22):2088–2097.

27. Edworthy SM, Baptie B, Galvin D, et al. Effects of an enhanced secondary prevention program for patients with heart
disease: a prospective randomized trial. *Can J Cardiol.* 2007;
23(13):1066–1072.

28. Faulkner MA, Wadibia EC, Lucas BD, Hilleman DE. Impact
of pharmacy counseling on compliance and effectiveness of
combination lipid-lowering therapy in patients undergoing
coronary artery revascularization: a randomized, controlled
trial. *Pharmacotherapy.* 2000;20:410–416.

29. Gould KA. A randomized controlled trial of a discharge
nursing intervention to promote self-regulation of care for
early discharge interventional cardiology patients. *Dimens
Crit Care Nurs.* 2011;30(2):117–125.

30. Guthrie RM. The effects of postal and telephone reminders
on compliance with pravastatin therapy in a national reg-

istry: Results of the first myocardial infarction risk reduction
program. *Clin Ther.* 2001;23(6):970–980.

31. Jiang X, Sit JW, Wong TK. A nurse-led cardiac rehabilitation
programme improves health behaviours and cardiac physiological risk parameters: Evidence from Chengdu, China. *J Clin
Nurs.* 2007;16(10):1886–1897.

32. Kotowycz MA, Cosman TL, Tartaglia C, Afzal R,
Natarajan MK, et al. Safety and feasibility of early hospital
discharge in ST-segment elevation myocardial infarction—a
prospective and randomized trial in low-risk primary percutaneous coronary intervention patients (the Safe-Depart Trial).
Am Heart J. 2010;159(1):117.

33. Kripalani S, Schmotzer B, Jacobson TA. Improving medication adherence through graphically enhanced interventions in
coronary heart disease (IMAGE-CHD): A randomized controlled trial. *J Gen Intern Med.* 2012;27(12):1609–1617.

34. Lehr BK. *A comparative study of self-management and
cognitive behavioral therapies in the treatment of cardiac
rehabilitation patients* [dissertation]. Milwaukee, WI: University of Wisconsin; 1986.

35. Muñiz J, Gómez-Doblas JJ, Santiago-Pérez MI, et al. The
effect of post-discharge educational intervention on patients
in achieving objectives in modifiable risk factors six months
after discharge following an episode of acute coronary syndrome, (CAM-2 Project): A randomized controlled trial. *Health
Qual Life Outcomes.* 2010;8:137.

36. Polack J, Jorgenson D, Robertson P. Evaluation of different
methods of providing medication-related education to patients
following myocardial infarction. *Can Pharm J.* 2008;141(4):
241–247.

37. Shemesh E, Koren-Michowitz M, Yehuda R, et al. Symptoms
of posttraumatic stress disorder in patients who have had a
myocardial infarction. *J Consult Liaison Psychiatry.* 2006;
47(3):231–239.

38. Sherrard H, Struthers C, Kearns SA, Wells G, Mesana T.
Using technology to create a medication safety net for cardiac
surgery patients: a nurse-led randomized control trial. *Can J
Cardiovasc Nurs.* 2009;19(3):9–15.

39. Smith DH, Kramer JM, Perrin N, et al. A randomized trial
of direct-to-patient communication to enhance adherence to
beta-blocker therapy following myocardial infarction. *Arch
Intern Med.* 2008;168(5):477–483.

40. Yilmaz MB, Pinar M, Naharci I, et al. Being well-informed
about statin is associated with continuous adherence and reach-
ing targets. *Cardiovasc Drugs Ther.* 2005;19(6):437–440.

41. Zuckerman IH, Weiss SR, McNally D, Layne B, Mullins CD,
Wang J. Impact of an educational intervention for secondary
prevention of myocardial infarction on Medicaid drug use
and cost. *Am J Manag Care.* 2004;10(7 part 2):493–500.

42. Miller P, Wikoff R, McMahon M, Garrett MJ, Ringel K.
Influence of a nursing intervention on regimen adherence and
societal adjustments postmyocardial infarction. *Nurs Res.*
1988;37(5):297–302.

43. Miller P, Wikoff R, McMahon M, et al. Personal adjustments
and regimen compliance 1 year after myocardial infarction.
Heart Lung. 1989;18(4):339–346.

44. Choudhry NK, Brennan T, Toscano M, et al. Rationale and
design of the Post-MI FREEE trial: a randomized evaluation
of first-dollar drug coverage for post-myocardial infarction secondary preventive therapies. *Am Heart J.* 2008;156(1):31–36.

45. Gould KA. A randomized controlled trial of a discharge
nursing intervention to promote self-regulation of care for
early discharge interventional cardiology patients. *Dimens
Crit Care Nurs.* 2009;30(2):117–125.

46. Conn VS, Enriquez M, Ruppar TM, Chan KC. Cultural relevance in medication adherence interventions with underrepresented adults: systematic review and meta-analysis of
outcomes. *Prev Med.* 2014;69:239–247.

47. Conn V. Packaging interventions to increase medication adherence: systematic review and meta-analysis. *Curr Med Res Opin.* 2015;31(1):145–160.

48. Burnier M, Schneider MP, Chioléro A, Stubi CL, Brunner HR. Electronic compliance monitoring in resistant hypertension: the basis for rational therapeutic decisions. *J Hypertens.* 2001; 19(2):335–341.

49. Lowy A, Munk VC, Ong SH, et al. Effects on blood pressure and cardiovascular risk of variations in patients' adherence to prescribed antihypertensive drugs: role of duration of drug action. *Int J Clin Pract.* 2011;65(1):41–53.

50. Westbrook JI, Duffield C, LiL, Creswick NJ. How much time do nurses have for patients? A longitudinal study quantifying hospital nurses' patterns of task time distribution and interactions with health professionals. *BMC Health Serv Res.* 2011;11:319.

51. Jones M, Johnston D. Understanding phenomena in the real world: the case for real time data collection in health services research. *J Health Serv Res Policy.* 2011;16(3):172–176.

52. Krantz MJ, Havranek EP, Haynes DK, Smith I, Bucher-Bartelson B, Long CS. Inpatient initiation of beta-blockade plus nurse management in vulnerable heart failure patients: a randomized study. *J Card Fail.* 2008;14(4):303–309.

53. Kirscht JP, Kirscht JL, Rosenstock IM. A test of interventions to increase adherence to hypertensive medical regimens. *Health Educ Q.* 1981;8(3):261–272.

54. Piette JD, Weinberger M, McPhee SJ, Mah CA, Kraemer FB, Crapo LM. Do automated calls with nurse follow-up improve self-care and glycemic control among vulnerable patients with diabetes? *Am J Med.* 2000;108(1):20–27.

55. Logan AG, Milne BJ, Achber C, Campbell WP, Haynes RB. Work-site treatment of hypertension by specially trained nurses. A controlled trial. *Lancet.* 1979;2(8153):1175–1178.

56. Rudd P, Miller NH, Kaufman J, et al. Nurse management for hypertension. A systems approach. *Am J Hypertens.* 2004; 17(10):921–927.

57. Chi MD, Vansomphone SS, Liu I-LA, et al. Adherence to statins and LDL-cholesterol goal attainment. *Am J Manag Care.* 2014;20(4):e105–e112.

58. Nag SS, Daniel GW, Bullano MF, et al. LDL-C goal attainment among patients newly diagnosed with coronary heart disease or diabetes in a commercial HMO. *J Manag Care Pharm.* 2007;13(8):652–663.

59. Coronary Heart Disease and Stroke Deaths—United States, 2006. http://www.cdc.gov/mmwr/preview/mmwrhtml/su6001a13.htm. Accessed June 6, 2014.

60. Gerber BS, Cho YI, Arozullah AM, Lee S-YD. Racial differences in medication adherence: A cross-sectional study of Medicare enrollees. *Am J Geriatr Pharmacother.* 2010;8(2): 136–145.

61. Rolnick SJ, Pawloski PA, Hedblom BD, Asche SE, Bruzek RJ. Patient characteristics associated with medication adherence. *Clin Med Res.* 2013;11(2):54–65.

62. Valentine JC. Judging the quality of primary research. In: Cooper HM, Hedges LV, Valentine JC, eds. *The Handbook of Research Synthesis and Meta-Analysis.* 2nd ed. Russell Sage Foundation; 2009:122–146.

63. Conn VS, Rantz MJ. Research methods: managing primary study quality in meta-analyses. *Res Nurs Health.* 2003;26(4): 322–333.

64. Dunbar-Jacob J, Sereika SM, Houze M, Luyster FS, Callan JA. Accuracy of measures of medication adherence in a cholesterol-lowering regimen. *West J Nurs Res.* 2012; 34(5):578–597.

65. Hansen RA, Kim MM, Song L, Tu W, Wu J, Murray MD. Comparison of methods to assess medication adherence and classify nonadherence. *Ann Pharmacother.* 2009;43(3): 413–422.

66. Zeller A, Ramseier E, Teagtmeyer A, Battegay E. Patients' self-reported adherence to cardiovascular medication using electronic monitors as comparators. *Hypertens Res.* 2008; 31(11):2037–2043.

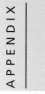

APPENDIX H

Lead Article

A Metaethnography of Traumatic Childbirth and its Aftermath: Amplifying Causal Looping

Qualitative Health Research
21(3) 301–311
© The Author(s) 2011
Reprints and permission:
sagepub.com/journalsPermissions.nav
DOI: 10.1177/1049732310390698
http://qhr.sagepub.com
⑤SAGE

Cheryl Tatano Beck[1]

Abstract

Integrating results from multiple analytic approaches used in a research program by the same researcher is a type of metasynthesis that has not often been reported in the literature. In this article the findings of one type of qualitative synthesis approach, a metaethnography, of six qualitative studies on birth trauma and its resulting posttraumatic stress disorder from my program of research are presented. This metaethnography provides a wide-angle lens to view and interpret the far-reaching, stinging tentacles of this often invisible phenomenon that new mothers experience. I used Noblit and Hare's seven-step approach for synthesizing the findings of qualitative studies. The original trigger of traumatic childbirth resulted in six amplifying feedback loops, four of which were reinforcing (positive direction), and two which were balancing (negative direction). Leverage points that identify where pressure in the amplifying causal loop can break the feedback loop where necessary are discussed.

Keywords

childbirth; metaethnography; metasynthesis; qualitative analysis; trauma

As Lisa recalled, "I am amazed that three and a half hours in the labor and delivery room could cause such utter destruction in my life. It truly was like being a victim of a violent crime of rape" (Beck, 2004a, p. 32). What happened to this mother that turned her birthing dream into a rape scene? The purpose of this article is to present the results of a metaethnography which focused not only on answering this question, but also on the repercussions of traumatic childbirth for women. By synthesizing the results of six qualitative studies on birth trauma and its resulting posttraumatic stress disorder (PTSD) from my research program, I used a wide-angle lens to view and interpret the far-reaching, stinging tentacles of this often invisible phenomenon. In two of the qualitative studies I examined the experience of a traumatic childbirth (Beck, 2004a, 2006b). My focus in the remaining four studies was the aftermath of birth trauma (Beck, 2004b; 2006a; Beck & Watson, 2008; Beck & Watson, 2010).

Metasynthesis

Metasynthesis is "an interpretive integration of qualitative findings that are themselves interpretive syntheses of data, including the phenomenologies, ethnographies, grounded theories, and other integrative and coherent descriptions or

explanations of phenomena, events, or cases that are the hallmarks of qualitative research" (Sandelowski & Barroso, 2007, p. 151). The aim of a metasynthesis is not to focus on the similarities of the results of the qualitative studies included in the metasynthesis, but instead to delve further into these findings to unearth new information to increase our understanding of the phenomenon (Paterson, Thorne, Canam, & Jillings, 2001). Sandelowski and Barroso differentiated between qualitative metasynthesis and qualitative metasummary. Qualitative metasummary is "a quantitative oriented aggregation of qualitative findings that are themselves topical or thematic summaries or surveys of data" (p. 151). Qualitative metasyntheses are more than just summaries. Their end product is a new interpretation of the findings.

Metasyntheses help to prevent what Glaser and Strauss (1971, p. 181) warned as qualitative research studies' results remaining as "respected little islands of knowledge separated from others and not helping to build a cumulative

[1]University of Connecticut, Storrs, Connecticut, USA

Corresponding Author:
Cheryl Tatano Beck, University of Connecticut School of Nursing,
231 Glenbrook Road, Storrs, CT 06269-2026, USA
Email: cheryl.beck@uconn.edu

187

body of knowledge in a substantive area." With more and more focus on metasynthesis, qualitative scholars are now delving further into its implications and applications (Thorne, Jensen, Kearney, Noblit & Sandelowski, 2004). Examples of recent metasyntheses span topics such as withdrawing life-sustaining treatments (Meeker & Jezewski, 2009), mothers' confidence in breastfeeding (Larsen, Hall, & Aagaard, 2008), diabetes in nine South Asian communities (Fleming & Gillibrand, 2009), healing from sexual violence (Draucker et al., 2009), and the hope experience of family caregivers of chronically ill persons (Duggleby et al., 2010).

Three types of metasyntheses are available to researchers (Sandelowski, Docherty, & Emden, 1997). The most frequently used type involves synthesizing results across studies on the same topic conducted by different researchers. A second type consists of using quantitative approaches to synthesize qualitative results from cases across different studies. Integrating results from multiple analytic approaches used in a research program by the same researcher is the third type. An example of this third kind of qualitative metasynthesis is a synthesis of the transition to parenthood of infertile couples (Sandelowski, 1995). This is the only metasynthesis located to date in which a series of qualitative research studies on a phenomenon conducted by the same researcher were synthesized.

Kearney (2001) described current approaches to the synthesis of findings of qualitative research studies into a new integrated whole as the meta family. Included in this meta family are such approaches as metastudy, metainterpretation, metaethnography, and grounded formal theory. Kearney placed these different synthesis approaches on an interpreting–theorizing continuum. On the theorizing end is formal grounded theory (Glaser, 2007), and on the interpretive end is metaethnography (Noblit & Hare, 1988).

Research Design

This metaethnography of birth trauma and its resulting PTSD resulting from childbirth was generated from the findings of six studies I conducted which were published between 2004 and 2010 (Beck 2004a, 2004b, 2006a, 2006b; Beck & Watson, 2008, 2010). Metaethnography is the synthesis of interpretive research. It involves a rigorous approach for constructing substantive interpretations about a group of qualitative studies. A metaethnographer compares and analyzes texts to create new interpretations by translating studies into one another. Noblit and Hare (1988) proposed that translating studies involves making analogies between the studies and also among the studies. An interpretive form of knowledge synthesis is achieved inductively. The aims of metaethnography are to enable:

1. More interpretive literature reviews
2. Critical examination of multiple accounts of an event, situation, and so forth
3. Systematic comparison of case studies to draw cross-case conclusions
4. A way of talking about our work and comparing it to the works of others
5. Synthesis of ethnographic studies (Noblit & Hare, 1988, p. 12)

Sample

These six studies are profiled in Tables 1 and 2. In the first study, "Birth Trauma: In the Eye of the Beholder," I focused on the experience of traumatic childbirth (Beck, 2004a). In the second study I examined PTSD following birth trauma (Beck, 2004b). In the third study I examined the anniversary of birth trauma (Beck, 2006a). These first three studies were phenomenological studies. The fourth study was a narrative analysis of birth trauma stories (Beck, 2006b). The fifth and sixth studies in my program of research were phenomenological studies looking at the impact of birth trauma on breastfeeding (Beck & Watson, 2008), and on the experience of subsequent childbirth after a previous traumatic birth (Beck & Watson, 2010). The total number of participants in these six studies was 175 mothers. Thirty-eight of the 40 mothers who participated in the first study on birth trauma (Beck, 2004a) also participated in the PTSD-following-childbirth study (Beck, 2004b). I achieved data saturation in each study. All the studies adhered to ethical standards. I received institutional review board approval for each study and informed consent was obtained from all participants.

Qualitative studies on traumatic childbirth have been conducted by researchers other than me, including Ayers (2007) and Nicholls and Ayers (2007). The studies conducted by these authors were not pertinent to the current metaethnography and thus were not included in it, because this metaethnography was a synthesis of results used in a program of research by the same researcher, that being myself.

Data Analysis

I used Noblit and Hare's (1988) seven-step approach for synthesizing the findings of qualitative studies. These steps overlapped and repeated as the synthesis was conducted, and included:

1. Choosing a phenomenon to be studied
2. Identifying which qualitative studies were pertinent
3. Reading the qualitative studies to be included in the synthesis

Table 1. Demographic Characteristics of Participants in the Individual Studies Included in the Metaethnography

Study	Sample Size	Country (N)	Age Range	Parity (N)	Marital Status (N)	Delivery Type (N)
Beck (2004a)	40	New Zealand (23) United States (8) Australia (6) United Kingdom (3)	25-40	Multiparas (24) Primiparas (16)	Married (34) Divorced (3) Single (3)	Vaginal (22) Cesarean (18)
Beck (2004b)	38	New Zealand (22) United States (7) Australia (6) United Kingdom (3)	25-44	Multiparas (26) Primiparas (12)	Married (34) Divorced (2) Single (2)	Vaginal (21) Cesarean (17)
Beck (2006a)	11	United States (6) New Zealand (3) Australia (1) United Kingdom (1)	26-38	Multiparas (8) Primiparas (3)	Married (11)	Vaginal (7) Cesarean (3) Both (1)
Beck (2006b)	37	United States (20) New Zealand (8) Australia (4) United Kingdom (4) Canada (1)	24-54	Multiparas (14) Primiparas (19) Missing (4)	Married (31) Divorced (1) Single (1) Missing (4)	Vaginal (18) Cesarean (13) Both (6)
Beck & Watson (2008)	52	New Zealand (28) United States (11) Australia (6) United Kingdom (4) Canada (3)		Multiparas (21) Primiparas (31)	Married (46) Living with partner (5) Separated (1)	Vaginal (26) Cesarean (25) Both (1)
Beck & Watson (2010)	35	United States (15) United Kingdom (8) New Zealand (6) Australia (5) Canada (1)	27-51	Multiparas (52)	Married (34) Divorced (1)	Vaginal (25) Cesarean (10)

4. Deciding how the studies were related to one another. Here the researcher lists the key metaphors in each study and how they are related to each other. Noblit and Hare use the term *metaphor* to refer to concepts, themes, or phrases when synthesizing studies. Three differing assumptions can be made regarding how studies are related: "(a) the accounts are directly comparable as 'reciprocal' translations; (b) the accounts stand in relative opposition to each other and are essentially 'refutational'; or (c) the studies taken together present a 'line of argument' rather than a reciprocal or refutational translation" (p. 36). In this metaethnography, the assumption was one of reciprocal translations.

5. Translating each study's metaphors into the metaphors of the others, and vice versa. Noblit and Hare described these translations as "especially unique syntheses because they protect the particular, respect holism, and enable comparison" (p. 28).

6. Synthesizing the translations, wherein a whole is created which is something more than the individual parts imply.

7. Expressing the synthesis, most often through the written word; however, plays, art, videos, or music are other options.

Care must be taken during the data analysis phase of a qualitative synthesis, as Sandelowski et al. warned:

Qualitative metasynthesis is not a trivial pursuit, but rather a complex exercise in interpretation: Carefully peeling away the surface layers of studies to find their hearts and souls in a way that does the least damage to them. Synthesists must analyze studies in sufficient detail to preserve the integrity of each study and yet not become so immersed in detail that no useable synthesis is produced. (1997, p. 370)

Table 2. Methodological Characteristics of the Qualitative Studies Included in the Metaethnography

Author	Year	Qualitative Research Design	Data Analysis
Beck	2004a	Phenomenology	Colaizzi
Beck	2004b	Phenomenology	Colaizzi
Beck	2006a	Narrative Analysis	Burke
Beck	2006b	Phenomenology	Colaizzi
Beck & Watson	2008	Phenomenology	Colaizzi
Beck & Watson	2010	Phenomenology	Colaizzi

Note. All studies had methodological characteristics of convenience sampling and Internet data collection.

Results

I constructed a detailed table of key metaphors from each of the six studies to facilitate the reciprocal translations (Table 3). These individual study metaphors were clustered into three overarching themes: stripped of protective layers, invisible wounds, and insidious repercussions. Under the theme of stripped of protective layers were the key metaphors that revealed that in birth trauma women perceived they were systematically stripped of essential protective layers, leaving them exposed and feeling very vulnerable. The overarching theme of invisible wounds addressed both the short- and long-term distressing emotions women struggled to cope with after experiencing a traumatic birth, such as fear, terror, grief, and feeling like a rape victim. Included under insidious repercussions were the often invisible detrimental effects of birth trauma on mothers' interactions with their infants.

Two of the six studies (Beck, 2004a; Beck, 2006b) included in the metaethnography uncovered the essence of what constituted traumatic childbirth for the women. The key metaphors in these two studies started the devastating domino effects that permeated mothers' lives as their dreams of motherhood were shattered. In my phenomenological study of traumatic childbirth (Beck, 2004a), a resounding characteristic of this phenomenon was that, just like beauty, birth trauma was in the eye of the beholder. What women perceived as a traumatic birth clinicians might have been viewed as a routine, normal delivery. Women felt abandoned, stripped of their dignity, and not cared for as an individual who deserved to be treated with respect. Obstetric staff neglected to communicate with mothers. Women often felt invisible, as Nicole explained:

> After an hour trying to deliver the baby with a vacuum extractor, the obstetrician said it was too late for an emergency cesarean. The baby was truly stuck. By now the doctors are acting like I'm not there. The attending physician was saying, "We

may have lost this bloody baby." The hospital staff discussed my baby's possible death in front of me, and argued in front of me just as if I weren't there. (Beck, 2004a, pp. 32-33)

Some women felt their trust in their respective obstetric care provider was betrayed, because they perceived that they received unsafe care but were powerless to rectify the dangerous situation. Mothers' traumatic experiences were pushed into the background as family and clinicians celebrated the birth of a live, healthy infant.

I later examined traumatic childbirth using a different qualitative research design, that being narrative analysis (Beck, 2006b). Using Burke's (1969) dramatistic pentad as the structure for viewing mothers' narratives, his ratio imbalance of act:agency appeared prominently in the narratives. Center stage in a woman's birth trauma narrative was how acts were performed during the birthing process. The manner in which obstetrical staff provided care to women during childbirth demonstrated a glaring absence of caring. The following is an excerpt from Michelle's narrative of the uncaring manner (agency) of the nurse who was present as the mother gave birth to her stillborn preterm infant:

> My husband went to get the nurse. The nurse said, you have only just had the gel, you couldn't be having IT yet. I said, yes. She is about to be born. The nurse checked and the head was visible. She looked shocked and said wait. I'll have to get a dish and returned with a green kidney shaped dish. The way she held the dish and the look on her face, I knew she did not want to be in the room. My husband held the dish for her. I then gave a little push and my daughter (still in her little sack) slipped quietly in the dish. The nurse took the dish from my husband and covered my daughter with a sheet. She then walked off without saying a word about where she was going. I called to her. Where are you taking her??? (I had not even seen her properly as she was still in her sack). The nurse said, I have to take IT to the doctor. She wants to see IT. Also the nurse continued to refer to me by my last name, not my first name. I said but I want to see my daughter. She said, Why? IT's dead. She then said I have to get someone to wash IT so IT can be examined. (Beck, 2006b, p. 461)

As the metaethnography progressed and more of the key metaphors were translated into each other, I had an "Aha!" moment. Operating in the aftermath of birth trauma—with its domino effects on various aspects of motherhood—was amplifying causal looping. In amplifying causal looping, "as consequences become continually causes and causes

Table 3. Individual Study Metaphors as Related to the Overarching Themes

Study	Stripped of Protective Layers	Invisible Wounds	Insidious Repercussions
Beck (2004a) Birth trauma: In the eye of the beholder	To care for me: Was that too much to ask? To communicate with me: Why was this neglected? To provide safe care: You betrayed my trust and I felt powerless	Fear Horror Terror Felt like a rape victim	The end justifies the means: At whose expense? At what price?
Beck (2004b) PTSD due to childbirth: The aftermath	Seeking to have questions answered and wanting to talk, talk, talk Isolation from world of motherhood	Going to the movies: Please don't make me go A shadow of myself: Too numb to try and change Dangerous trio of anger, anxiety, and depression: Spiraling downward	World of motherhood: Dreams shattered
Beck (2006a) Anniversary of birth trauma: Failure to rescue	Failure to rescue Lack of caring Lack of communication	The prologue: An agonizing time The actual day: A celebration of a birthday or torment of an anniversary	The epilogue: A fragile state Subsequent anniversaries: For better or worse Emotional bonding with infant missing
Beck (2006b) Pentadic cartography: Mapping birth trauma narratives	Act: agency ratio imbalance Powerless	Terrified Shock Loss Grief Flashbacks Like being raped	Suicidal thoughts
Beck & Watson (2008) Impact of birth trauma on breastfeeding		Proving oneself as a mother: Sheer determination Making up for an awful arrival: Atonement to the baby Just one more thing to be violated: Mother's breasts Intruding flashbacks: Stealing anticipated joy	Disturbing detachment: An empty affair
Beck & Watson (2010) Subsequent childbirth after a previous traumatic birth	Frighteningly alone	Riding the turbulent wave of panic during pregnancy Fear Anxiety Dread Terror Denial	Numbness to fetus Still elusive: The longed-for healing experience Grieving for what could have been Past can never be changed

continually consequences one sees either worsening or improving progressions or escalating severity" (Glaser, 2005, p. 9). Causal loops involve feedback behavior in which the effects of a change serve to intensify or oppose the original change. Feedback is an important concept to consider. A change in one factor can impact another factor, which then can affect the first factor. When feedback decreases the impact of a change, it is sometimes referred to as a balancing loop. In contrast, a reinforcing loop occurs when feedback increases the impact of a change. This causal looping can amplify in either a positive or negative direction. The term *positive* does not necessarily mean that the changes are good; it only means that the changes are reinforced. *Negative* only indicates that changes are resisted; it does not necessarily mean the effects or changes are bad.

The amplifying feedback loops that emerged from this metaethnography of the five phenomenological studies and one narrative analysis on traumatic childbirth are illustrated in Figure 1. A successive series of amplifying feedback loops occurred. The original trigger of traumatic childbirth resulted in six amplifying feedback loops, four of which were reinforcing (positive direction), and two of which were balancing (negative direction).

Reinforcing Loop #1

The first reinforcing feedback loop focused on the detrimental effects that the posttraumatic stress symptoms resulting from childbirth can have on mothers' breastfeeding experiences. When attempting to breastfeed, some women suffered with uncontrollable flashbacks to their traumatic birth. As Molly revealed:

> I had flashbacks to the birth every time I would feed him. When he was put on me in the hospital, he wasn't breathing and he was blue. I kept picturing this; and could still feel what it was like. Breastfeeding him was a similar position as to the way he was put on me. (Beck & Watson, 2008, p. 234)

For some mothers, these intruding flashbacks were so distressing that they made a decision to stop breastfeeding. Angie admitted that, "The flashbacks to the birth were terrible. I wanted to forget about it and the pain, so stopping breastfeeding would get me a bit closer to my 'normal' self again" (Beck & Watson, 2008, p. 234).

Avoidance of triggers to the recollection of the original trauma, in this case traumatic birth, permeated mothers' lives. Their infants were constant reminders of their birth trauma. For some mothers, feeling detached from their babies and distancing themselves from this trigger hindered their breastfeeding. Rachael shared,

> Breastfeeding my son in the first few months, certainly the first 6 but possibly as much as 9 months, was an empty affair. I felt nothing at all. Breastfeeding was just one of the many things I did while remaining totally detached from my baby. (Beck & Watson, 2008, p. 234)

Nancy, who had an emergency cesarean birth under general anesthesia, revealed, "I didn't feel like a real mother, as I was unable to give my daughter a normal birth. I felt very disconnected from this baby as I breastfed her" (Beck & Watson, 2008. p. 235).

Women traumatized during childbirth often felt like victims of rape: violated and stripped of their dignity. Hypervigilance is one of the clusters of symptoms of posttraumatic stress. Some women became vigilant about protecting their bodies from being violated yet again. This hypervigilance focused on their breasts and hindered their breastfeeding. Jeanne, whose labor had been induced and who had a failed vacuum extraction followed by a cesarean birth, shared the following:

> When I breastfed my baby, I felt like it was one more invasion up on my body and I couldn't handle that after the labor I had suffered. Whenever I put her to breast, I wanted to scream and vomit at the same time. (Beck & Watson, 2008, p. 233)

In the following comment Leslie was referring to the staff in the neonatal intensive care unit who were trying to help her breastfeed her preterm infant: "I was sick of everyone grabbing my breasts like they didn't belong to me. My breasts were just another thing to be taken away and violated" (Beck & Watson, 2008, p. 233).

In this first amplifying causal loop the posttraumatic stress symptoms of birth trauma had a positive (reinforcing) effect on breastfeeding experiences, which in turn intensified women's distress and posttraumatic stress symptoms, creating a vicious cycle of trauma and distress.

Balancing Loop #1

The first balancing loop, like the first reinforcing loop, involved the feedback between posttraumatic stress and breastfeeding. In this causal loop, some factors related to breastfeeding opposed the original effects of posttraumatic stress from birth trauma and helped to diminish these distressing symptoms. One of the themes in my phenomenological study with Watson (2008) on the impact of birth trauma on breastfeeding was "Helping to heal mentally: Time out from the pain in one's head." For some women, breastfeeding helped to heal them. *Soothing* was a term used by some mothers to describe breastfeeding. Karen, who had experienced a terrifying postpartum hemorrhage, explained:

> Breastfeeding was a timeout from the pain in my head. It was a "current reality"—a way to cling onto some "real life," whereas all the trauma that continued to live on in my head belonged to the past, even though I couldn't seem to keep it there. (Beck & Watson, 2008, p. 233)

Reinforcing Loop #2

This second reinforcing causal loop involved the feedback between posttraumatic stress following childbirth and mother–infant interaction. This positive amplifying loop was operating in all the studies included in this metaethnography. In my study on PTSD resulting from childbirth (Beck, 2004b), a disturbing theme revealed that posttraumatic stress choked off lifelines to the world of motherhood. Women's dreams of how motherhood would be were shattered. With PTSD, some women distanced themselves from their infants. Their infants were triggers to intensifying their posttraumatic stress symptoms, such as flashbacks and nightmares. As Linda described,

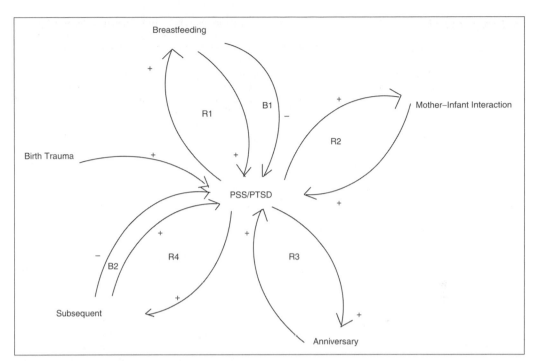

Figure 1. Amplifying causal loop diagram illustrating traumatic childbirth and its aftermath
R = reinforcing loop; B = balancing loop; PSS/PTSD – posttraumatic stress symptoms/posttraumatic stress disorder.

At night I tried to connect/acknowledge in my heart that this was my son, and I cried. I knew that there were great layers of trauma around my heart. I wanted to feel motherhood. I wanted to experience and embrace it. Why was I chained up in the viselike grip of this pain? (Beck, 2004b, p. 222)

The disturbing detachment from their infants of mothers suffering with posttraumatic stress symptoms was confirmed in the breastfeeding study (Beck & Watson, 2008).

In the anniversary-of-birth-trauma study (Beck, 2006a), some mothers revealed that the traumatic effects of birth left them feeling like they were not real mothers, and that an emotional bond with their infants was missing. Debbie recalled the following about her child's first birthday:

I wanted to die. I felt nothing for her and found it hard to celebrate the joy of this child that meant so little to me. I took excellent care of her, but it was as if I was babysitting; the emotional bond just wasn't there. (Beck, 2006a, p. 386)

From the subsequent childbirth-after-previous-traumatic-birth study results (Beck & Watson, 2010), we now are privy to the reinforcing effect—this time the effect on mother–fetus bonding. During their pregnancies women experienced terror, panic, and fear as they waited for 9 months for the dreaded labor and delivery. Some women turned to denial of their pregnancy to "survive" this period. Laurie shared that, throughout her pregnancy, she "felt numb to my baby" (p. 245).

Reinforcing Loop #3

The third reinforcing feedback loop in this metaethnography concerned the anniversary-of-birth trauma (Beck, 2006a). Feedback from the yearly anniversary increased the impact of the posttraumatic stress symptoms and amplified distress in mothers. It was not just the actual day of the anniversary that amplified this distress, but also the prologue of weeks and sometimes months leading up to the anniversary of traumatic birth. Fear, grief, anxiety, dread, depression, and guilt were just some of the distressing emotions women struggled with as the anniversary approached. The calendar, seasons, and clock times were all triggers to flareups of posttraumatic stress symptoms. Anna, whose birth trauma occurred near Halloween, explained:

> There is also a distinct smell of dead leaves in the air that screams, "October!" Hearing the word, October, and seeing the word in writing gives me chills. When I would see decorations for Halloween, fear rushed through my body. (Beck, 2006a, p. 385)

Women also struggled with the actual day: Was it a celebration of their child's birthday, or the torment of an anniversary? The birthday of Shannon's child triggered the following flashback of this mother's emergency cesarean birth: "I can't stop seeing images of a woman drugged and strapped down and being gutted like a fish. I can't get those or my own images out of my mind. I didn't know how to celebrate my daughter's birthday" (Beck, 2006a, p. 386).

Women often paid a heavy toll as a result of their surviving the actual anniversary. One of the themes in my phenomenological study (2006a) was "The epilogue: A fragile state." Mothers vividly shared how they felt at anniversary time, as the invisible wounds from their traumatic births were reopened. Women needed time to heal their raw wounds. Christine described this reinforcing effect:

> As hard as I try to move away from the trauma, at birthday anniversary time I am pulled straight back as if on a giant rubber band into the midst of it all and spend MONTHS AFTER trying to pull myself away from it again. (Beck, 2006a, p. 387)

Reinforcing Loop #4

Results of the phenomenological study of subsequent childbirth after a previous traumatic birth (Beck & Watson, 2010) provided data upon which the fourth reinforcing causal loop was based. During pregnancy, women rode a turbulent wave of panic and other distressing emotions as their posttraumatic stress symptoms increased in intensity. Nicole revealed the following about the entire period of her pregnancy: "My 9 months of pregnancy were an anxiety filled abyss which was completely marred as an experience due to the terror that was continually in my mind from my experience 8 years earlier" (Beck & Watson, 2010, p. 245).

Women employed numerous strategies during pregnancy to break the reinforcing cycle of one traumatic birth followed by another traumatic birth. Examples of various strategies include exercise, yoga, relaxation techniques, keeping a journal, hypobirthing (a method of natural childbirth

using relaxation and self-hypnosis to eliminate fear and tension), reading about the birth process, and creating birth-oriented art. Sadly, for some women, their longed-for healing birth experience remained elusive. The amplifying feedback loop was reinforced. An example of one such instance of this positive feedback was from Carol, who had opted for a homebirth. Because of postpartum hemorrhage she had to be transported by ambulance to the hospital, all the while terrified she would not live to raise her baby. She vividly described her experience on the operating table:

> With my legs held in the air by two strangers while a third mopped the blood between my legs, I felt raped all over again. I wanted to die. I had failed as a woman. My privacy had been invaded again. I felt sick. (Beck & Watson, 2010, p. 247)

Balancing Loop #2

Three fourths of the women in my (2010) study with Watson described that their subsequent childbirth was a "healing experience," or at least "a lot better" than their prior traumatic birth had been. The second balancing feedback loop captures this opposing change to the feedback loop. A reverence was brought to their subsequent birthing processes, and the women felt empowered. What helped to initiate this balancing feedback loop? Some reasons mothers gave included (a) being treated with respect, dignity, and compassion; (b) having pain relief taken seriously; (c) improved communication with labor and delivery staff; and (d) not feeling rushed to deliver. Kathryn described this negative (balancing) feedback loop:

> It was as healing and empowering as I had always hoped for. I did not want any high tech management. My homebirth was the proudest day of my life and the victory was sweeter because I overcame so very much to come to it. (Beck & Watson, 2010, p. 247)

Discussion

Leverage points identify where pressure in the amplifying causal loop can produce desired outcomes, namely breaking the feedback loop where necessary (Newell, Proust, Dyball, & McManus, 2007). Obviously, with birth trauma, the ideal intervention is to prevent it, to treat each woman during the birthing process as if she were a survivor of previous trauma (Crompton, 2003). Highley and Mercer (1978) expressed it best, as they reminded clinicians of the reverence that needs to be provided to women in labor:

Being able to assist a woman in one of the greatest tasks of her life—giving birth to and mothering a baby—is a privilege and challenge that touches every nurse who assists in her care. The challenge extends not only to the concrete physical help that the mother needs, but to the subtle consideration and attention which help her maintain her self-control and thus her self-respect. (p. 41)

The panoramic view provided by this metaethnography (see Figure 1) clearly illustrates the multiple, repetitive, reinforcing, amplifying causal loops that permeate mothers' lives as they struggle with the long-term aftermath of traumatic childbirth. Four of the six amplifying loops are reinforcing, thus intensifying posttraumatic stress symptoms in mothers. Leverage points abound for interrupting these positive amplifying causal loops. Clinicians fail to rescue women with birth trauma time and time again: during breastfeeding, during their interactions with their infants, during yearly anniversaries, and in subsequent childbirth. Many precious opportunities to balance these causal loops are lost. Obstetric care providers need to ensure that women are surrounded with protective layers during the birthing process. These protective layers include feeling cared for, being communicated with, being treated with respect and dignity, allowing some control when appropriate, supporting women, and providing assurance.

To help prevent the four reinforcing causal loops from coming into play, clinicians need to be vigilant in observing women for any symptoms indicating that they might have experienced a traumatic birth. Instruments are available to screen women in the postpartum period for posttraumatic stress symptoms. One such instrument is the Post-Traumatic Stress Symptoms Scale (Foa, Riggs, Dancu & Rothbaum, 1993). If women screen positive for elevated symptom levels, referrals to mental health professionals can be made. Treatment options, such as eye movement desensitization reprocessing, have been shown to be effective in women with posttraumatic stress symptoms resulting from traumatic childbirth (Sandstrom, Wiberg, Wikman, Willman, & Hogberg, 2008).

Regarding Reinforcing Loop #1, an example of one leverage point is providing intensive one-on-one support for traumatized women as they initiate breastfeeding. For the second reinforcing loop, periodic routine assessment of mother–infant interactions during the postpartum period can be one leverage point. These assessments can provide an opportunity to identify women struggling with posttraumatic stress symptoms.

Yearly physical exams for children provide a golden opportunity for clinicians to try and interrupt Reinforcing Loop #3. At these well-child checkups, mothers should also be the focus of health care providers. Women need to be asked if they are struggling around the yearly anniversary of their children's birth.

Leverage points to address Reinforcing Loop #4 can and should occur throughout the 9 months of pregnancy. If a woman is a multipara, an essential component of her initial prenatal visit should be a discussion of the mother's perception of her previous births. Were any of these births perceived as traumatic births? England and Horowitz (1998) urged clinicians to encourage wounded mothers to grieve their prior traumatic births so as to lift the burden of their invisible pain. To try and prevent another traumatic birth, clinicians can share with women the strategies other mothers used (Beck & Watson, 2010).

Some of the amplifying causal loops discovered in this metaethnography confirmed results reported in qualitative studies conducted by other researchers. For example, Reinforcing Loop #2, mother–infant interactions, supported findings from Nicholls and Ayers' (2007) study of PTSD in six couples. The women commented on poor bonding with their infants, "putting on an act" with their babies because they did not have any positive feelings toward their babies. Overprotective/anxious bonding and avoidant/rejecting bonding were reported by these mothers.

The essence of what constituted traumatic childbirth identified in this metaethnography confirmed results of previous qualitative studies. For example, in Ayers' (2007) study with 25 mothers with posttraumatic stress symptoms, women used adjectives like *panicky*, *alarmed*, *scared*, and *helpless* to describe their traumatic births. Some mothers shared that they dissociated and had thoughts of death during labor.

Ideas for further research can be gleaned from this metaethnography. Some of the "domino effects" of traumatic childbirth are apparent from this synthesis, but more qualitative research can be conducted to discover what other insidious effects of birth trauma permeate women's lives. For example, are mothers' interactions with their older children also affected? Additional research to identify more balancing feedback loops is also warranted. Since all six studies included in this metaethnography were conducted via the Internet, replication of these qualitative studies with non-Internet samples is needed.

The reinforcing amplifying feedback loops discovered in this metaethnography provide compelling evidence to help bring visibility to this mostly invisible phenomenon. A mother in one of my studies (Beck, 2004b) said it best when describing her PTSD following childbirth: "It's like an invisible wall around the sufferer" (p. 221). In the recent United States national survey, Listening to Mothers II, 9% of new mothers screened positive for meeting the *DSM-IV* (American Psychiatric Association, 2000) criteria for a diagnosis of PTSD following childbirth

(Declercq, Sakala, Corry, & Applebaum, 2008). The qualitative results of this metaethnography of traumatic childbirth "put the flesh on the bones" of this sobering quantitative statistic of the state of new mothers in the United States (Patton, 1990).

Declaration of Conflicting Interests

The author declared no conflicts of interest with respect to the authorship and/or publication of this article.

Funding

The author received no financial support for the research and/or authorship of this article.

References

American Psychiatric Association. (2000). *Diagnostic and statistical manual of mental disorders* (4th ed.). Washington, DC: Author.

Ayers, S. (2007). Thoughts and emotions during traumatic birth: A qualitative study. *Birth, 34*, 253-263. doi:10.1111/j.1523-536x2007.0018.x

Beck, C. T. (2004a). Birth trauma: In the eye of the beholder. *Nursing Research, 53*, 28-35. doi:10.1097/00006199-20040 1000-00005

Beck, C. T. (2004b). Post-traumatic stress disorder due to childbirth: The aftermath. *Nursing Research, 53*, 216-224. doi:10.1097/00006199-200407000-00004

Beck, C. T. (2006a). The anniversary of birth trauma: Failure to rescue. *Nursing Research, 55*, 381-390. doi:10.1097/0000 6199-200611000-00002

Beck, C. T. (2006b). Pentadic cartography: Mapping birth trauma narratives. *Qualitative Health Research, 16*, 453-466. doi:10.1177/1049732305285968

Beck, C. T, & Watson, S. (2008). Impact of birth trauma on breastfeeding: A tale of two pathways. *Nursing Research, 57*, 228-236. doi:10.1097/01.nnr.0000313494.87282.90

Beck, C. T, & Watson, S. (2010). Subsequent childbirth after a previous traumatic birth. *Nursing Research, 59*, 241-249. doi:10.1097/nnr.06013e3181e501fd

Burke, K. (1969). *A grammar of motives*. Berkley, CA: University of California Press.

Crompton, J. (2003, summer). Post-traumatic stress disorder and childbirth. *Childbirth Educators New Zealand Education Effects*, 25-31.

Declercq, E. R., Salaka, C., Corry, M. P., & Applebaum, B. O. (2008). *New mothers speak out: National survey results highlight women's postpartum experiences*. New York: Childbirth Connection. Retrieved from Childbirth Connection Web site at http://www.childbirthconnection.org/listeningtomothers/

Draucker, C. B., Martsolf, D. S., Ross, R., Cook, C. B., Stidham, A. W., & Mweemba, P. (2009). The essence of healing from sexual violence: A qualitative metasynthesis. *Research in Nursing & Health, 32*, 366-378. doi:10.1002/nur.20333

Duggleby, W., Holtslander, L., Kylma, J., Duncan, V., Hammond, C., & Williams, A. (2010). Metasynthesis of the hope experience of family caregivers of persons with chronic illness. *Qualitative Health Research, 20*, 148-158. doi:10.1177/1049732309358329

England, P., & Horowitz, R. (1998). *Birthing from within*. Albuquerque, NM: Partera Press.

Fleming, E., & Gillibrand, W. (2009). An exploration of culture, diabetes, and nursing in the South Asian community. *Journal of Transcultural Nursing, 20*, 146-155. doi:10.1177/1043659608330058

Foa, E. B., Riggs, D. S., Dancu, C. V., & Rothbaum, B. O. (1993). Reliability and validity of a brief instrument for assessing posttraumatic stress disorder (PSS-SR). *Journal of Traumatic Stress, 6*, 459-473. doi:10.1002/jts.2490060405

Glaser, B. G. (2005). *The grounded theory perspective III: Theoretical coding*: Mill Valley, CA: Sociology Press.

Glaser, B. G. (2007). *Doing formal grounded theory: A proposal*. Mill Valley, CA: Sociology Press.

Glaser, B. G., & Strauss, A. L. (1971). *Status passage*. Chicago: Aldine-Atherton.

Highley, B., & Mercer, R. T. (1978). Safeguarding the laboring woman's sense of control. *MCN: The American Journal of Maternal Child Nursing, 4*, 39-41. doi:10.1097/00005721-197801000-00013

Kearney, M. H. (2001). New directions in grounded formal theory (pp. 227-246). In R. S. Schreiber & P. N. Stern (Eds.), *Using grounded theory in nursing*. New York: Springer.

Larsen, J. S., Hall, E. O. C., & Aagaard, H. (2008). Shattered expectations: When mothers' confidence in breastfeeding is undermined—A metasynthesis. *Scandinavian Journal of Caring Science, 22*, 653-661. doi:10.1111/j.1471-6712.2007.00572.x

Meeker, M. A., & Jezewski, M. A. (2009). Metasynthesis: Withdrawing life-sustaining treatments. The experience of family decision-makers. *Journal of Clinical Nursing, 18*, 163-173. doi:10.111/j.1365-2702.2008.02465.x

Newell, B., Proust, K., Dyball, R., & McManus, P. (2007). Seeing obesity as a systems problem. *NSW Public Health Bulletin, 18*, 214-218. doi:10.1071/nb07028

Nicholls, K., & Ayers, S. (2007). Childbirth-related post-traumatic stress disorder in couples: A qualitative study. *British Journal of Health Psychology, 12*, 491-509. doi:10.1348/135910706x120627

Noblit, G. W., & Hare, R. D. (1988). *Meta-ethnography: Synthesizing qualitative studies*. Newbury Park, CA: Sage.

Paterson, B. L., Thorne, S. E., Canam, C., & Jillings, C. (2001). *Meta-study of qualitative health research*. Thousand Oaks, CA: Sage.

Patton, M. Q. (1990). *Qualitative evaluation and research methods*. Newbury Park, CA: Sage.

Sandelowski, M. (1995). A theory of the transition to parenthood of infertile couples. *Research in Nursing & Health, 18*, 123-132. doi:10:1002/nur.4770180206

Sandelowski, M., & Barroso, J. (2007). *Handbook for synthesizing qualitative research*. New York: Springer.

Sandelowski, M., Docherty, S., & Emden, C. (1997). Qualitative metasynthesis: Issues and techniques. *Research in Nursing & Health, 20*, 365-371. doi:10.1002/(sici)1098-240x(199708)

Sandstrom, M., Wiberg, B., Wikman, M., Willman, A. K., & Hogberg, U. (2008). A pilot study of eye movement desensitization and reprocessing treatment (EMDR) for post-traumatic stress after childbirth. *Midwifery, 24*, 62-73. doi:10-1016/j.midw.2006.07.008

Thorne, S., Jensen, L., Kearney, M. H., Noblit, G., & Sandelowski, M. (2004). Qualitative metasynthesis: Reflections on methodological orientation and ideological agenda. *Qualitative Health Research, 14*, 1342-1365. doi:10.1177/1049732304269888

Bio

Cheryl Tatano Beck, DNSc, CNM, FAAN, is a distinguished professor at the University of Connecticut School of Nursing in Storrs, Connecticut, USA.

Answers to Selected Study Guide Exercises

CHAPTER 1

A. FILL IN THE BLANKS

1. paradigm
2. constructivism
3. Positivism
4. applied
5. clubs
6. clinical
7. generalizability
8. cause
9. assumption
10. Empirical
11. determinism
12. Replication
13. methods
14. qualitative
15. biases
16. Quantitative
17. identification
18. explanation
19. therapy
20. meaning

B. MATCHING EXERCISES

1. a	2. b	3. d	4. b	5. a
6. b	7. d	8. b	9. c	10. a

D. APPLICATION EXERCISES

Exercise D.1: Questions of Fact (Appendix A)

a. Yes, this was a systematic study that tested the efficacy of a behaviorally based smartphone intervention designed to promote weight loss in young adults aged 18 to 25 years.

b. It was a quantitative study. The researchers systematically measured several outcomes (e.g., weight, body mass index, waist circumference, self-efficacy for healthy eating) using measures that yielded quantitative information.

c. The underlying paradigm was positivism/postpositivism.

d. Yes, the study involved the collection of information through the senses (i.e., through scrutiny of study participants' responses to series of questions and observation of physical attributes).

e. This study was applied research—there was a practical problem that the researchers wanted to solve (i.e., a problem relating to weight management in young adults).

f. Yes, this study was concerned with evaluating whether the intervention *caused* weight loss among the study participants exposed to the intervention. In this and most studies, there is an underlying assumption that phenomena are multiply determined. Thus, the participants' weight is *caused* by a number of factors, and the one being tested in this study is whether one of the causes is participation in a special intervention.

g. The purposes of the study could be described as prediction and control—the investigators examined possible methods of controlling (improving) weight and weight-related outcomes.

h. Yes, this study directly addressed a question relevant to the *treatment* of young adults—a therapy question. The results of this study, together with those from other similar studies, could provide guidance about evidence-based ways to help young adults manage their weight.

Exercise D.2: Questions of Fact (Appendix B)

a. Yes, this was a systematic study of breastfeeding promotion in a neonatal intensive care unit (NICU).

b. It was a qualitative study. The researcher used loosely structured methods to capture in an in-depth fashion the experiences of nurses and mothers with high-risk infants in the NICU, relative to the promotion of breastfeeding.

c. The underlying paradigm is constructivism (naturalism).

d. Yes, the study involved the collection of information through the senses (e.g., through conversations with nurses, through direct observation of practices in the NICU, and through scrutiny of documents in the NICU).

e. This study is best described as basic—to gain a better understanding of the structure and processes of the culture in a particular NICU. Interventions could, however, be designed that are based on the study findings.

f. No, this study is not cause-probing per se. Qualitative studies seldom focus on causes and effects, although in-depth scrutiny of phenomena can sometimes suggest causal linkages.

g. The purpose of the study can be described as exploration into the everyday world of NICU processes and transactions, with emphasis on actions and interactions relating to breastfeeding.

h. This study addresses the EBP question described in the textbook as "Meaning and Processes," that is, developing an in-depth understanding of the NICU environment and processes.

CHAPTER 2

A. FILL IN THE BLANKS

1. guideline
2. Systematic
3. pilot
4. Cochrane
5. outcome
6. population
7. therapy
8. AGREE
9. PICO
10. Meta-analysis
11. comparison
12. evidence hierarchy
13. intervention (or influence)
14. metasynthesis
15. Evidence-based practice (EBP)
16. quality improvement

B. MATCHING EXERCISES

1. c	2. b	3. c	4. b	5. d
6. a	7. a	8. b		

C. STUDY QUESTIONS

C.1.

a. I	b. P	c. C	d. I
e. O	f. P	g. I	h. O
i. C	j. O		

D. APPLICATION EXERCISES

Exercise D.1: Questions of Fact (Appendix C)

a. The purpose of the evidence-based practice project was to develop, implement, and evaluate the effectiveness of a standardized nursing procedure to increase the identification of depression in family members of active duty soldiers.

b. The setting for the project was a military family practice clinic located on a U.S. Army infantry post in Hawaii.

c. The project was guided by the Iowa Model of Evidence-Based Practice to Promote Quality Care.

d. The authors described the project as having *both* a problem-focused trigger and a knowledge-focused trigger. Regarding the former, the introduction indicated that "the absence in this clinic of a systematic method to screen family members of deployed soldiers for depression and the inability to estimate rates of depression in this clinical population were the problem-focused triggers for this project." They cited national standards and guidelines calling for the screening of all adults for depression in primary care settings as the knowledge-focused triggers.

e. There were three authors of this report, and presumably they were major team members on this project. Two authors were masters-prepared officers in the U.S. Army Nurse Corps, and the third was an instructor at the University of Hawaii. The article also indicates that a "multidisciplinary panel of stakeholders," which included advance practice registered nurses (APRNs), physicians, certified nurse assistants, RNs, a psychologist, and clinic administrators, formed the EBP team. It is not unusual for EBP project teams to comprise research and clinical staff and to be multidisciplinary.

f. The report did not discuss implementation at length, but it did state that the project team was led by a change champion (an APRN) and an opinion leader (a physician), who were persuasive and influential in the clinic. The article stated that "the EBP project received enthusiastic support throughout the organization and at the highest levels of nursing leadership."

g. Yes, the report described the study that was undertaken as a pilot study.

h. Yes, one of the purposes of this pilot study was to evaluate the effectiveness of the newly developed practice guideline for screening for depression.

Exercise D.2: Questions of Fact (Appendix G)

a. Yes, the article by Chase and colleagues described a systematic review undertaken to summarize evidence on the effectiveness of interventions designed to promote medication adherence among patients with coronary artery disease. Systematic reviews are an especially important type of pre-appraised evidence. The particular type of systematic review in this example is a meta-analysis.

b. The meta-analysis in this study integrated information from several studies, including randomized controlled trials (RCTs), and so evidence from this study would be at the top rung of the evidence hierarchy portrayed in Figure 2.1.

c. The researchers stated that "the purpose of this meta-analysis was to determine the overall effectiveness of interventions designed to improve medication adherence among adults with CAD." The researchers also stated a secondary purpose—to examine whether certain features of the study "moderated" intervention effectiveness. This means that the researchers looked for evidence not only of whether interventions are effective in increasing medication adherence but also whether certain features of the intervention (e.g., whether the intervention was delivered by nurses or others) increased the benefits.

CHAPTER 3

A. FILL IN THE BLANKS

1. dependent
2. entrée
3. data
4. sample
5. operational
6. theory
7. statistical
8. literature
9. emergent
10. experimental
11. trial
12. phenomenology
13. ethnography
14. saturation
15. population
16. grounded
17. construct
18. effect
19. design
20. causal (cause-and-effect)
21. themes
22. construct
23. subject
24. variable
25. independent
26. relationship
27. observational

B. MATCHING EXERCISES

B.1.   1. a   2. c   3. b   4. a
            5. b   6. b   7. c   8. c
            9. b   10. c

B.2.   1. b   2. c   3. a   4. c
            5. c   6. b   7. d   8. d

B.3.   1. a   2. b   3. a   4. c
            5. b   6. c   7. d   8. c
            9. b   10. a

C. STUDY QUESTIONS

C.2.

a. Independent variable (IV) = participation versus nonparticipation in assertiveness training; dependent or outcome variable (DV) = psychiatric nurses' effectiveness
b. IV = patients' postural positioning; DV = respiratory function
c. IV = amount of touch by nursing staff; DV = patients' psychological well-being
d. IV = frequency of turning patients; DV = incidence of decubitus
e. IV = history of parents' abuse during their childhood; DV = parental abuse of their own children
f. IV = patients' age and gender; DV = tolerance for pain
g. IV = pregnant women's number of prenatal visits; DV = labor and delivery outcomes
h. IV = children's experience (vs. absence of experience) of a sibling death; DV = levels of depression
i. IV = gender; DV = compliance with a medical regimen
j. IV = participation versus nonparticipation in a support group among family caregivers of patients with AIDS; DV = coping
k. IV = time of day; DV = elders' hearing acuity
l. IV = location of giving birth—home versus other; DV = parents' satisfaction with the childbirth experience
m. IV = type of diet in the outpatient setting among patients undergoing chemotherapy; DV = incidence of positive blood cultures

C.5.

a. An ethnographic study would not be experimental—no intervention would be introduced.
b. The independent variable is relaxation therapy (the intervention), and the dependent or outcome variable is pain.
c. Grounded theory studies are not clinical trials, which involve an intervention.
d. Study participants would not be exposed to an intervention in phenomenological studies.
e. In experimental studies, decisions about data collection would be made well before implementing the intervention.

C.6.   a. Ethnographic
            b. Phenomenological
            c. Grounded theory

D. APPLICATION EXERCISES

Exercise D.1: Questions of Fact (Appendix D)

a. All five researchers were doctorally prepared nurses.
b. The study participants were patients diagnosed with heart disease.
c. Participants were recruited from one of two cardiology clinics. One clinic served primarily minority urban patients and the other served primarily Caucasian patients from a small city in a rural setting. The clinics are presumably located in the State of Illinois in the United States because all researchers are affiliated with institutions in that state. The data were collected during routine clinic appointments.
d. The central variable in this study is patients' level of *fatigue*. The authors did not specifically label any variables as *dependent* or *independent*, but the research questions indicate that fatigue was both an independent and dependent variable in the researchers' analyses. As stated in the abstract, one study objective was to assess whether demographic (age, education, income), physiological (hypertension, hyperlipidemia), or psychological variables (depressive symptoms) were correlated with fatigue. For this

objective, fatigue is the outcome—the researchers considered the other factors as independent variables that were potentially associated with or that influenced levels of fatigue. A third objective was to examine whether fatigue was associated with the patients' quality of life. For this objective, it can be inferred that the researchers conceptualized levels of fatigue (the independent variable) as potentially influencing patients' quality of life (the outcome variable).

e. Fatigue was conceptually defined in the very first sentence of the report. Fatigue was operationally defined by scores on a scale called the Fatigue Symptom Inventory or FSI. The FSI consists of 14 questions that ask about fatigue intensity, duration, and interference with activities of daily living. Each question is answered on an 11-point scale, from 0 (*not at all fatigued*/no interference) to 10 (*as fatigued as I could be*/extreme interference). The report also provided information on how responses to the 14 questions are scored to produce an overall score.

f. The data in this study were both quantitative and qualitative. The researchers administered a number of scales that yielded numeric information (e.g., fatigue, quality of life) but also asked in-depth questions, such as "Describe your fatigue." Responses to these questions were in narrative form and were analyzed qualitatively.

g. For the second study objective, the researchers investigated the relationship between the various demographic, physiological, and psychological factors on the one hand and fatigue on the other. In the context of this study, it is best to consider the relationships associative rather than causal— although it is certainly plausible that certain factors *caused* fatigue. The authors' conceptual model suggests the possibility of causal pathways, but the researchers judiciously noted (in the Discussion section) that "it remains to be determined if depression is the cause or consequence of fatigue." For their third objective, the researchers studied the relationship between

fatigue and quality of life. Again, the model shown in their Figure 1 suggests the possibility that fatigue levels affect patients' quality of life, but the authors did not explicitly infer a causal connection between fatigue and quality of life.

h. There was no intervention in this study. The researchers captured characteristics of the study participants at one point in time without intervening in any way.

i. The study involved the statistical analysis of the quantitative data and qualitative analysis of the narrative data.

Exercise D.2: Questions of Fact (Appendix F)

a. There was only one researcher in this study—which is fairly rare in quantitative studies but more common in qualitative ones. Jeanne Cummings, a doctorally prepared nurse was (at the time the article was published) a visiting professor at the City University of New York.

b. The study participants were 12 dyads of *storytellers* and *listeners*. The storytellers were people who had been involved in a widely publicized disaster—the crash landing of U.S. Airways Flight 1549 into the Hudson River in January 2009. The listeners were people with whom the storytellers had shared the story of the traumatic event.

c. The context of the study was the crash landing of the airplane into the Hudson River. There was, however, no specific setting for the storytelling (which would have occurred in multiple, varied settings). Almost all study participants were interviewed in person (only three were interviewed over the telephone), but information about where the interviews took place was not provided.

d. The key concept was the storytelling aspect of a particular traumatic event.

e. No, there were no *independent variables* or *dependent variables* in this qualitative study.

f. The data for this study were qualitative.

g. Although this study did not explicitly focus on relationships, the analysis revealed that the nature of the relationship between the storyteller and listener did "color" or affect the listener's and storyteller's experience during the telling of the story (Theme 5).

h. This study was described as an interpretive phenomenological study.

i. This study was nonexperimental.

j. There was no intervention in this study.

k. The study did not report any statistical information (e.g., the average age of the participants). The study involved the qualitative analysis of rich, narrative data.

CHAPTER 4

A. FILL IN THE BLANKS

1. bias
2. title
3. reflexivity
4. level
5. trustworthy
6. significant
7. IMRAD
8. blinding (or masking)
9. abstract
10. confounding
11. journal
12. valid
13. inference
14. Reliability
15. control
16. Randomness
17. Transferability

B. MATCHING EXERCISES

1. c	2. d	3. b	4. a	5. c
6. e	7. d	8. b	9. c	10. e
11. b	12. d			

D. APPLICATION EXERCISES

Exercise D.1: Questions of Fact (Appendix A)

a. Yes, the structure of the Stephens and colleagues' article follows the IMRAD format. There is an Introduction that begins with the first words ("Overweight and obesity are major public health concerns"). Then there are Methods, Results, and Discussion sections. The Methods and Results sections have several subsections. For example, the Methods section has subsections labeled Setting and Participants, Outcome Measures, Interventions, and Statistical Analysis.

b. Yes, the abstract to this article includes all this information, organized into sections called Background, Objective, Methods, Results, and Conclusions.

c. The study methods were described mainly using the passive voice. For example, the first paragraph indicates that "participants were randomly assigned to intervention or control." In the active voice, this could have been "We randomly assigned participants to intervention or control."

d. This study is experimental. The researchers intervened by offering a smartphone intervention to some young adults but not to others.

e. Yes, the abstract stated that 62 young adults were *randomized* to receive either the smartphone application and health coach intervention and counseling or to a control group (right after the bolded Methods heading).

Exercise D.2: Questions of Fact (Appendix E)

a. Yes, the report by Byrne and colleagues basically followed the IMRAD format. The first part of the article is the introduction, with a subsection labeled "Literature Review." The next section is called Methodology. The "Results" are labeled "Findings" in this article, and the final section is the Discussion.

b. The abstract indicated the study purpose in the first sentence (to "develop a theoretical framework about caregivers' experiences . . . "). Then there was a brief statement about methods (a grounded theory approach was used, and data were collected at three points in time with 18 caregivers). Key findings were then highlighted, and the last sentence noted that the findings have important implications for clinicians, researchers, educators, and decision makers.

c. The presentation was in both the active and the passive voice. As an example of the passive voice, the first sentence of the Methodology section stated that "a constructivist grounded theory methodology *was used*." The authors used the active voice in the first paragraph under the Data Collection subsection: "The first author conducted 45 face-to-face interviews . . . "

d. Yes, this study was a grounded theory study, which is appropriate for understanding social processes relating to a phenomenon. Here, the researchers were interested in understanding the processes in which spousal caregivers engaged during their spouses' transition from a geriatric rehabilitation unit to home.

CHAPTER 5

A. FILL IN THE BLANKS

1. codes
2. Anonymity
3. risk
4. Beneficence
5. Process consent
6. stipend
7. Belmont
8. implied
9. assent
10. confidentiality
11. disclosure
12. Institutional Review Board (IRB)
13. dilemma
14. vulnerable groups
15. Informed consent
16. Debriefing
17. minimal

B. MATCHING EXERCISES

1. d	2. b	3. c	4. b	5. a
6. d	7. b	8. a	9. c	10. a
11. b	12. d			

D. APPLICATION EXERCISES

Exercise D.1: Questions of Fact (Appendix D)

a. Yes, in the last paragraph of the "Sample and Setting" subsection under Methods, the researchers indicated that the study protocol was reviewed and approved by the IRBs of both cardiology clinics from which participants were recruited for the study.

b. No, the study participants were adults with a chronic illness (coronary heart disease) and would not be considered "vulnerable."

c. There is no reason to suspect that participants were subjected to any physical harm or discomfort or psychological distress. Only people who were medically stable were eligible to participate in the study. The content of the questionnaire and interview does not appear stressful.

d. It does not appear that participants were deceived in any way.

e. There is no reason to suspect any coercion was used to force unwilling people to participate in the study. There is no information in the report concerning the number of prospective participants who declined to participate, but presumably some people who were recruited did not agree to take part in the study.

f. The report indicated that written informed consent was obtained from all participants. It is not possible to determine the extent to which disclosure was "full," but there does not appear to be any reason to conceal information in this study.

g. The report did not provide information about where data collection actually took place or how the privacy and confidentiality of participants were protected. Adequate protections were likely in place, however, given that approval for the study protocols was given by two IRBs. Presumably, statements regarding privacy and confidentiality were made in the informed consent form.

Exercise D.2: Questions of Fact (Appendix B)

a. Yes, the report indicates that approval for the study was granted by the "Human Subjects' Committees," presumably the committee in the children's hospital where the study took place and perhaps also (because *committees* is plural) the committee of Cricco-Lizza's institutional affiliation at the time of the research.

b. The focus of the study was nurses in the NICU, not the mothers or their infants. The nurses would not be considered vulnerable.

c. Participants were not subjected to any physical harm or discomfort. Nurses were observed performing their normal duties. It is possible that there was a certain degree of self-consciousness when the study started, but it is likely that the nurses became accustomed to the presence of the researcher who was probably considered a colleague.

d. Participants were probably not deceived. The article states that "information was provided to the nurses through the intranet, staff meetings, and individual encounters in the NICU." It might be noted, though, that observations were made "unobtrusively," meaning that nurses were not always aware that their interactions with families were under direct scrutiny—and presumably families were not aware either. Notification about the observations undoubtedly would have affected the very interactions of interest, and behaviors would likely have been atypical, undermining the study purpose. The nurses under observation knew that Cricco-Lizza was a nurse researcher who was interested in learning about their perspectives on infant feeding.

e. It does not appear that any coercion was involved.

f. The report stated that the researcher obtained written informed consent from the 18 key informants who were formally interviewed. Informed consent was not obtained from the 114 nurses who were considered "general informants" or from any family members.

g. Cricco-Lizza stated that the interviews with key informants took place in a private room near the NICU. She did not explicitly discuss who had access to the audiotaped interviews or the transcripts, but it seems safe to presume that they were safeguarded. No names

were used in the report. When verbatim quotes were presented in the report, she said things such as "one nurse said" or "one key informant stated."

CHAPTER 6

A. FILL IN THE BLANKS

1. problem
2. statement of purpose
3. question
4. hypothesis
5. relationship
6. test
7. independent
8. nondirectional
9. proof
10. two
11. research
12. null

B. MATCHING EXERCISES

B.1.

1. b	2. c	3. a	4. b
5. a	6. c	7. b	8. a

B.2.

1. a	2. c	3. d	4. a
5. b	6. d	7. a	8. c
9. b	10. d	11. b	12. c
13. b	14. a	15. c	

C. STUDY QUESTIONS

C.4. Independent variable = I; dependent/outcome variable = O

2a. I = type of stimulation (tactile vs. verbal); O = physiological arousal

2b. I = infants' birthweight; O = hypoglycemia in term newborns

2c. I = use versus nonuse of isotonic sodium chloride solution; O = oxygen saturation

2d. I = patients' fluid balance; O = success in weaning patients from mechanical ventilation

2e. I = patients' gender; O = amount of narcotic analgesics administered by nurses

3a. I = prior blood donation versus no prior donation; O = amount of anxiety

3b. I = amount of conversation initiated by nurses; O = patients' ratings of nursing effectiveness

3c. I = ratings of nurses' informativeness; O = amount of preoperative stress

3d. I = pregnancy status (pregnant vs. not pregnant); O = incidence of peritoneal infection

3e. I = type of delivery (vaginal vs. cesarean); O = incidence of postpartum depression

D. APPLICATION EXERCISES

Exercise D.1: Questions of Fact (Appendix D)

a. The first four paragraphs of this report stated the essence of the problem that the researchers addressed. In brief, the problem may be summarized as follows: Fatigue has been found to be a frequent symptom in patients with chronic health problems, including acute myocardial infarction and chronic heart failure. However, the severity and characteristics of fatigue in patients with stable coronary heart disease (CHD) has not been explored. It is important to better understand fatigue in this population, because fatigue may be an indicator of a new onset or of progressive CHD.

b. The authors stated three objectives in the study abstract as well as in the introduction to the report. The purposes were to "1. Describe fatigue (intensity, distress, timing, and quality) in patients with stable CHD; 2. Determine if specific demographic (gender, age, education, income), physiological (hypertension, hyperlipidemia), or psychological (depressive symptoms) variables were correlated with fatigue; and 3. Determine if fatigue was associated with health-related quality of life (HRQoL)." The authors used the verb "describe" for the first purpose, indicating that the study had a descriptive intent. The verb "describe" is appropriate in both quantitative and qualitative studies—and in this study, both types of data were collected. The researchers used the verb "determine" for the

next two purposes, which suggest a quantitative approach. However, given the limitations of any single study—particularly the reliance on relatively small samples from local populations—a verb such as "examine" or "assess" would probably have been preferable to "determine," which suggests a degree of definitiveness that is not attainable.

c. The report did not explicitly state research questions, although they could be inferred from the purpose statement. For example, the question corresponding to the first descriptive aim might be: What are the characteristics of fatigue—in terms of intensity, distress level, timing, and quality—among patients with stable CHD? A question corresponding to the second purpose might be: What factors, including demographic, physiological, and psychological, are associated with fatigue in patients with stable CHD? And a question corresponding to the third purpose would be: Is fatigue associated with HRQoL in patients with stable CHD?

d. No hypotheses were formally stated in the body of the article. However, there are footnotes at the bottom of Tables 3 and 4 that indicate that the researchers *did* have hypotheses about factors that were related to fatigue intensity and fatigue interference, respectively. Based on the information in these tables, one research hypothesis could be stated as follows: We predict that a patient's age will be correlated with their level of pain intensity and pain interference. This is stated as a non-directional hypothesis. A directional hypothesis might be the following: We predict that older patients will have higher levels of pain intensity and pain interference than younger patients.

e. Yes, the researchers used hypothesis-testing statistical tests. These are described in the Results section, under the subheading "Fatigue Intensity/Severity" and HRQoL and Fatigue. For example, the researchers tested the hypothesis that fatigue intensity was related to a patient's gender. They found that fatigue intensity was significantly higher in women than in men ($p = .003$). The probability is less than 3 in 1,000 that this result is spurious.

Exercise D.2: Questions of Fact (Appendix B)

a. The first paragraph of this report indicated that the research focused on the problem of breastfeeding promotion in neonatal intensive care units (NICUs). The next two paragraphs elaborate on the problem, noting that maternity practices in the United States often impede breastfeeding and the uptake of evidence-based practice guidelines.

b. Cricco-Lizza stated the purpose in the abstract: "Purpose: This study explored the structure and process of breastfeeding promotion in the NICU." This statement is reiterated in the very first sentence of the report and again in the last sentence of the introduction.

c. Specific research questions were not articulated. We could state a question as follows, which is simply the purpose rephrased interrogatively: What are the structure and process of breastfeeding promotion in the NICU?

d. No hypotheses were stated—or would one have been appropriate in this qualitative study.

e. No, no hypotheses were tested. Qualitative studies do not use statistical methods to test hypotheses.

CHAPTER 7

A. FILL IN THE BLANKS

1. primary
2. secondary
3. ancestry
4. descendancy
5. electronic (bibliographic)
6. mapping
7. keywords
8. CINAHL
9. Boolean
10. MeSH
11. PubMed
12. author

B. MATCHING EXERCISES

B.1.   1. d   2. b   3. c   4. b
            5. a   6. c   7. b   8. d

D. APPLICATION EXERCISES

Exercise D.1: Questions of Fact (Appendix G)

a. This review was a systematic review—a meta-analysis.

b. Yes, the introduction described a research problem that the researchers addressed. The problem might be stated as follows: Medication therapy provides known benefits for the secondary prevention of coronary artery disease (CAD). Yet many patients do not adhere to prescribed medication regimens and such nonadherence has been linked to poor health outcomes. Interventions to improve adherence in patients with CAD have been developed and tested but findings about their effectiveness have not been systematically integrated.

c. Yes, there was a statement of purpose in the abstract: The purpose of this meta-analysis was to determine the overall effectiveness of interventions designed to improve medication adherence (MA) among adults with CAD. In addition, sample, study design, and intervention characteristics were explored as potential moderators to intervention effectiveness." Additionally, two research questions were stated at the end of the Introduction: (1) What is the overall effectiveness of MA interventions on MA outcomes among patients with CAD? (2) Does intervention effectiveness vary based on intervention, sample, or design characteristics?" For students who do not yet understand what the researchers meant by "moderators" in the purpose statement, the questions may be easier to understand. The researchers were interested in exploring whether beneficial effects on interventions were different for different types of people, for different types of interventions, and when the research designs were different.

d. The researchers used 13 different electronic databases in their literature search, including ones we discussed in Chapter 7 (PubMed, CINAHL) and others we did not.

e. The authors used many key words (and MeSH terms) that included the following: *patient compliance, medication adherence, drugs, prescription drugs, pharmaceutical preparations, generic dosage, compliant, compliance, adherent, adherence, noncompliant, noncompliance, nonadherent, nonadherence, medication(s), regimen(s), prescription(s), prescribed, drug(s), pill(s), tablet(s), agent(s), improve, promote, enhance, encourage, foster, advocate, influence, incentive, ensure, remind, optimize, increase, impact, prevent, address, decrease.*

f. Yes, the report indicated that "ancestry searches of prior reviews' bibliographies were conducted."

g. The report did not state that their search was restricted to English-language publications. It is unclear if there were any language restrictions—although it seems unlikely that studies described in *all* languages would have been included.

h. This meta-analysis included 24 studies.

i. All studies included in the review were quantitative; meta-analyses integrate quantitative findings.

Exercise D.2: Questions of Fact (Appendix H)

a. Beck undertook a systematic review of qualitative studies relating to birth trauma—a type of metasynthesis that is called a meta-ethnography, as explained in more detail in Chapter 18. In this case, the metasynthesis involved integrating results from multiple analytic approaches in studies by the same researcher (Beck).

b. The purpose of this metasynthesis was to integrate and amplify findings from qualitative studies on birth trauma and resulting posttraumatic stress disorder. Beck indicated her purpose in the first paragraph of the report.

c. This particular synthesis integrated information from qualitative studies on traumatic births that had previously

been conducted by Beck herself in her extensive program of research on traumatic births.

d. Six of Beck's prior studies were included in this metasynthesis.

e. The six studies in the review included five phenomenological studies and one narrative analysis (see Chapter 11).

CHAPTER 8

A. FILL IN THE BLANKS

1. framework
2. conceptual
3. descriptive
4. middle
5. model
6. human beings, environment, health, nursing
7. Pender
8. Parse
9. Adaptation
10. self-efficacy
11. stages, change
12. Planned Behavior

B. MATCHING EXERCISES

B.1.   1. c   2. e   3. c   4. e
           5. d   6. a   7. b   8. d

B.2.   1. c   2. d   3. e   4. a
           5. b   6. f

D. APPLICATION EXERCISES

Exercise D.1: Questions of Fact (Appendix D)

a. Eckhardt and colleagues stated that they used the Theory of Unpleasant Symptoms as the organizing framework for their study.

b. The Theory of Unpleasant Symptoms was not described in the textbook but it is a theory that has been used by other nurse researchers.

c. The theory is not described in detail, but this likely reflects space constraints in the journal rather than the authors' neglect.

d. Yes, the article states that the Theory of Unpleasant Symptoms was the basis for the researchers' framework but that they adapted it for this study. The report did not specify what specific adaptations were made.

e. Yes, a schematic model of the organizing framework used in this research was presented in Figure 1.

f. The key concepts in the model are (1) physiological factors (e.g., hypertension, comorbid conditions), (2) psychological factors (e.g., depressed mood), (3) situational factors (e.g., age, sex, education), (4) symptom experiences (fatigue severity, fatigue interference), and (5) performance (quality of life and functional status).

g. The schematic model did not show connections among concepts in a traditional manner, namely, with arrows between boxes. However, it seems reasonable to conclude that the model is intended to be read from the top down. That is, the physiological, psychological, and situational factors are presumed to affect patients' symptom experience, which in turn influences performance concepts.

h. The report did not articulate formal conceptual definitions of each construct in the model. For example, there is no conceptual definition of "quality of life." However, operational definitions of all concepts were provided.

i. No, the researchers did not state formal hypotheses deduced from the conceptual framework—although they tested some, and these are consistent with our reading of the model, as explained in question g. For example, one hypothesis they tested was that fatigue intensity is related to situational factors (age, income), psychological factors (depression), and physiological factors (e.g., hypertension).

Exercise D.2: Questions of Fact (Appendix E)

a. No, the authors did not describe any a priori framework or theory that guided this research. For example, there was no mention of symbolic interactionism. Given space constraints in journals, however, this does not mean that the study lacked a conceptual framework.

b. Yes, the purpose of the study was to generate a theory that was grounded in the experiences of the study participants. The authors referred to their grounded theory as *reconciling in response to fluctuating needs*.

c. Yes, Figure 1 of the report was a schematic model depicting the researchers' grounded theory. The figure was a good way to illustrate three overlapping phases of reconciling (*getting ready, getting into it,* and *getting on with it*) as well as three subprocesses of reconciliation: *navigating, safekeeping,* and *repositioning.*

d. Inasmuch as this was a grounded theory study, no hypotheses were tested. A grounded theory study sometimes results in the identification of hypotheses that can be tested in a subsequent quantitative study.

CHAPTER 9

A. FILL IN THE BLANKS

1. validity
2. crossover
3. attrition
4. selection
5. random
6. blinding
7. control
8. Mortality
9. prospective (or cohort)
10. statistical
11. internal
12. external
13. cross-sectional
14. counterfactual
15. case-control
16. longitudinal
17. Matching
18. power
19. history
20. wait
21. baseline (or pretest)
22. quasi-experiments
23. relationships (or associations)
24. retrospective

B. MATCHING EXERCISES

B.1.   1. b   2. b   3. a   4. d
5. b   6. a   7. d   8. a
9. b   10. d

C. STUDY QUESTIONS

C.2.   2a. Both   2b. Nonexperimental
2c. Both   2d. Nonexperimental
2e. Nonexperimental
3a. Nonexperimental
3b. Both   3c. Nonexperimental
3d. Nonexperimental
3e. Nonexperimental

D. APPLICATION EXERCISES

Exercise D.1: Questions of Fact (Appendix A)

a. Yes, the purpose of the study was to evaluate the effects of a weight loss intervention that used smartphone technology plus text messaging from a health coach.

b. The design for this study was experimental.

c. The independent variable was participation versus nonparticipation in the special intervention that was being evaluated for its efficacy. The dependent variables included body weight, body mass index, waist circumference, physical activity, and self-efficacy for healthy eating and exercise.

d. Yes, randomization was used. Eligible participants were enrolled and then randomly assigned to either the intervention group or a control group, in blocks of four. Sixty-two participants were enrolled in the study—31 in each group.

e. The control group strategy in this study was the absence of a special intervention. The control group completed questionnaires but did not receive any special services. Control group members were asked not to use any smartphone applications focused on weight loss during the study. However, they were given the smartphone application used in the intervention

(Lose It!), but not the text messages from a health coach, after the follow-up data were collected.

f. In this study, data were collected from experimental and control group members both before and after the intervention. Thus, we could call the design a pretest–posttest experimental design.

g. The article did not say anything about blinding, which usually means that no blinding was used.

h. The data were collected twice (before the intervention and 3 months later). This study could, therefore, be described as longitudinal.

i. Stephens and colleagues used randomization to groups to control confounding characteristics, which is the most effective strategy possible. It could also be said that they used another method, namely, homogeneity—although this method was not explicitly used as a control method. All of the study participants were between the ages of 18 and 25 years, were not diabetic, were not taking weight loss medications, and were not pregnant.

j. Through randomization, virtually all participant characteristics (e.g., sex, income, grade point average, weight, etc.) would have been controlled. Additionally, through homogeneity, age, pregnancy status, and so on were controlled (i.e., held constant).

k. Yes, there was modest attrition. As shown in Figure 1, 2 people out of 31 in the intervention group and 1 person out of 31 in the control group were not included in the final analyses. Thus, the overall rate of attrition was 4.8% ($3 \div 62$). This is a very modest rate of attrition for a 3-month study.

l. Selection was not a threat in this study because random assignment was used to equalize the groups. Table 2 shows that the two groups were not significantly different at baseline in terms of age, race, sex, and—most importantly—weight-related outcomes. That is, in the far right-hand column the probability values (p) are all greater than .05, which means that the group differences on these baseline variables were probably a function of chance.

m. No, the rate of attrition in this study was quite low and so the mortality threat would not likely undermine the study's internal validity.

Exercise D.2: Questions of Fact (Appendix D)

a. No, there was no intervention in this study.
b. The study design was nonexperimental. It had both descriptive components (e.g., What was fatigue like in patients with coronary heart disease?) and correlational components (What factors—demographic, physiological, psychological—were associated with [predictive of] fatigue? Is fatigue correlated with health-related quality of life?).
c. The article did not articulate a cause-probing intent. The stated purpose was to *describe* fatigue in patients with stable coronary heart disease (CHD) and to examine factors *correlated with* fatigue. The authors were careful to avoid causal language. Indeed, they specifically noted that, regarding the observed relationship between fatigue and depression, it could not be ascertained whether fatigue caused depression, or depression caused fatigue. They also specially noted in their conclusion that it would be desirable to undertake longitudinal studies that might shed more light on the nature of the relationship between these variables.
d. The main dependent variable in this study was levels of fatigue; the independent variables were demographic variables (gender, age, education, income), physiological variables (hypertension, hyperlipidemia), and psychological variable (depression). However, the authors looked at fatigue as an independent variable potentially affecting quality of life.
e. None of the variables in the study could be experimentally manipulated.
f. No, randomization was not used. This was a nonexperimental study.
g. This is a descriptive correlational study. It could also be described as retrospective: Eckhardt and colleagues were interested in identifying predisposing factors that could predict levels of fatigue.

h. No, blinding was not used in this study.
i. No, this study was cross-sectional, and it was not prospective. Data were collected at a single point in time, and the factors examined as possible predictors of fatigue could be considered retrospective in nature—that is, as potentially existing prior to fatigue.

CHAPTER 10

A. FILL IN THE BLANKS

1. Consecutive
2. eligibility
3. size
4. population
5. strata
6. Quota
7. probability
8. representativeness
9. Convenience
10. random
11. bias
12. systematic
13. power analysis
14. self
15. closed
16. open
17. scale
18. Likert
19. visual
20. set
21. observational
22. checklist
23. Time
24. Measurement
25. Reliability
26. internal consistency
27. test–retest
28. Validity
29. Criterion
30. groups

B. MATCHING EXERCISES

B.1.
1. c	2. a	3. d	4. b
5. d	6. b	7. c	8. d
9. a	10. b		

B.2.
1. a, c	2. a, b	3. b, c	4. b
5. b	6. a, b, c	7. a, b, c	8. a

B.3.   1. b   2. a   3. c   4. d
5. b   6. b

C. STUDY QUESTIONS

C.1.   a. Simple random
b. Convenience
c. Systematic
d. Quota
e. Purposive
f. Consecutive

C.2.   The sampling interval is 20. After the first element (23) is selected, the next three would be 43, 63, and 83.

C.6.   C—internal consistency reliability is only relevant for multi-item scales

D. APPLICATION EXERCISES

Exercise D.1: Quantitative Appendix Studies

a. None of the studies in the appendices used probability samples of participants. However, in the Yackel et al. study, one outcome (compliance with documentation) was measured by means of an audit of randomly sampled charts.
b. The quantitative studies in Appendices A and E used convenience sampling.
c. It appears that the pilot test of the EBP project described in Appendix C used consecutive sampling—that is, all eligible patients within a certain timeframe.

Exercise D.2: Quantitative Appendix Studies

a. All three studies in these appendices used structured self-reports as a method of data collection. Stephens and colleagues used self-administered questionnaires that incorporated several psychosocial scales (to measure activity levels, 24-hour food consumption, and self-efficacy for healthy eating and exercise). Yackel and colleagues gathered data on the satisfaction of providers and nursing staff regarding the screening program using a self-report item, measured on a Likert scale (described in the "Results" section). Eckhardt and colleagues administered several psychosocial scales, presumably in a self-administered format (although specifics of data collection procedures were not described). Key variables were measured using multi-item self-report scales (e.g., fatigue, depressive symptoms, and health-related quality of life).
b. In the Yackel et al. studies, it appears that observational methods were used to monitor intervention fidelity, although these methods were not described in detail and the data were not used to capture independent or dependent variables.
c. Stephens and colleagues collected anthropomorphic data on height, weight, body mass index, and waist circumference.
d. Records were used extensively in the Yackel study. For example, the primary outcome was how many patients were screened positive for depression before and after the screening program was implemented and these data were obtained from records. Nurse compliance in documentation was assessed by means of an audit of randomly selected charts. Time-and-motion data for the length of time it took to screen patients were also obtained through records.

Exercise D.3: Questions of Fact (Appendix D)

a. The target population in Eckhardt et al.'s study could perhaps be described as community-dwelling patients with stable coronary heart disease (CHD) in the United States (or in Midwestern United States). The accessible population was patients in cardiology clinics in the state of Illinois.
b. The eligibility criteria for the study included (a) a diagnosis of stable CHD, (b) the ability to speak and read English, and (c) living independently. Exclusion criteria included (a) heart failure with reduced ejection fraction (<40%), (b) terminal illness with prediction of less than 6 months to live,

(c) myocardial infarction or a CABG in the previous 2 months, (d) unstable angina, (e) symptoms reflecting worsening or exacerbation of cardiac disease, and (f) hemodialysis. The exclusion criteria were intended to eliminate patients with a recent acute event, those with worsening symptoms, and those with comorbid conditions associated with fatigue.

c. The sampling method was nonprobability, specifically, sampling by convenience. However, recruitment in two sites serving different demographic groups greatly enhanced the representativeness of the sample. One clinic served primarily urban minority patients with CHD, whereas the second clinic served Caucasian patients from a more rural setting. The authors noted in the Discussion section that a possible limitation of the study was the use of a convenience sample.

d. Specific recruitment strategies were not discussed in the article (e.g., who did the recruiting, what prospective participants were told, how they were screened for eligibility, what percentage of those approached actually participated).

e. The researchers increased the likelihood that their sample would be diverse and more representative by recruiting from two sites serving very different demographic and residential groups. In the section of the article labeled "Strengths and Limitations," the authors specifically noted that "sampling an urban and rural population resulted in ethnic and geographic diversity, thus increasing the generalizability of findings."

f. The total sample size was 102 participants.

g. The report made no mention of having performed a power analysis to estimate sample size needs. No explanation was provided regarding why a sample of 102 patients was selected, nor is sample size discussed in the Discussion section of the report.

h. Demographic characteristics of the study participants were described in the Results section and summarized in Table 1. Participants ranged in age from 34 to 86 years; the average age was 65 years. The majority of participants were non-Hispanic white (56%), male (64%), married (59%), and retired (52%). About 45% of the sample had at least some college education.

i. The researchers relied on preexisting scales developed by other researchers to measure the key variables of fatigue (using the 14-item Fatigue Symptom Inventory), depressive symptoms (using the 9-item Patient Health Questionnaire-9), and health-related quality of life (using the 36-item SF-36). The researchers also measured many other background variables, such as comorbid conditions and smoking history. It is possible the researchers developed their own questions, but it is also possible they used or adapted questions from previous studies.

j. The researchers used existing scales for which evidence about internal consistency reliability and validity was available. For example, for the SF-36 that was used to measure health related quality of life (HRQoL), the researchers noted that "the SF-36 has been extensively used to measure HRQoL and has established reliability and validity in numerous populations." In addition to *selecting* measures known to have good psychometric properties, the researchers computed internal consistency coefficients using data from their own sample. For example, for the SF-36, they found that reliability was good for seven of the eight SF-36 subscales. The coefficients ranged from .79 to .88.

CHAPTER 11

A. FILL IN THE BLANKS

1. emergent
2. Ethnonursing
3. participant
4. informants
5. focused
6. lived
7. essence
8. Interpretive, hermeneutics
9. bracketing
10. basic
11. Glaser, Strauss

12. constant
13. historical
14. case
15. narrative
16. critical
17. Feminist
18. action

B. MATCHING EXERCISES

B.1.   1. b   2. a   3. d   4. c
            5. b   6. a   7. b   8. c
            9. d   10. c   11. a   12. d

C. STUDY QUESTIONS

C.1.   a. Grounded theory
            b. Ethnography
            c. Phenomenology
            d. Hermeneutics (phenomenology)

D. APPLICATION EXERCISES

Exercise D.1: Questions of Fact (Appendix E)

a. The research by Byrne and colleagues was a grounded theory study.

b. The researchers used the Charmaz approach to grounded theory, a constructivist approach, as described in the first paragraph under "Methodology." However, the researchers cited two of Glaser's writings in the section on data analysis.

c. The central phenomenon studied was the care transition experiences of spousal caregivers, when their spouses moved from a geriatric rehabilitation unit to home.

d. Yes, the study was longitudinal. Byrne and colleagues collected data from most study participants (15 out of 18) at multiple points in time to better understand the transition experience. The intent was to interview participants three times: 48 hours after discharge from the geriatric unit, 2 weeks after discharge, and 4 to 6 weeks after discharge.

e. This study was conducted in Ontario, Canada. Families were recruited through a long-term care hospital. Data were collected in the participants' homes.

f. Yes, in the Analysis subsection, the researchers stated that they used "the constant comparative method with all units of data." They also elaborated: "Constant comparison entailed comparing incident to incident and comparing incidents over time between and within participants."

g. Yes, Byrne and colleagues identified the basic social process as *reconciling in response to fluctuating needs*. (The authors did not, however, identify the basic concern or problem that caregivers experience during the spouses' transition from the geriatric rehabilitation unit to home.)

h. The methods used in this study were congruent with a grounded theory approach. The researchers conducted lengthy conversational interviews at multiple points in time with 18 caregivers whose spouse was transitioning from a geriatric rehabilitation unit. In addition, the researchers made observations of the interactions between the spouses and care recipients prior to, during, and after the interviews. As noted previously, constant comparison was used in analyzing the rich data.

i. No, this study did not have an ideological perspective. Even if all of the study participants had been female (which they were not), gender was not a key construct in helping the researchers interpret the data—although the authors did discuss gender differences in the Discussion section of their article.

Exercise D.2: Questions of Fact (Appendix F)

a. The study by Cummings was a phenomenological study, based on the interpretive phenomenological school of inquiry.

b. The central phenomenon of this study was the experience of listeners and storytellers when a traumatic event is being communicated within the dyad.

c. This study was not longitudinal. Interviews were conducted at a single point in time with the storytellers and the listeners.

d. The context for the study was the crash landing of U.S. Airways Flight

1549 in the Hudson River on January 15, 2009. The researcher conducted interviews with 12 people who were on the flight (storytellers) and 12 friends or family members to whom they told their stories, mostly face-to-face. The settings and locations of the interviews were not described.

e. Even though the study involves two groups of people, storytellers and listeners, the focus was not on comparing their experiences—the focus was on the *sharing* of a traumatic event.

f. The in-depth interviewing methods used in this study were well suited to answering the research questions and were congruent with interpretive phenomenology. The researcher noted that she reached saturation (obtained redundant information) after interviewing nine dyads, but interviews with an additional three dyads helped to confirm saturation.

g. No, there was no ideological perspective in this study.

CHAPTER 12

A. FILL IN THE BLANKS

1. Snowball (Network)
2. Theoretical
3. purposive
4. maximum variation
5. data saturation
6. topic
7. semi
8. grand tour
9. Photovoice
10. focus group
11. key informants
12. field, log

B. MATCHING EXERCISES

B.1.
1. b	2. c	3. a	4. d
5. a	6. b	7. a	8. a
9. b	10. d		

B.2.
1. a	2. b	3. c	4. a
5. b	6. c	7. a	8. b
9. a	10. a		

D. APPLICATION EXERCISES

Exercise D.1: Questions of Fact (Appendix B)

a. Specific eligibility criteria were not stated in this report. All of the study participants were nurses who worked "in a level IV NICU in a freestanding children's hospital in the Northeastern United States."

b. The article stated that study information was provided to the nurses through staff meetings, the hospital's intranet, and individual encounters in the NICU. The article did not discuss specific recruitment procedures.

c. The article implies that maximum variation was used in sampling nurses: Informants "were selected for maximal variety of infant feeding and NICU experiences." There is a further statement that nurses were "purposively selected to provide a wide angle view of breastfeeding promotion."

d. The sample included 114 nurses who were general informants, out of 250 nurses employed in the NICU. From this general sample, 18 key informants were chosen who were followed more intensively and interviewed in-depth.

e. The article did not mention data saturation.

f. The article described background characteristics of the nurses in the sample. For example, of the 114 general informants, 96 were white, and all but one were female. Among the 18 key informants, the mean age was 33 years, with a range between 22 and 51 years. There was also diversity in terms of education (from diploma to a master's degree) and level of expertise (from novice to clinical expert).

g. Yes, the study involved in-depth unstructured interviews with the 18 key informants in this study who were nurses working in the NICU. In addition to formal interviews, the key informants were informally interviewed several times over the course of the study.

h. The article did not describe the interviews in detail. The formal interviews involved "open-ended questions," which presumably means that a semistructured format was used—that is, the interviewer asked a set of pre-determined questions. It seems likely that for the informal interviews, an unstructured format was used—that is, questioning was probably more ad hoc and was triggered by an event or activity that the researcher had observed.

i. No, examples of the questions asked in the interviews were not provided.

j. The article stated that the formal interviews lasted 1 hour.

k. The interviews were recorded and subsequently transcribed verbatim.

l. Yes, participant observation was an important source of data in this study. There were a total of 128 observation sessions that lasted between 1 and 2 hours. The observations focused on "the nurses' behaviors during interactions with babies, families, nurses, and other health care professionals throughout everyday NICU activities." Examples included infant feedings, shift reports, and nurse-led breastfeeding support groups.

m. The article stated that "all observational and informal interview data were documented immediately after each session," presumably onto a computer file or in a handwritten set of notes.

n. The researcher gathered additional data through documents, such as breastfeeding standards of care, teaching plans, and written policies and procedures.

o. Cricco-Lizza herself collected the study data. The article stated that "the investigator introduced herself as a nurse researcher" and that her role "evolved from observation to informal interviews over time."

Exercise D.2: Questions of Fact (Appendix E)

a. The article indicated that the caregivers who were the participants had to be returning home from the geriatric rehabilitation unit (GRU) with a husband or wife who did not have cognitive impairment or dementia.

b. Participants were recruited at the long-term care hospital through a GRU team member who was not affiliated with the study. Then, those who were willing to participate were approached by Byrne.

c. The researchers referred to "initial" sampling (presumably convenience sampling) and theoretical sampling that was used to guide data collection. Byrne and colleagues provided the readers with a specific example of their theoretical sampling having to do with how and when caregivers shifted the boundaries.

d. The sample consisted of 18 caregivers: 9 men and 9 women.

e. The report mentioned theoretical saturation of categories. The authors noted that "in accordance with theoretical sampling, the categories noted to be relevant to the development of the emerging theoretical framework guided the sampling process rather than particular sample characteristics such as demographics."

f. There is no mention of sampling confirming or disconfirming cases.

g. Characteristics of the 18 couples were briefly described. The caregivers' mean age was 77.4 years, and they had been married for 47 years, on average. Care recipients, who were on average slightly older, had had a mean length of stay on the GRU of 41 days.

h. Yes, the primary form of data collection was via self-report. The questions focused on "sensitizing concepts" from prior-related research (e.g., changes in the relationship since returning home, social supports available).

i. In-depth face-to-face interviews in the participants' homes were used to collect self-report data. The goal was to conduct interviews longitudinally, at three points in time, but not all participants were able to adhere to this schedule.

j. The researchers gave examples of questions (e.g., "Participants were asked how they would describe their relationship with their spouse currently . . . in comparison to before they were admitted to the GRU and about who had been especially helpful to them in caring for their spouse.")

k. Interviews lasted between 35 and 120 minutes.

l. All interviews were audio recorded and transcribed verbatim by an experienced transcriptionist.

m. Yes, the researcher also observed and recorded interactions between the spouses. The report noted that the researcher (the first author) was "'finely tuned in' to look for interactions that would help elucidate processes and categories emerging from the data."

CHAPTER 13

A. FILL IN THE BLANKS

1. mixed methods
2. sequence, priority
3. qualitative
4. qualitative
5. sequential
6. concurrent
7. pragmatism
8. clinical trial
9. effectiveness
10. randomized
11. intervention theory
12. process
13. survey
14. Outcomes
15. structure
16. quality improvement (QI)
17. secondary
18. methodological

B. MATCHING EXERCISES

1. a, b   2. d   3. c   4. a   5. b
6. d   7. b   8. a, b, c, d

D. APPLICATION EXERCISES

Exercise D.1: All Studies in the Appendices

a. Clinical trial:
   • The Stephens et al. study in Appendix A could be described as a clinical trial—a randomized design was used to test an innovative intervention with clinical applications.
b. Economic analysis:
   • None of the studies in the appendices involved an economic analysis (or, if they did, that part of the study was not presented in the reports).

c. Outcomes research:
   • None of the studies in the appendices could be described as outcomes research.
d. Survey research:
   • The Eckhardt et al. study (Appendix D) is the closest thing to a survey in the appendices, although it is not truly an example of survey research. Surveys typically gather self-report data from a broad population of respondents—like in an opinion poll—rather than from patients with a particular health problem who were receiving services at a particular institutions.
e. Secondary analysis:
   • All of the reports in the appendices (except for the systematic reviews in Appendixes G and H) described studies that collected original data; there are no secondary analyses.
f. Methodological research:
   • None of the studies in the appendices could be described as methodological research.

Exercise D.2: Questions of Fact (Appendix D)

a. Yes, this was a mixed methods study. As described in the introduction, the study had three purposes: (1) to describe fatigue (intensity, distress, timing, and quality) in patients with stable coronary heart disease (CHD); (2) to determine if specific demographic, physiological, or psychological variables were correlated with fatigue; and (3) to determine if fatigue was associated with health related quality of life. Quantitative information played a particularly important role in addressing the second and third purposes but was also used to address the first. The qualitative strand was used to enrich the description of fatigue, that is, the first purpose. No specific mixed methods purpose or question was stated.
b. The quantitative strand had priority in the study design.
c. The design was sequential—data for the quantitative strand were gathered, followed by the collection of qualitative data.
d. The design used in this study would be described as an explanatory design,

using Creswell's terminology. Qualitative data were used to explain and elaborate on the results of the quantitative analyses. The authors themselves used a different name for their design: a partially mixed sequential dominant status design. They referenced different authors for their design typology.

e. The authors themselves used notation to depict their design: QUAN → qual.

f. Eckhardt and colleagues used nested sampling. There were 102 CHD patients in the QUAN strand. Using patients' scores on a measure of fatigue (the FSI-Interference Scale), the researchers identified participants with high, moderate, and low levels of interference from fatigue. Thirteen patients in these three groups participated in an in-depth interview in which they were asked to describe their daily lives and the fatigue they experienced.

g. The report did not provide much detail about how the actual integration took place. The report states that the two strands of data "were compared to determine patterns, enhance description, and address any discrepancies. Qualitative data were used to expand the overall depth of quantitative findings and provide a more thorough description of fatigue." The authors also noted that they paid particular attention to discrepancies and viewed discrepancies as potentially "generative." In their results section, they provided a good example of a discrepancy and how this led to further ideas. One 81-year-old participant in the qualitative strand was in the low fatigue group—a score of 0 on scored on the FSI-Interference Scale—and yet in the in-depth interview he stated, "I just get tired. Some days I almost start crawling." The researchers speculated that this incongruence might "represent an accommodation to decreased physical capacity because of CHD."

CHAPTER 14

A. FILL IN THE BLANKS

1. ordinal
2. ratio
3. nominal
4. interval
5. continuous
6. negative, positive
7. unimodal, bimodal
8. normal
9. mean
10. mode
11. standard
12. crosstabs
13. odds ratio
14. Inferential
15. Alpha
16. Type I
17. Type II
18. power
19. level
20. *t*-test
21. confidence
22. analysis of variance (ANOVA)
23. *d* statistic
24. Pearson's *r*
25. positive
26. chi-squared
27. regression
28. predictor
29. square
30. covariate
31. Logistic
32. Coefficient (Cronbach's) alpha
33. intraclass correlation
34. Cohen's kappa
35. sensitivity

B. MATCHING EXERCISES

B.1.   1. d   2. a   3. d   4. b
            5. c   6. a   7. b   8. d
            9. c   10. b   11. b   12. a

B.2.   1. b   2. a   3. c   4. d
            5. b   6. b   7. a   8. a
            9. c   10. a

C. STUDY QUESTIONS

C.1.   Unimodal around the mode of 51, fairly symmetric

C.2.   Mean: 81.8; Median: 83; Mode: 84

C.3.

OBSERVED FREQUENCIES FOR CHILDREN WITH LACTOSE INTOLERANCE						
	Gender				Total	
	Girls		Boys			
Status	n	%	n	%	N	%
Lactose intolerant	16	26.7	12	20.0	28	23.3
Not lactose intolerant	44	73.3	48	80.0	92	76.7
Total	60	100.0	60	100.0	120	100.0

For the sample as a whole, nearly one out of four children were lactose intolerant. In this sample, boys were less likely than girls to be lactose intolerant (20.0% vs. 26.7%, respectively). To learn if this difference is statistically significant, we would need to perform a chi-squared test.

C.4. a. $-.13$
b. Yes, at $p < .01$
c. Number of doctor visits, physical functioning scores
d. Women who had lower physical functioning scores had significantly more doctor visits than women with higher scores.

C.5. a. Chi-squared
b. t-test
c. Pearson's r
d. ANOVA

C.6. a. Logistic regression
b. ANCOVA
c. Multiple regression

D. APPLICATION EXERCISES

Exercise D.1: Studies in Appendices A, C, and D

a. All three of the studies reported some percentages. Stephens et al. reported some demographic characteristics of their sample as percentages in Table 2 (e.g., percentage of white, 38.7% in both the intervention and control groups). Yackel et al. reported satisfaction with the screening program in percentages (e.g., 95% of nurses strongly agreed that screening enhanced quality of care 1 year after program implementation). Eckhardt et al. reported many background and clinical characteristics of their sample as percentages. In fact, all of the statistics in Table 1 were percentages (e.g., 86.3% of the sample used aspirin).

b. Stephens et al. did not report means and standard deviations (*SD*s). The researchers did not state their rationale for using alternative descriptive indexes in the report itself, but Stephens informed us (in a personal communication) that their decision was based on their relatively small sample size. (Their decision was reasonable, but the rationale is too complex to explain here.) Yackel and colleagues reported some means but not *SD*s; for example, they reported that the mean time added per patient encounter after the screening program introduced was 2 minutes, 53 seconds. Eckhardt et al. reported a few means and *SD*s. For example, in the "Demographic Characteristics" subsection of the Results section, they reported that the mean age of participants was 65 years (*SD* = 11). They also presented some of their findings with means and *SD*s. For example, for the scores on the fatigue scale, women had a mean of 4.38 (*SD* = 2.16), whereas men had a mean of 3.43 (*SD* = 2.16). This information was presented in the text, not in tables.

c. Yackel et al. and Eckhardt et al. did not report medians but the Stephens' research team did. In fact, Stephens and colleagues reported medians rather than means for all outcomes. For example, for the demographic characteristics reported in Table 11, the median age was 20.0 years in both the intervention and control group. Tables 3 and 4 present results of the randomized trial, and again, median values (and ranges) were reported. For example, the median pre- and post-intervention weight of those in the intervention group were 82.8 and 80.1, respectively.

d. None of the articles reported modes.

Exercise D.2: Studies in Appendices A, C, and D

a. Neither Yackel et al. nor Stephens et al. used *t*-tests in their analyses. (Stephens and colleagues did, however, use a repeated measures ANOVA for some analyses). Eckhardt reported the results of several *t*-tests. For example, men and women were compared with respect to fatigue-related outcomes using *t*-tests. The researchers noted that women reported significantly more interference from fatigue than men ($t = 2.74$, $p = .007$).

b. Stephens and colleagues used chi-squared tests for some of their analyses, as noted in the subsection labeled "Statistical Analysis." The actual test values were not, however, reported. For example, in Table 2, it is likely that chi-squared tests were used to compare the proportion of male and female in the two study groups. The difference was not statistically significant ($p = .6322$). Yackel did not perform any chi-squared analyses. Eckhardt and colleagues reported that they used chi-squared tests in their analysis of demographic data, but the results were not presented in the article.

c. Stephens et al. undertook analyses that examined, for the intervention group, the relationship between the number of days logged for exercise activity and the amount of weight lost. However, the researchers did not report the actual values of the correlation coefficients.

(In a personal communication, Stephens informed us that they did use Pearson's *r* in this analysis.) Yackel and colleagues did not report any correlation coefficients or *any* type of inferential statistics. Eckhardt and colleagues used correlation procedures extensively. They noted in their subsection labeled "Quantitative Analysis" that Pearson's *r* (and Spearman's rho) were used "to identify factors associated with fatigue." In Table 2, for example, the researchers presented values of *r* for fatigue intensity and fatigue interference with several independent variables. The highest correlations for both outcomes were with scores on a measure of depressive symptoms ($r = .56$ and $.66$, respectively, both $p < .0001$).

Exercise D.3: Questions of Fact (Appendix D)

a. Referring to Table 1:
  - Nominal level: Gender, race/ethnicity, marital status, employment status, presence of comorbid condition, and types of medications taken
  - Ordinal level: As operationalized in this article, education was measured on an ordinal scale.
  - Interval level: None
  - Ratio level: None. Education *could* have been measured on a ratio scale, as the number of years of schooling completed. However, ordinal categories such as the ones used actually are more informative than presenting mean years of schooling completed.
  - The typical study participant was a white (non-Hispanic) male who was married and retired, with at least 12 years of education.
  - 12.7% of the sample had a graduate degree.
b. Referring to Table 2:
  - Fatigue intensity scores were significantly correlated with the following variables: gender, PHQ-9 (depressive symptoms) score, income, and smoking history.
  - The correlation between education and fatigue intensity was $-.16$. This suggests that people who had more

education were slightly *less* likely to have high fatigue intensity scores than those with less education. However, this correlation was not statistically significant ($p = .12$) and so it cannot be concluded that education was correlated with fatigue intensity at all.

- Table 2 suffers from a flaw that is very common in research reports—the table does not indicate how the variable gender was coded. If men were coded with a higher value than women (e.g., 1 vs. 0), then the positive and significant correlation of .22 would indicate higher scores for men than for women because the correlation is positive. But if women were coded with a higher value than men (e.g., 2 vs. 1), then the reverse would be true. We know from the text (but not the table) that women had higher fatigue scores. The researchers should have provided coding information for gender, race, and several other variables in Table 2, because without such information, the table by itself fails to communicate important information.

c. Eckhardt and colleagues used multiple regression analysis in this study.

d. Yes, in Tables 3 and 4, the researchers presented the results of multiple regression analyses and reported the values of R^2. For example, in Table 4, in the multiple regression equation that involved the prediction of fatigue interference scores on the basis of gender, age, and scores on the measure of depressive symptoms, the value of R^2 was .46.

CHAPTER 15

A. FILL IN THE BLANKS

1. interpretation
2. correlation
3. Effect
4. CONSORT
5. limitations (weaknesses)
6. hypothesis
7. precision

8. Discussion
9. significant
10. clinical
11. minimal important change
12. responder

B. MATCHING EXERCISES

1. b   2. a   3. e   4. d   5. c
6. a, d   7. a   8. e

D. APPLICATION EXERCISES

Exercise D.1: Questions of Fact (Appendix A)

a. Yes, Figure 1 was a CONSORT-type flow chart that showed that 87 young adults were screened for the study and 62 were randomized. The chart then shows the number in intervention and control group who were allocated to each group, the number who dropped out, and the number who completed the study and were included in the analysis ($N = 59$).

b. Baseline values on the key demographic and outcome variables were presented in Table 2 for both intervention and control group members, and the last column presents information about the statistical significance of group differences on these variables. None of the group differences was statistically significant at the .05 level, suggesting the absence of selection biases. When randomization is used as in this study, selection bias is seldom a threat to the internal validity of a study—and when differences do occur, it is purely a function of chance.

c. There was little attrition, and the difference in rates of attrition between the two groups was small (6.4% in the intervention group and 3.2% in the control group)—only 2 and 1 persons, respectively, dropped out of the study by the time of the 3-month follow-up. The researchers did not do an analysis of potential attrition biases, but such an analysis would not have yielded useful information because the Ns were too small. It should be noted that the researchers did a power analysis to estimate their sample size needs, and in that power analysis they assumed an attrition rate of 15%. Thus, their attrition rate (overall, 4.8%) was lower than expected. It does not seem likely that their results were biased by attrition.

d. Hypotheses about the effects of the intervention were not formally stated, although they were clearly implied. There were statistically significant differences between the intervention and control groups for the three main outcomes—weight, body mass index (BMI), and waist circumference. For example, the change in median values for weight was +1.5 kg for the control group and −2.7 kg for the intervention group, $p = .026$, as shown in Table 3. Both groups had improvements in self-efficacy and physical activity over the 3-month period, but group differences were not statistically significant. In terms of participants' diet (Table 4), only 37 study participants (15 in the intervention group and 22 in the control group) provided information about their diets. The only significant group difference was for the consumption of fiber, which was higher in the intervention group. It is possible that more of the dietary differences would have been significant with a larger sample. For example, those in the intervention group consumed less added sugars ($p = .077$) and more protein ($p = .080$). For these dietary outcomes, the analyses were likely insufficiently powered to detect differences at significant levels.

e. The article did not provide confidence intervals around values for the main outcomes (e.g., differences between group means or medians). In Table 5, 95% CIs are shown around values for the b coefficients for the relationships between the consistency of logging physical activity and weight change. We did not explain b coefficients in the textbook—although they were discussed in the Supplement to Chapter 14.

f. Effect size estimates summarizing the magnitude of the intervention effects were not presented in the report.

g. There was no explicit discussion about internal validity in the Discussion section, but the authors did note, correctly, that a major strength of this study was the use of a randomized design. Such a design provides a basis for an inference of causality—that is, that participation in the intervention *caused* improvements in weight, waist circumference, and BMI. There do not appear to be any threats to the internal validity of the study. In experimental designs, attrition can be a major threat, but the rate of attrition in this study was low.

h. Yes, the authors did note in the Discussion that generalizability was limited because the study participants were all attending college at an east coast university in the United States. Generalizing the results to, for example, low-income young adults living in a poor urban neighborhood in Texas would not be warranted without a replication.

i. There was no explicit discussion about statistical conclusion validity in the Discussion section. The researchers did, however, note in their Discussion that the sample size was small and this in turn could have resulted in Type II errors for some of the outcomes—especially those relating to diet.

j. Yes, some of the findings were discussed vis-à-vis findings from earlier research. For example, the researchers stated that "these results are promising when examining other similar research," and then cited two earlier studies.

k. Yes, several limitations of the study were discussed. These included the small sample size, the constraints on generalizability, and the inability to identify whether the intervention effects are attributable to the smartphone part of the intervention, or to the health coach. Regarding sample size, we note that in the power analysis, the researchers assumed an effect size of $d = .80$ based on a previous study. However, this is a very large and probably unrealistic effect size estimate. In any event, there was sufficient power for the main outcomes but not for the secondary ones.

l. No, the researchers did not say anything specifically about the clinical significance of their findings. They came to a broad conclusion that the trial provided "valuable information" about the intervention and did say that it had a "meaningful impact" on weight, BMI, and waist circumference. However, they did not define what constituted a "meaningful" effect.

Exercise D.2: Questions of Fact (Appendix D)

a. The researchers mentioned bias twice. First, they stated that they timed the in-depth qualitative interview 3 to 5 weeks after enrollment in the study, specifically to avoid the risk of *recall* biases. Second, participants for the qualitative interviews were purposively selected from patients who were high, moderate, or low on a key research variable, level of interference from fatigue. To avoid bias, the researchers analyzed the qualitative data without knowing which of the three fatigue groups the people were in. Thus, they made efforts to avoid something akin to *expectation bias*.

b. Hypotheses were not formally stated in the introduction of this article, and yet hypotheses were implied (by virtue of the researchers' conceptual model) and tested statistically. For example, the framework (Figure 1) implies that fatigue would affect quality of life, and Table 5 shows that both fatigue intensity and fatigue interference were significantly and negatively correlated with all dimensions on the quality of life scale in this sample.

c. In this cross-sectional study, the issue of temporal ambiguity (i.e., whether one variable preceded or followed another) makes it difficult to infer a causal connection. The researchers specifically made a point about this in their Discussion section: " . . . it remains to be determined if depression is the cause or consequence of fatigue."

d. Precision was not addressed—that is, there were no confidence intervals. CIs around correlation coefficients are almost never presented, and most of the analyses in this study were correlational.

e. The researchers did not specifically use effect-size language in discussing their results. However, the value of r and R^2 can be directly interpreted as effect size indexes. For example, the value of $R^2 = .46$ (the prediction of fatigue interference) would be considered high. (The standard convention for a "large" R^2 is .30.) Thus, the three predictors shown in Table 4 (age, gender, and depression scores) had a fairly strong relationship with fatigue interference.

f. Yes, the researchers explicitly noted that the generalizability of their findings was likely enhanced by including a diverse mix of participants in terms of urban/rural residence and ethnicity.

g. Yes, some limitations of the study were explicitly noted in the Discussion section as well as some strengths. The limitations included the use of a convenience sample and the potential inclusion of patients with undiagnosed heart failure.

h. Yes, the researchers did discuss clinical significance at the individual level. They noted (in the section on "Quantitative measurement—Fatigue") that a previous researcher had established a fatigue intensity score of 3 or higher on the Fatigue Symptom Inventory (FSI) as reflective of clinically meaningful fatigue. The researchers then reported that 57% of the men and 78% of the women in their sample had clinically meaningful levels of fatigue. This finding was the first thing they discussed in their Discussion because this represents very high levels of fatigue. Indeed, categorizing participants as having or not having clinically significant levels of fatigue is more useful information than simply reporting that the mean fatigue intensity score was 4.4 for women and 3.4 for men. Thus, this study illustrates the value of defining clinical significance at the individual level and using a benchmark to classify patients.

CHAPTER 16

A. FILL IN THE BLANKS

1. coding
2. content

3. domain
4. taxonomic
5. descriptive
6. line-by-line
7. metaphor
8. circle
9. exemplars
10. Paradigm
11. open
12. selective
13. memo
14. emergent
15. constructivist

B. MATCHING EXERCISES

1. a, b, c   2. a   3. b   4. a, b, c   5. a
6. c   7. b   8. d

C. STUDY QUESTIONS

C.1.

a. A grounded theory analysis would not yield themes—a phenomenological study involves a thematic analysis.
b. Texts from poetry are used by interpretive phenomenologists, not by ethnographers (unless the poetry is a product of the culture under study, which it is not in this case).
c. Phenomenological studies do not focus on domains, ethnographies do.
d. Grounded theory studies do not yield taxonomies, ethnographies do.
e. A paradigm case is a strategy in a hermeneutic analysis, not in an ethnographic one.

D. APPLICATION EXERCISES

Exercise D.1: Questions of Fact (Appendix E)

a. Yes, Byrne and colleagues audiotaped the interviews with the 18 spousal caregivers. The audiotapes were transcribed by an experienced transcriptionist. The article did not indicate how many pages of transcription resulted, but it did say that interviews were between 35 and 120 minutes long. In total, there were 45 interviews. This likely resulted in hundreds of pages in the data set that had to be read and reread, coded, and analyzed.
b. Yes, at the end of the subsection labeled "Data Collection," the authors indicated that "data generation and data analysis occurred simultaneously, which supported follow-ups with participants about emerging codes and categories."
c. It does not appear that computer software was used in the analysis of data for this study.
d. No, Byrne and colleagues did not use metaphors, although they used rich and colorful language to describe features of their framework (e.g., "getting into it, getting on with it").
e. Yes, the report indicated that Byrne (the first author) wrote memos during the analysis: "When a code was raised to the level of a category, the first author created a memo describing the category, the elements contained in the category, illustrative quotes that reflected the category, and further ideas on which to follow-up to ensure theoretical saturation of the category. These memos were shared and discussed among authors."
f. The report stated that Byrne engaged in line-by-line coding and then all authors contributed to focused and theoretical coding. The researchers noted that moving from line-by-line to focused coding was not a linear process. Excellent examples of the coding process were provided in the section labeled "Analysis."

Exercise D.2: Questions of Fact (Appendix F)

a. Yes, Cummings' interviews were audiotaped and transcribed verbatim by a transcriptionist who had completed special training relating to the protection of the rights of study participants.
b. The report did not mention that Cummings used computer software to organize and manage her data. Her statement about making marginal notes using different color highlighters strongly suggests that she relied exclusively on manual methods of organization and coding.

c. Cummings reported that she used van Manen's phenomenological approach.

d. The article stated that Cummings maintained a journal "to record additional observations and personal reflections."

e. Cummings discussed the analytic process in terms of steps she attributed to van Manen: holding preconceived beliefs in abeyance; undertaking a holistic reading of each transcript to get a sense of it as a whole; rereading the transcripts to identify statements or phrases that best represented participants' experiences; identifying categories; and dwelling with the data to identify key themes. (Cummings did not follow van Manen's approach strictly, however, perhaps because of the sensitive nature of the inquiry.) In van Manen's interpretive approach, researchers typically go back and forth with participants to have them reflect on the experiences, typically using the transcript of the first interview as a starting point in a subsequent conversation.

f. Cummings' analysis revealed five essential themes: (1) The story has a purpose; (2) the story may continue to change as different parts are revealed; (3) the story is experienced physically, mentally, emotionally, and spiritually; (4) Imagining the "what" as well as the "what if"; and (5) the nature of the relationship colors the experience of the listener and storyteller.

g. Yes, Cummings provided rich supportive evidence for her themes in the form of direct quotes from the interviews. For example, here is a quote from theme 4, from a listener: "There is no way you can understand; there's no way, even if you had a similar experience, that you can put yourself in their shoes."

CHAPTER 17

A. FILL IN THE BLANKS

1. Credibility
2. triangulation
3. dependability

4. transferability
5. audit
6. thick description
7. confirmability
8. internal
9. observation
10. negative
11. member
12. Investigator
13. Authenticity
14. peer
15. prolonged

B. MATCHING EXERCISES

1. a   2. b   3. c   4. a   5. b

D. APPLICATION EXERCISES

Exercise D.1: Questions of Fact (Appendix E)

a. Yes, Byrne and colleagues devoted an entire subsection of their report to describing their approach to quality enhancement labeled "Criteria for Rigor."

b. The researchers used several types of triangulation. First, there was method triangulation. The primary source of data was from interviews with the spouse caregivers, but these data were augmented with observations of the interactions between caregivers and their spouses. They noted that they "used triangulation not to confirm existing data but rather to enhance completeness." Another form of triangulation was investigator triangulation. Byrne did much of the preliminary coding and analysis but shared her work with her coauthors, and all researchers contributed to the final framework. It might be said that time triangulation was used, given the multiple points of data collection, but the researchers were less interested in verification in later interviews than they were in understanding how the process of reconciliation evolved over time.

c. Many strategies were used to enhance rigor in this study:
  • We might conclude that both persistent observation (the researchers' very thorough and in-depth scrutiny

of the reconciliation process) and prolonged engagement (continuing to gather data and observe over participants a 6-week period) were used as quality-enhancement strategies in this study.

- The report indicated that the preliminary theoretical framework was shared with five caregivers as a member-checking strategy. The authors noted that "caregivers reported being able to 'see' their own experience of transition in the processes presented." Moreover, the authors stated that the framework was modified based on feedback from participants.
- The report did not discuss any efforts to search for disconfirming evidence although this does not necessarily mean it did not occur.
- The report indicated that the researcher maintained a reflexive journal and that entries were made on an electronic notebook for each interview.
- The report stated that an audit trail was maintained, although details were not provided, except to note that an electronic field notebook was used to record audit trail details.

Exercise D.1: Questions of Fact (Appendix F)

a. No, Cummings did not have a section of her report specifically describing quality-enhancement strategies. Her strategies were presented in the second paragraph of the "Data Analysis" section.

b. Triangulation was not a key part of Cummings' quality-enhancement strategies. It is true that she gathered data from both storytellers and listeners, but this is not really data source triangulation because the experiences of listener and storyteller were considered separately (i.e., the point of including the listeners was not to triangulate information from the storytellers but to understand their parallel experience). Investigator triangulation was not really used either—that is, a *team* of investigators did not undertake the analysis.

c. Several strategies were used to enhance rigor in this study:

- Cummings does not appear to have used persistent observation in her research. Although she gathered data from both parties to storytelling episodes, she did not (for example) go back to participants and ask them to reflect on transcripts and co-interpret them.
- Cummings used peer debriefing. She "collaborated with two professional colleagues and expert qualitative researchers who reviewed transcripts and findings."
- Regarding member checks, Cummings noted that "findings were presented and clarified with participants to assess whether the transcripts were accurate and whether identified themes resonated with them." The report did not indicate whether both listeners and storytellers were involved in the member checks or how many participants were asked to contribute.
- There was no mention of searching for disconfirming evidence.
- Reflexivity was used in this study. The report indicated that a journal was kept to record observations and personal reflections. Cummings also noted that the first step in the analysis process was to put aside preconceived notions and beliefs about the phenomenon under study.
- The report did not state that an audit trail was maintained, although this does not mean that it did not happen.
- The researcher is a doctorally trained nurse practitioner. She noted in the introduction that the issue of listening to traumatic events is crucial for nurse practitioners and that little is known about the impact of listening to stories of traumatic events on nurses. The acknowledgment at the end of the article suggests that Cummings herself was a listener to the story about the crash landing— her brother was onboard the United Airlines plane that crashed into the Hudson River.

CHAPTER 18

A. FILL IN THE BLANKS

1. meta-analysis
2. scoping
3. hand
4. grey
5. publication
6. quality
7. heterogeneity
8. difference
9. subgroup
10. forest plot
11. metasynthesis
12. meta-ethnography
13. meta-summary
14. frequency
15. intensity

B. MATCHING EXERCISES

1. c   2. d   3. b   4. a   5. b
6. a   7. d   8. b

D. APPLICATION EXERCISES

Exercise D.1: Questions of Fact (Appendix G)

a. The purpose of Chase and colleagues' meta-analysis was "to determine the overall effectiveness of interventions designed to improve medication adherence (MA) among adults with CAD (coronary artery disease)." The independent variable was receipt versus nonreceipt of a special intervention, and the dependent (outcome) variable was MA. Chase and colleagues articulated two specific research questions: (1) What is the overall effectiveness of MA interventions on MA outcomes among patients with CAD? and (2) Does intervention effectiveness vary as a function of characteristics of the intervention, the sample, or the study design?

b. To be eligible for this meta-analysis, a primary study had to be a two-group treatment versus control group study that tested the effectiveness of an intervention to increase MA in adult patients aged 18 years or older with a diagnosis of CAD. A total of 24 studies (but 28 comparisons) met these criteria. Note that this meta-analysis is similar to the Conn et al. study summarized at the end of Chapter 18 in the textbook—and both Vicki Conn and Todd Ruppar were authors on both articles. However, the meta-analysis in this *Study Guide* did not have as an inclusion criterion that the patients had to have a MA problem.

c. The reviewers relied primarily on electronic database searches. They searched in about a dozen databases and searched using a wide array of terms. They also used hand searching of 57 relevant journals, author searches of key researchers in the field, and ancestry searches using the bibliographies of identified studies.

d. No, this study did not present a flow chart summarizing the search and selection process. No information was provided about how many studies were initially identified through their search strategies and how many were eliminated for various reasons. Recent guidelines for reporting meta-analyses indicate that a flow chart should be provided, much like a CONSORT-type flow chart described in the textbook.

e. It was noted in the abstract and in the Results section that a total of 18,839 people participated in the primary studies.

f. Participants in the primary studies were on average 62.9 years old; this was the median of the study mean ages. The majority of study participants were male and, in studies for which ethnicity was reported, white. Many studies reported that their participants had additional chronic diseases, such as hypertension and hyperlipidemia.

g. According to the Table 4, 20 of the 28 comparisons involved random assignment to a treatment or a control group. Thus, the review included studies with both experimental ($n = 20$) and quasi-experimental ($n = 8$) designs.

h. Study quality was assessed using a domain approach, rather than a scale approach. Each study was coded for the presence or absence of certain features, including randomization, use of a theory, the blinding of data collectors, and the use of the recommended analytic approach called *intention to treat*. All of the coding was performed by two independent research specialists and then compared and discussed until there was 100% agreement.

i. Studies were not excluded on the basis of quality, per se, but they were excluded if used a very weak one-group pretest–posttest design.

j. The effect size used in this study was the standardized mean difference, which we referred to in the textbook as *d*.

k. Yes, the researchers tested for heterogeneity. They opted to use a random effects model, even before learning that the test for heterogeneity was statistically significant because they expected variation of effects across studies.

l. Yes, Figure 1 presented the main effects on a study-by-study basis in a forest plot.

m. The overall effect size comparing adherence outcomes for those in an intervention group compared to a control group was .229. As shown in Table 2, the 95% confidence interval around this value was .138 to .321, which is significant because the interval does not include zero. We can be 95% confident that the true beneficial effect lies somewhere in the interval between .14 and −.32 (rounded values).

n. Regarding Figure 1:
- The study with the largest effect size was a small study published in 1985 at the bottom of the forest plot. The ES for this study was 2.521, favoring those in the intervention group.
- Yes, there were many studies for which intervention effectiveness was nonsignificant—all those where the lines for the 95% CI crosses the vertical line for 0.00. Indeed, this was true for most of the studies in Figure 1.
- Yes, there were five studies for which the value of *d* was negative, indicating outcomes favoring the control group. However, in none of these cases was the result statistically significant. This can be

seen by examining the values of the lower and upper limits of the 95% CI. For these five studies where the value of *d* was negative, the lower limit was negative but the upper limit was positive, thus indicating the possibility that the value of *d* could be 0.

o. Yes, numerous exploratory subgroup analyses were undertaken to assess factors contributing to the heterogeneity of effects across studies. One particularly interesting finding was that MA interventions delivered by nurses were especially effective. Another finding was that interventions in which health care providers were given information about patients' adherence were more effective than interventions without this component. Also, interventions initiated in inpatient settings were especially effective. Many of the subgroup analyses, however, yielded nonsignificant results. It should be noted that the small number of studies in the sample would make it especially difficult to find significant subgroup effects.

Exercise D.2: Questions of Fact (Appendix H)

a. Beck undertook a metasynthesis of six of her own studies in her program of research on traumatic births and did not search for other qualitative studies on the same or a related topic. Beck's was, thus, a special type of metasynthesis. (Of course, as an expert in the area of traumatic birth, Beck is thoroughly familiar with the literature in her field.)

b. Beck did not explicitly discuss this controversy, although her approach would have integrated any of her studies on the topic of traumatic births, regardless of tradition. Her metasynthesis combined five phenomenological studies and one narrative analysis.

c. The data in the primary studies were all derived from self-reports—from Internet-based self-reports.

d. A total of 175 mothers participated in Beck's six primary studies.

e. Beck used Noblit and Hare's approach to doing a metasynthesis, which they called meta-ethnography. Beck provided an excellent description of the seven phases of the approach.

f. No, a meta-summary is a strategy developed by Sandelowski and colleagues, and Beck did not follow this approach.

g. Beck identified three overarching themes in her studies of birth trauma: (1) stripped of protective layers, (2) invisible wounds, and (3) insidious repercussions. Beck also discovered that traumatic childbirth had a domino effect on various aspects of new motherhood, which she identified as *amplifying causal looping*.

h. Yes, Beck included some powerful verbatim quotes from the primary studies in support of her thematic integration.